Dosage Calculations: A Ratio-Proportion Approach

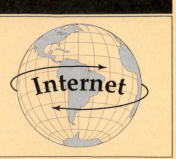
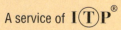

Dosage Calculations: A Ratio-Proportion Approach

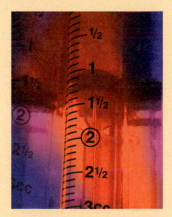

first edition

Gloria D. Pickar, RN, EdD
Seminole Community College
Sanford, Florida

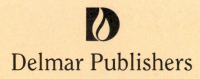

Delmar Publishers

I(T)P An International Thomson Publishing Company

Albany • Bonn • Boston • Cincinnati • Detroit • London • Madrid • Melbourne
Mexico City • New York • Pacific Grove • Paris • San Francisco • Singapore • Tokyo
Toronto • Washington

NOTICE TO THE READER

Cover Design: Cummings Advertising

Delmar Staff:
Publisher: William Brottmiller
Developmental Editor: Marah Bellegarde
Project Editor: Patricia Gillivan
Production Coordinator: Barbara A. Bullock
Art and Design Coordinator: Timothy J. Conners
Editorial Assistant: Diane Biondi

Printed in the United States of America
3 4 5 6 7 8 9 10 XXX 05 04 03 02 01

For more information, contact Delmar, 3 Columbia Circle, PO Box 15015, Albany, NY 12212-0515; or find us on the World Wide Web at http://www.delmar.com

International Division List

Japan:
Thomson Learning
Palaceside Building 5F
1-1-1 Hitotsubashi, Chiyoda-ku
Tokyo 100 0003 Japan
Tel: 813 5218 6544
Fax: 813 5218 6551

UK/Europe/Middle East:
Thomson Learning
Berkshire House
168-173 High Holborn
London
WC1V 7AA United Kingdom
Tel: 44 171 497 1422
Fax: 44 171 497 1426

Canada:
Nelson/Thomson Learning
1120 Birchmount Road
Scarborough, Ontario
Canada M1K 5G4
Tel: 416-752-9100
Fax: 416-752-8102

Spain:
Thomson Learning
Calle Magallanes, 25
28015-MADRID
ESPANA
Tel: 34 91 446 33 50
Fax: 34 91 445 62 18

Australia/New Zealand
Nelson/Thomson Learning
102 Dodds Street
South Melbourne, Victoria 3205
Australia
Tel: 61 39 685 4111
Fax: 61 39 685 4199

Latin America:
Thomson Learning
Seneca, 53
Colonia Polanco
11560 Mexico D.F. Mexico
Tel: 525-281-2906
Fax: 525-281-2656

Asia:
Thomson Learning
60 Albert Street, #15-01
Albert Complex
Singapore 189969
Tel: 65 336 6411
Fax: 65 336 7411

Library of Congress Cataloging-in-Publication Data
Pickar, Gloria D., 1946-
    Dosage calculations: a ratio-proportion approach / Gloria D.
Pickar. — 1st ed.
        p.   cm.
    Includes index.
    ISBN 0-7668-0630-8
    1. Pharmaceutical arithmetic. I. Title.
    [DNLM: 1. Pharmaceutical Preparations—administration & dosage.
2. Mathematics. QV748 P594d 1998]
RS57.P533   1998
615'.14—dc
DNLM/DLC   98-3830
for Library of Congress   CIP

table of contents

preface

introduction

In our continued efforts to meet educational needs, we are pleased to release *Dosage Calculations: A Ratio-Proportion Approach.* This text is based upon the popular *Dosage Calculations,* fifth edition, by Gloria Pickar. This text was developed for instructors and health care professionals who prefer using the ratio-proportion method, and continues our tradition of leading innovations in the teaching and learning of dosage calculations. *Dosage Calculations: A Ratio-Proportion Approach* offers a clear and concise method of calculating medication (drug) dosages and is directed to the student or professional who feels uncomfortable with mathematics.

This method has been extensively classroom-tested and reviewed by over 300,000 faculty and students, who state that it helps them allay math anxiety and master accurate dosage calculations.

The only math prerequisite is the ability to do basic arithmetic. For those who need a review, Chapter 1 offers an overview of basic arithmetic procedures with extensive exercises for practice. The student is encouraged to use a 3-step method for calculating dosages:

1. convert measurements to the same system and same size units;
2. consider what dosage is reasonable; and
3. calculate using ratio-proportion.

Full color is used to make the text user friendly. Chapter elements such as rules, notes, remember, quick review boxes, and examples are color-coded for easy recognition and use. Color also highlights review sets and practice problems. All drug labels are reproduced in full color to provide greater clarity and readability for reference in solving problems.

All syringes are drawn to full size to provide accurate scale renderings to help students master the reading of injectable dosages. An amber color has been added to selected syringe drawings throughout the text to *simulate a specific amount of medication,* as indicated in the example or problem. Because the color used may not correspond to the actual color of the medications named, *it must not be used as a reference for identifying medications.*

In addition to the detailed table of contents, an extensive index has been added as a tool to support the student's review of concepts and skills.

organization of content

The text is organized in a natural progression of basic to more complex information. Students gain self-confidence as they master content in small increments with ample review and reinforcement.

chapter 1 provides a review of basic arithmetic procedures, with numerous examples and practice problems to ensure that students can apply the procedures. A pretest is included to determine student comprehension of basic arithmetic skills.

chapters 2 and 3 deal with the three systems of measurement (metric, apothecaries', and household) and conversion from one system of measurement to another. Both ratio-proportion and the formula method of performing conversions are included, as well as international or 24-hour time, and temperature conversions.

The metric system of measurement is stressed because of its increased standardization in the health care field. (The use of apothecaries' and household systems is further deemphasized.)

In *chapter 4* students learn to recognize and select appropriate equipment for the administration of medications based on the drug, dosage, and the method of administration. Emphasis is placed on interpreting syringe calibrations to ensure that the dosage to be administered is accurate. All photos and drawings have been enhanced for improved clarity.

chapter 5 presents the common abbreviations used in health care so that students can become proficient in interpreting medical orders. Additionally, the section on computerized medication administration records has been updated and expanded.

It is essential that students be able to read medication labels to calculate dosages accurately. This ability is developed by having students interpret the medication labels provided beginning in *chapter 6*. These labels represent current commonly prescribed medications and are presented in full color and actual size (except in a few instances where the label is enlarged to improve readability).

chapters 7 and 8 guide the student to apply all the skills mastered to achieve accurate oral and injectable drug dosage calculations. Students learn to think through the problem logically for the right answer and then to apply ratio-proportion to double-check their thinking. When this logical but unique system is applied every time to every problem, experience has shown that decreased math anxiety and increased accuracy result.

Insulin types, species, and manufacturers have been introduced with a description of insulin action time. 70-30 insulin is also thoroughly explained.

chapter 9 presents the formula method of calculating dosages. Ample review sets and practice problems provide the opportunity to apply this method. The formula method is also applied in Chapters 10, 11, and 12 as an alternative calculation method.

chapter 10 covers the calculation of pediatric dosages and concentrates on the body weight and body surface area (BSA) methods. Ample practice is provided for both methods. Combination drugs and safe dosage ranges are introduced.

Intravenous administration calculations are presented in *chapters 11 and 12*. Coverage reflects the greater application of IVs in drug therapy. Shortcut calculation methods are presented and explained fully. More infusion devices, such as electronic and patient-controlled pumps, are emphasized. Heparin and saline locks, types of IV solutions, IV monitoring, IV administration records, and blood transfusions are included in Chapter 11. Pediatric, obstetric, heparin, and critical care IV calculations are presented in Chapter 12. Ample problems help students master the necessary calculations.

Procedures in the text are introduced using several examples. Key concepts are summarized and highlighted before the practice problems to give students an opportunity to review the concepts prior to working through the problems. Learning is reinforced by review questions that immediately follow the topic covered. The importance of calculation accuracy is emphasized by patient scenarios that apply critical thinking skills.

posttests at the end of the text serve to evaluate the student's progress and skills in dosage calculations. Posttest 2 is presented in a case study format to simulate actual clinical calculations.

An *answer key* at the back of the text provides answers and selected solutions to problems in the Review Sets, Practice Problems, and Posttests.

features

- Critical thinking skills are applied to real-life patient care situations to emphasize the importance of accurate dosage calculations and the avoidance of medication errors.
- Photos and drug labels are presented in full color; color is used to highlight and enhance the visual presentation of content to improve readability. Special attention is given to visual clarity.
- A math review (Chapter 1) brings students up to the required level of basic math competency.
- Measurable objectives at the beginning of each chapter emphasize the content to be learned.
- SI conventional metric system notation is used (apothecaries' and household system of measurement are deemphasized).
- International (24-hour) time, Celsius and Fahrenheit temperature, and conversion problems are included.
- RULE boxes highlight and draw the student's attention to pertinent instructions.
- REMEMBER boxes highlight information to be memorized.
- QUICK REVIEW boxes precede review sets and summarize critical information in each section.
- Content is presented from simple to complex concepts in small increments followed by Review Sets of problems for better understanding and to reinforce learning.
- Many problems are included involving the interpretation of syringe scales to ensure that the proper dosage is administered. Once the dosage is calculated, the student is directed to draw an arrow on a syringe at the proper value.
- Many labels of current and commonly prescribed medications are included to help students learn how to select the proper information required to determine correct dosage.
- Solved examples are included to demonstrate the ratio-proportion method of calculating dosages; practice problems provide opportunities for students to master skills.
- Photographs of equipment commonly used in administering medications and IVs are included.
- The formula method is included, giving students and instructors a choice of which method they prefer to use.
- The section on types of insulin and insulin dosage has been expanded.
- Computer medication and IV administration records have been added and expanded.
- The chapter on calculating pediatric dosages uses both the body weight and body surface area (BSA) methods, emphasizing the requirement for accurate dosages to prevent over- or under-medication of the pediatric patient.

- IV equipment and calculations are included. IV solutions are thoroughly discussed and blood transfusions are introduced. Pediatric, obstetric, heparin, and critical care IV calculations have been expanded.
- Clear instructions are included for calculating IV medications administered in mg or mcg per kilogram per minute.
- Clinical situations are simulated using actual medication labels, syringes, physician order forms, and medication administration records.
- Case study format of Posttest 2 simulates actual clinical calculations.
- The index facilitates student and instructor access to content and skills.

computer software

With this edition of *Dosage Calculations: A Ratio-Proportion Approach*, Delmar introduces a companion study guide and testing CD-ROM for Windows™. The CD-ROM is an interactive multimedia presentation that includes the complete text of the book, sample problems, review questions, and a testing component. The program provides scoring, helpful hints, animations, and color photos and illustrations. It is designed for individual, self-paced learning at home or in the computer lab.

supplement

An *Instructor's Guide* is available for this text. The *Instructor's Guide* includes solutions for all Review Sets, Practice Problems, and Posttests. In addition, extra problems are given for each chapter for testing purposes. Transparency masters are also provided to help instructors highlight important concepts.

acknowledgments

reviewers

The following people devoted considerable time and effort to reviewing this text in various stages. Appreciation is expressed to the instructors who reviewed the revised manuscript, provided problem solutions, or served as technical proofreaders.

Maureen Tremel, MSN, ARNP: Seminole Community College, Sanford, FL

Beverly Meyers, BA, MEd: Jefferson College, Hillsboro, MO

Rita Berry, RN, MSN: West Virginia Northern Community College, Wheeling, WV

Kay Cummins, RN: Cloud County Community College, Concordia, KS

Janett L. Stuart, RN, BSN: Lenoir Community College, Kinston, NC

Annice D. Conaway, RN, MS: J. F. Drake State Technical College, Huntsville, AL

Patricia S. Sandoe, RN, MSN, FNP: Wythe Medical Associates, Wytheville, VA

Susan Karm Wieczorek, RN, MSN: Fortson, GA

Marjean Corry, RN, BSN: Sanford-Brown College, St. Charles, MO

Alan Nelms, MS: Aiken Technical Community College, Aikin, SC

Marsha E. Nickerson, MN, RN, PHN: Santa Monica Community College, Santa Monica, CA

Special appreciation and recognition is given to Maureen Tremel, nursing instructor at Seminole Community College, Sanford, FL, who directly assisted the author with content research, updating of clinical information, and field testing.

manufacturers

The following companies provided technical data, photographs, syringes, drug labels, package inserts, package labels, or packaging to illustrate examples, problems, and posttests.

Abbott Laboratories, North Chicago, IL 60064

Apothecon, Princeton, NJ 08543

BASEL Pharmaceuticals Division of CIBA-GEIGY Corp., Summit, NJ 07901

Baxter Healthcare Corporation, Deerfield, IL 60015

Becton Dickinson, Rutherford, NJ 07070

Beecham Laboratories, Bristol, TN 37620

Boots Pharmaceuticals, Inc., Lincolnshire, IL 60069

Bristol Laboratories, Bristol-Myers Pharmaceutical and Nutritional Group, Evansville, IN 47221

Bristol-Myers Oncology Division, Evansville, IN 47721

Burroughs Wellcome Co., Research Triangle Park, NC 27709

CIBA Pharmaceutical Company, Division of CIBA-GEIGY Corporation, Summit, NJ 07901

Dista Products Company, Division of Eli Lilly & Co., Indianapolis, IN 46285

The DuPont Merck Pharmaceutical Company, Wilmington, DE 19880

Elkins-Sinn, Inc., Cherry Hill, NJ 08003

GEIGY Pharmaceuticals, Division of CIBA-GEIGY Corporation, Ardsley, NY 10502

Glaxo Pharmaceuticals, Division of Glaxo Inc., Research Triangle Park, NC 27709

Hoechst-Roussel Pharmaceuticals Inc., Somerville, NJ 00876

Hoffman-LaRoche Inc., Nutley, NJ 07110

ICI Pharma, Division of ICI Americas Inc., Wilmington, DE 19897

Lakeside Pharmaceuticals, Cincinnati, OH 45215

Lederle Parenterals, Inc., Carolina, Puerto Rico 00630

Eli Lilly and Company, Indianapolis, IN 46285

McNeil Pharmaceutical, Spring House, PA 19477

Marion Laboratories, Inc., Pharmaceutical Division, Kansas City, MO 64137

Marion Merrill Dow, Inc., Kansas City, MO 64134

Mead Johnson Oncology Products, A Bristol-Myers Squibb Co., Evansville, IN 47721

Medex Inc., Dublin, OH 43017

Novo Nordisk Pharmaceuticals Inc., Princeton, NJ 08540

Parke-Davis Division of Warner-Lambert Company, Morris Plains, NJ 07950

Pfizer Laboratories Division, New York, NY 10017

Reed & Carnrick, Division of Block Drug Company, Inc., Jersey City, NJ 07302

Roche Products Inc., Manati, Puerto Rico 00701

Roerig Pfizer, A Division of Pfizer Inc., New York, NY 10017

Rorer Consumer Pharmaceuticals, A Division of Rorer Pharmaceutical Corporation, Fort Washington, PA 19034

Roxane Laboratories, Inc., Columbus, OH 43216

Russ Pharmaceuticals, Inc., Birmingham, AL 35242

Sanofi Winthrop Pharmaceuticals, New York, NY 10016

Schiapparelli Searle, Chicago, IL 60680

G. D. Searle & Co., Chicago, IL 60680

SmithKline Beecham Pharmaceuticals, Philadelphia, PA 19101

Summit Pharmaceuticals, Division of CIBA-GEIGY Corporation, Summit, NJ 07901

Syntex Corporation, Palo Alto, CA 94303

Taylor Pharmacal Company, Decatur, IL 62525

The Upjohn Company, Kalamazoo, MI 49001

Wallace Laboratories Division, Carter-Wallace, Inc., Cranbury, NJ 08512

Winthrop Pharmaceuticals, New York, NY 10016

Wyeth-Ayerst Laboratories, Philadelphia, PA 19101

from the author

I wish to thank my many students and colleagues who have provided inspiration and made contributions to the production of the text. I am particularly grateful to Eve Grey for her careful attention to typing, to Maureen Tremel for her careful attention to researching and updating information, to Marah Bellegarde for her careful attention to deadlines and details, to Greg Vis for the vision to see the necessity of this text, and to Roger Pickar for his careful attention to me and our children.

Gloria D. Pickar, EdD

introduction to the student

The accurate calculation of drug dosages is an essential skill in health care. Serious harm to the patient can result from a mathematical error when calculating a drug dosage. It is the responsibility of those administering drugs to precisely and efficiently carry out drug orders.

Learning to calculate drug dosages need not be a difficult or burdensome process. *Dosage Calculations: A Ratio-Proportion Approach* provides an uncomplicated, easy-to-learn, easy-to-recall, 3-step method of dosage calculations. Once you master this method, you will be able to consistently compute dosages with accuracy, ease, and confidence.

The text is a self-study guide. The only mathematical prerequisite is the basic ability to add, subtract, multiply, and divide whole numbers. A review of fractions, decimals, percents, ratios, proportions, and Roman numerals is included. You are encouraged to work at your own pace and seek assistance from a qualified instructor as needed.

Each procedure in the text is introduced by several examples. Key concepts are summarized and highlighted before the practice problems. This gives you an opportunity to review the concepts before working the problems. Ample review and practice problems are given to reinforce your skill and confidence.

Before calculating the dosage, you are asked to consider the reasonableness of the computation. More often than not, the correct amount can be estimated in your head. Many errors can be avoided if you approach dosage calculation in this logical fashion. The mathematical computation can then be used to double-check your thinking. Answers to all problems and step-by-step solutions to select problems are included at the back of the text.

Many photos and drawings are included to demonstrate key concepts and equipment. Drug labels and measuring devices (for example, syringes) are included to give a simulated "hands on" experience outside of the clinical setting or laboratory. New critical thinking skills emphasize the importance of dosage calculation accuracy.

My earlier text has helped many thousands of students just like you to feel at ease about math and to master dosage calculations. I am interested in your feedback to this new version. Please write to me to share your reactions and success stories.

Gloria D. Pickar, EdD
Seminole Community College
100 Weldon Boulevard
Sanford, FL 32773-6199

using this book . . .

■ Content is presented from simple to complex concepts in small increments followed by a quick review and solved examples. Review sets and practice problems provide opportunities to reinforce learning.

■ All syringes are drawn to full size to provide accurate scale renderings to help students master the reading of injectable dosages.

Draw an arrow to indicate the calibration that corresponds to the dose to be administered.

11. Administer 0.75 cc

12. Administer 1.33 cc

13. Administer 2.2 cc

14. Administer 1.3 cc

15. Administer 0.33 cc

16. Administer 66 U of U-100 insulin

Administer 27 U of U-100 insulin

Generic and brand names of the drug:
By law the generic name must be identified on all drug labels. The brand name is followed by the sign ® meaning the name is registered. Occasionally, only the generic name appears.

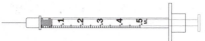

Generic Name (penicillin G potassium)

NDC 0078-0098-05
100 CAPSULES
RESTORIL®
(temazepam) C IV
15 mg

CAUTION: Federal law prohibits dispensing without prescription.

SANDOZ PHARMACEUTICALS CORPORATION
EAST HANOVER, NJ 07936

LOT SPECIMEN

Brand Name (Restoril) and Generic Name (temazepam)

■ Photos and drug labels are presented in full color; color is used to highlight and enhance the visual presentation of content and to improve readability. Special attention is given to visual clarity.

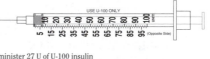

Fig. 7–1 Tablets, Caplets, and Gelcaps

- **critical thinking** skills are applied to real-life patient care situations to emphasize the importance of accurate dosage calculations and the avoidance of medication errors.
- **rule** boxes highlight and draw the students' attention to pertinent instructions.
- **remember** boxes highlight information to be memorized.
- **quick review** boxes summarize critical information.

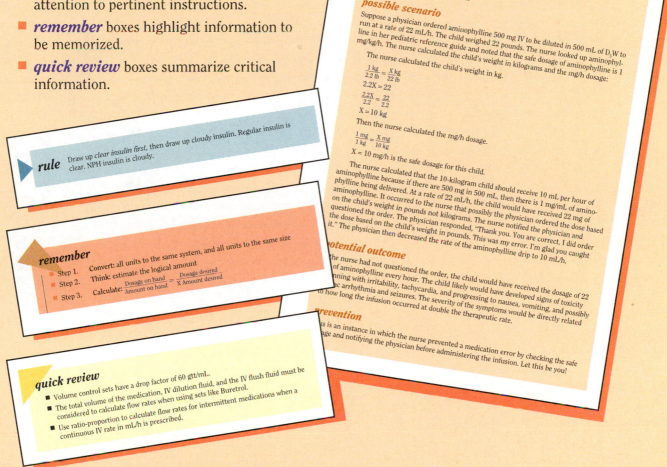

rule

Draw up *clear insulin first*, then draw up cloudy insulin. Regular insulin is clear. NPH insulin is cloudy.

remember

- Step 1.   Convert: all units to the same system, and all units to the same size
- Step 2.   Think: estimate the logical amount
- Step 3.   Calculate: $\frac{\text{Dosage on hand}}{\text{Amount on hand}} = \frac{\text{Dosage desired}}{\text{X Amount desired}}$

quick review

- Volume control sets have a drop factor of 60 gtt/mL.
- The total volume of the medication, IV dilution fluid, and the IV flush fluid must be considered to calculate flow rates when using sets like Buretrol.
- Use ratio-proportion to calculate flow rates for intermittent medications when a continuous IV rate in mL/h is prescribed.

---

critical thinking skills

Let's look at an example in which the nurse *prevents* a medication error by calculating the safe dosage of a medication before administering the drug to a child.

■ error 2

Dosage that is too high for a child.

possible scenario

Suppose a physician ordered aminophylline 500 mg IV to be diluted in 500 mL of D$_2$W to run at a rate of 22 mL/h. The child weighed 22 pounds. The nurse looked up aminophylline in her pediatric reference guide and noted that the safe dosage of aminophylline is 1 mg/kg/h. The nurse calculated the child's weight in kilograms and the mg/h dosage:

The nurse calculated the child's weight in kg.

$\frac{1 \text{ kg}}{2.2 \text{ lb}} = \frac{X \text{ kg}}{22 \text{ lb}}$

$2.2X = 22$

$\frac{2.2X}{2.2} = \frac{22}{2.2}$

$X = 10 \text{ kg}$

Then the nurse calculated the mg/h dosage.

$\frac{1 \text{ mg}}{1 \text{ kg}} = \frac{X \text{ mg}}{10 \text{ kg}}$

$X = 10$ mg/h is the safe dosage for this child.

The nurse calculated that the 10-kilogram child should receive 10 mL per hour of aminophylline because if there are 500 mg in 500 mL, then there is 1 mg/mL of aminophylline being delivered. At a rate of 22 mL/h, the child would have received 22 mg of aminophylline. It occurred to the nurse that possibly the physician ordered the dose based on the child's weight in pounds not kilograms. The nurse notified the physician and questioned the order. The physician responded, "Thank you. You are correct. I did order the dose based on the child's weight in pounds. This was my error. I'm glad you caught it." The physician then decreased the rate of the aminophylline drip to 10 mL/h.

potential outcome

If the nurse had not questioned the order, the child would have received the dosage of 22 mg of aminophylline every hour. The child likely would have developed signs of toxicity beginning with irritability, tachycardia, and progressing to nausea, vomiting, and possibly cardiac arrhythmia and seizures. The severity of the symptoms would be directly related to how long the infusion occurred at double the therapeutic rate.

prevention

This is an instance in which the nurse prevented a medication error by checking the safe dosage and notifying the physician before administering the infusion. Let this be you!

CD-ROM included!

   With the first edition of Pickar's *Dosage Calculations: A Ratio-Proportion Approach*, Delmar Publishers introduces a comprehensive learning program on CD-ROM for Windows™. The CD-ROM is an interactive multimedia presentation that has been designed to enhance self-paced learning.

Features include:

- Complete text
- Tutorial to help you get started
- 300-word glossary
- Audio pronunciation of drug names, including common sound-alike drug names
- Testing assessment tool with scoring capabilities
- Section review questions with answers and rationales
- Chapter practice problems with answers and rationales

- Critical thinking skills
- Animations
- Color photographs
- 160 drug labels
- Intuitive and attractive interface
- Help feature
- Toll-free technical support
- Plus Flash!, an electronic flash card program

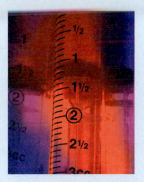

Mathematics Review for Dosage Calculations

As a prerequisite objective, *Dosage Calculations* takes into account that you can add, subtract, multiply, and divide whole numbers.

objectives

Upon mastery of Chapter 1, you will be able to perform the basic mathematical computations essential for calculating drug dosages. To accomplish this, you will also be able to:

- Express the whole Arabic numbers 1–30 in Roman numerals.
- Add, subtract, multiply, and divide fractions, decimals, percents, and ratios.
- Reduce fractions to lowest terms.
- Round a decimal to a given place value.
- Interpret values expressed in ratios.
- Convert among fractions, decimals, percents, and ratios.
- Determine the value of X in simple equations.
- Set up proportions for solving problems.
- Cross-multiply to find the value of X in a proportion.

Set aside $1\frac{1}{2}$ hours in a quiet place to complete the 50 items in the following diagnostic test. You will need scratch paper to work the problems.

Use your results to determine your current computation strengths and weaknesses to guide your review. A minimum score of 86 is recommended as an indicator of readiness for dosage calculations; in which case, you may proceed directly to Chapter 2. However, note any problems that you answered incorrectly, and use the related review material to refresh yourself.

The aim of this diagnostic test and the review that follows is to enhance your confidence in your arithmetic skill and to avoid careless mistakes later when you perform dosage calculations.

Good luck.

Mathematics Diagnostic Test

Directions:
1. Carry answers to three decimal places and round off to two places.
   (Examples: 5.175 = 5.18; 5.174 = 5.17)

2. Express fractions in lowest terms.

   (Example: $\frac{6}{10} = \frac{3}{5}$)

Time Limit: 90 minutes

1. $1517 + 0.63 =$ _____

2. Express the value of XIX + VIII in Arabic numerals. _____

3. $9.5 + 17.06 + 32 + 41.11 + 0.99 =$ _____

4. $\$19.69 + \$304.03 =$ _____

5. $93.2 - 47.09 =$ _____

6. $1005 - 250.5 =$ _____

7. Express the value of $6003 - 5995$ in Roman numerals. _____

8. $509 \times 38.3 =$ _____

9. $\$4.12 \times 42 =$ _____

10. $17.16 \times 23.5 =$ _____

11. $972 \div 27 =$ _____

12. $2.5 \div 0.001 =$ _____

13. Express the value of $176 \div 16$ in Roman numerals. _____

14. Express $\frac{1500}{240}$ as a decimal. _____

15. Express 0.8 as a fraction. _____

16. Express $\frac{2}{5}$ as a percent. _____

17. Express 0.004 as a percent. _____

18. Express 5% as a decimal. _____

19. Express $33\frac{1}{3}\%$ as a ratio in lowest terms. _____

20. Express $1:50$ as a decimal. _____

21. $\frac{1}{2} + \frac{3}{4} =$ _____

22. $1\frac{2}{3} + 4\frac{7}{8} =$ _____

23. $1\frac{5}{6} - \frac{2}{9} =$ _____

24. Express the value of $\frac{1}{100} \times 60$ as a fraction. _____

25. Express the value of $4\frac{1}{4} \times 3\frac{1}{2}$ as a fraction. _____

26. Identify the fraction with the greatest value: $\frac{1}{150}, \frac{1}{200}, \frac{1}{100}$ _____

27. Identify the decimal with the least value: $0.009, 0.19, 0.9$ _____

28. $\frac{6.4}{0.02} =$ _____

29. $\frac{0.02 + 0.16}{0.4 - 0.34} =$ _____

30. Express the value of $\frac{3}{12 + 3} \times 0.25$ as a decimal. _____

31. 8% of $50 =$ _____

32. $\frac{1}{2}\%$ of $18 =$ _____

33. 0.9% of $24 =$ _____

Find the value of X. Express your answer as a decimal.

34. $\frac{500}{125} = \frac{1.25}{X}$ _____

35. $\frac{300}{150} \times 2 = X$ _____

36. $\frac{5}{1.5} = \frac{2.5}{X}$ _____

37. $\frac{1,000,000}{250,000} \times X = 12$ _____

38. $\frac{1.7}{X} = \frac{0.51}{150}$ _____

39. $X = (82.4 - 52)\frac{3}{5}$ _____

40. $\dfrac{\frac{1}{150}}{\frac{1}{300}} \times 1.2 = X$ _____

41. Express 2:10 as a fraction in lowest terms. _____

42. Express 2% as a ratio in lowest terms. _____

43. If 5 equal medication containers contain 25 tablets total, how many tablets are in each container? _____

44. If 1 pound of sugar equals 4 cups, how many pounds of sugar are in 1 cup? _____

45. If 1 kilogram equals 2.2 pounds, how many kilograms does a 66 pound child weigh? _____

46. If 1 kilogram equals 2.2 pounds, how many pounds are in 1.5 kilograms? (Express your answer as a decimal.) _____

47. If 1 centimeter equals $\frac{3}{8}$ inch, how many centimeters are in $2\frac{1}{2}$ inches? (Express your answer as a decimal.) _____

48. If you have a roll of quarters and you must pay $1.25, how many quarters will you use? _____

49. This diagnostic test has a total of 50 problems. If you incorrectly answer 5 problems, what percentage will you have answered correctly? _____

50. For every 5 female student nurses in a nursing class, there is 1 male student nurse. What is the ratio of female to male student nurses? _____

After completing these problems, see pages 287 and 288 to check your answers. Give yourself two points for each correct answer.

Perfect score = 100   My score = _____
Readiness score = 86 or higher

Roman Numerals

Some of the medications you will administer will be ordered and measured by amounts expressed in Roman numerals, whereas others will be expressed as Arabic numbers. Interpreting Roman numerals is probably nothing new to you, as you most likely have used them frequently when reading chapter headings or preparing an outline.

We are going to consider only the Roman numerals up to the value of 30, since these are the ones you will use in reading drug orders and drug labels.

In the Roman system of counting, letters are used to designate numbers. Learn the following common Roman numerals and their Arabic equivalents.

remember

Roman Numeral	Arabic Number	Roman Numeral	Arabic Number
I	1	VII	7
II	2	VIII	8
III	3	IX	9
IV	4	X	10
V	5	XX	20
VI	6	XXX	30

A simple set of rules governs the Roman system of notation. The position of one letter to another is very important and determines the value of the Roman numeral.

 rule To repeat a Roman numeral twice doubles its value; to repeat a Roman numeral three times triples its value.

EXAMPLES: I = 1 and II = 2
X = 10 and XXX = 30

 rule Roman numerals may not be repeated more than three times in succession.

EXAMPLES: III = 3 is a correct notation; however, IIII = 4 is incorrect.
The Arabic number 4 is correctly written IV in Roman numerals.

 rule When a Roman numeral of a smaller value *follows* one of a larger value, they are *added*.

EXAMPLE: VI = 5 + 1 = 6

 rule When a Roman numeral of a smaller value *precedes* one of a larger value, the smaller is *subtracted* from the larger.

EXAMPLE: IV = 5 − 1 = 4

 rule When a Roman numeral of a smaller value comes between two of larger values, the subtraction rule is applied *first*, then the addition rule.

EXAMPLES: XIV = 10 + (5 − 1) = 10 + *4* = 14
XXIX = 10 + 10 + (10 − 1) = 10 + 10 + *9* = 29

quick review

When interpreting Roman numerals:

- Letters are used to designate numbers. Example: I = 1, V = 5, X = 10
- Repeating a letter twice, doubles its value. Example: II = 2
- Repeating a letter three times triples its value. Example: III = 3
- Roman numerals are only repeated up to three times. Example: III YES! IIII NO!
- When a smaller Roman numeral follows a larger, add. Example: XI = 10 + 1 = 11
- When a smaller Roman numeral comes before a larger, subtract.
  Example: IX = 10 − 1 = 9
- When a smaller Roman numeral comes between two larger ones, subtract then add. Example: XIX = 10 + (10 − 1) = 19

review set 1

Convert the following Arabic numbers to Roman numerals.

1. 28 = _____   4. 15 = _____
2. 13 = _____   5. 9 = _____
3. 17 = _____

Perform the indicated operations and record the results in Arabic numbers.

6. VII + XXIII = _____   9. XII × II = _____
7. XXVII − IV = _____   10. XXIV ÷ VI = _____
8. XIX − XIV = _____

Perform the indicated operations and record the results in Roman numerals.

11. 5 × 4 = _____   14. 625 ÷ 125 = _____
12. 18 + 12 = _____   15. 17 + 14 − 11 + 4 = _____
13. 16 ÷ 4 = _____

After completing these problems, see page 288 to check your answers.

Fractions

A *fraction* indicates a portion of a whole number. There are two types of fractions: *common fractions*, such as $\frac{1}{2}$ (usually referred to simply as fractions) and *decimal fractions*, such as 0.5 (usually referred to simply as decimals).

A fraction is an expression of division with one number placed over another number ($\frac{1}{4}$, $\frac{2}{3}$, $\frac{4}{5}$). The bottom number or *denominator* indicates the total number of parts into which the whole is divided. The top number or *numerator* indicates how many of those parts are considered. The fraction may also be read as the "numerator *divided* by the denominator."

EXAMPLE: $\frac{1}{4}$ $\frac{\text{numerator}}{\text{denominator}}$ 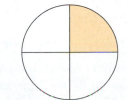   The whole is divided into four equal parts (denominator), and one part (numerator) is considered.

$\frac{1}{4}$ = 1 part of 4 parts or $\frac{1}{4}$ of the whole.
The fraction $\frac{1}{4}$ may also be read as "1 divided by 4."

HINT: The *denominator* begins with *d* and is *down* below the line in a fraction.

There are four types of common fractions.

1. *Proper fractions*—in which the value of the numerator is *less* than the value of the denominator. The value of the proper fraction is also *less* than 1.

    EXAMPLE: $\dfrac{5}{8}\ \dfrac{\text{numerator}}{\text{denominator}}$ = less than 1

HINT: Whenever the numerator is less than the denominator, the value of the fraction must be less than 1.

2. *Improper fractions*—in which the value of the numerator is *greater* than or *equal* to the value of the denominator. The value of the improper fraction is *greater* than or *equal* to 1.

    EXAMPLES: $\dfrac{8}{5}$ = more than 1

    $\dfrac{5}{5} = 1$

NOTE: Whenever the numerator is greater than the denominator, the value of the fraction must be greater than 1. When the numerator and denominator are equal, the value of the improper fraction is always 1; since a nonzero number divided by itself is 1.

3. *Mixed number*—in which a whole number and a proper fraction are combined. The value of the mixed number is always *greater* than 1.

    EXAMPLE: $1\dfrac{5}{8} = 1 + \dfrac{5}{8}$ = more than 1

4. *Complex fractions*—in which the numerator or the denominator, or both, may be a whole number, proper fraction, or mixed number. The value may be *less* than, *greater* than, or equal to 1.

    EXAMPLES: $\dfrac{\frac{5}{8}}{\frac{1}{2}}$ = greater than 1 $\dfrac{1\frac{5}{8}}{\frac{1}{5}}$ = greater than 1

    $\dfrac{\frac{5}{8}}{2}$ = less than 1

    $\dfrac{\frac{1}{2}}{\frac{2}{4}} = 1$

To perform dosage calculations you must be able to convert among different types of fractions as described previously and reduce fractions to lowest terms. You must also apply the operations of addition, subtraction, multiplication, and division. Review these simple rules of working with fractions. Stay with it until the concepts are crystal clear and automatic.

Conversion

It is important to be able to convert among different types of fractions. Conversion allows you to perform various calculations with greater ease, and permits you to express answers in simplest terms.

Converting Mixed Numbers to Improper Fractions

▶ *rule*   To change or convert a mixed number to an improper fraction with the same denominator *multiply the whole number by the denominator and add the numerator.* Put that value in the numerator and use the denominator of the fraction part of the mixed number.

EXAMPLE: $1\frac{5}{8} = (1 \times 8) + 5 = 13$ eighths or $\frac{13}{8}$.

Converting Improper Fractions to Mixed Numbers

▶ **rule**   To change or convert an improper fraction to an equivalent mixed number or whole number, *divide the numerator by the denominator*. Any remainder is expressed as a proper fraction and reduced to lowest terms.

EXAMPLE: $\frac{8}{5} = 8 \div 5 = 1\frac{3}{5}$

Equivalent Fractions

The value of a fraction can be expressed in several ways. This is called *finding an equivalent fraction*. In finding an equivalent fraction both terms of the fraction (numerator and denominator) are either multiplied or divided by the *same number*. The form of the fraction is changed but the value of the fraction remains the same.

When calculating dosages it is usually easier to work with fractions of the smallest numbers possible. This concept of finding equivalent fractions is called *reducing the fraction to the lowest terms* or simplifying the fraction.

Reducing Fractions to Lowest Terms

▶ **rule**   To reduce a fraction to lowest terms, *divide the largest whole number* that will go evenly into *both* the numerator and the denominator.

EXAMPLE: Reduce $\frac{6}{12}$ to lowest terms.

6 is the largest number that will divide evenly into both 6 (numerator) and 12 (denominator).

$6 \div 6 = 1, 12 \div 6 = 2$

$\frac{6}{12} = \frac{1}{2}$ in lowest terms

NOTE: If *both* the numerator and denominator *cannot* be divided evenly by a whole number, then the fraction *is* in lowest terms.

Enlarging Fractions

▶ **rule**   To find an equivalent fraction in which both terms are larger, *multiply both* the numerator and the denominator by the *same number*.

EXAMPLE: Enlarge $\frac{3}{5}$ to the equivalent fraction in tenths.

$3 \times 2 = 6; 5 \times 2 = 10$

$\frac{3}{5} = \frac{6}{10}$

Comparing Fractions

In calculating some drug dosages, it is helpful to know when the value of one fraction is greater or less than another. The relative sizes of fractions can be determined by comparing the numerators when the denominators are the same or comparing the denominators if the numerators are the same.

> **rule** If the numerators are the same, the fraction with the smaller denominator has the greater value.

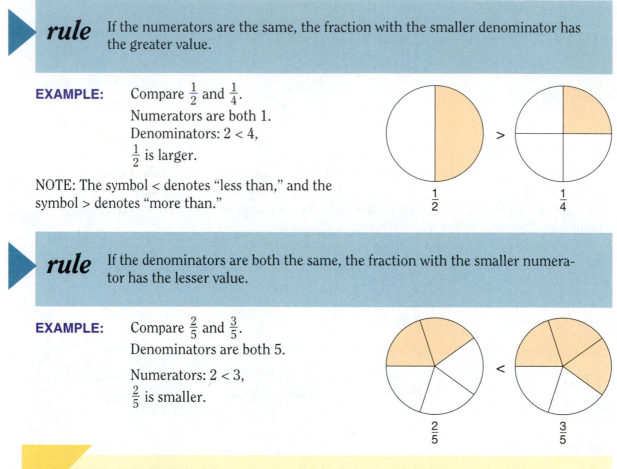

EXAMPLE: Compare $\frac{1}{2}$ and $\frac{1}{4}$.
Numerators are both 1.
Denominators: 2 < 4,
$\frac{1}{2}$ is larger.

NOTE: The symbol < denotes "less than," and the symbol > denotes "more than."

> **rule** If the denominators are both the same, the fraction with the smaller numerator has the lesser value.

EXAMPLE: Compare $\frac{2}{5}$ and $\frac{3}{5}$.
Denominators are both 5.

Numerators: 2 < 3,
$\frac{2}{5}$ is smaller.

quick review

- To convert a mixed number to an improper fraction, multiply the whole number by the denominator and add the numerator. Example: $1\frac{1}{3} = \frac{4}{3}$.
- To convert an improper fraction to a mixed number, divide the numerator by the denominator. Example: $\frac{20}{9} = 2\frac{2}{9}$.
- To reduce a fraction to lowest terms, divide both terms by the largest whole number that will divide evenly. Value remains the same. Example: $\frac{6}{10} = \frac{3}{5}$.
- To enlarge a fraction, multiply both terms by the same number. Value remains the same. Example: $\frac{1}{12} = \frac{2}{24}$.

review set 2

1. Circle the *improper* fraction(s).

$$\frac{2}{3}, \quad 1\frac{3}{4}, \quad \frac{6}{6}, \quad \frac{7}{5}, \quad \frac{16}{17}, \quad \begin{array}{c}\frac{1}{9}\\\frac{2}{3}\end{array}$$

2. Circle the *complex* fraction(s).

$$\frac{4}{5}, \quad 3\frac{7}{8}, \quad \frac{2}{2}, \quad \frac{9}{8}, \quad \frac{8}{9}, \quad \frac{\frac{1}{100}}{\frac{1}{150}}$$

3. Circle the *proper* fraction(s).

$$\frac{1}{4}, \quad \frac{1}{14}, \quad \frac{14}{1}, \quad \frac{14}{14}, \quad \frac{1\frac{1}{4}}{14}$$

4. Circle the *mixed* number(s) *reduced to the lowest terms.*

$$3\frac{4}{8}, \quad \frac{2}{3}, \quad 1\frac{2}{9}, \quad \frac{1}{3}, \quad 1\frac{1}{4}, \quad 5\frac{7}{8}$$

5. Circle the pair(s) of *equivalent* fraction(s).

$$\frac{3}{4} = \frac{6}{8}, \quad \frac{1}{5} = \frac{2}{10}, \quad \frac{3}{9} = \frac{1}{3}, \quad \frac{3}{4} = \frac{4}{3}, \quad 1\frac{4}{9} = 1\frac{2}{3}$$

Change the following mixed numbers to improper fractions.

6. $6\frac{1}{2} =$ _____   9. $7\frac{5}{6} =$ _____

7. $1\frac{1}{5} =$ _____   10. $102\frac{3}{4} =$ _____

8. $10\frac{2}{3} =$ _____

Change the following improper fractions to whole numbers or mixed numbers; reduce to lowest terms.

11. $\frac{24}{12} =$ _____   14. $\frac{100}{75} =$ _____

12. $\frac{8}{8} =$ _____   15. $\frac{44}{16} =$ _____

13. $\frac{30}{9} =$ _____

Enlarge the following fractions to the number of parts indicated.

16. $\frac{3}{4}$ to eighths _____   19. $\frac{2}{5}$ to tenths _____

17. $\frac{1}{4}$ to sixteenths _____   20. $\frac{2}{3}$ to ninths _____

18. $\frac{2}{3}$ to twelfths _____

Circle the correct answer.

21. Which is larger? $\frac{1}{150}, \quad \frac{1}{100}$

22. Which is smaller? $\frac{1}{1000}, \quad \frac{1}{10,000}$

23. Which is larger? $\frac{2}{9}, \quad \frac{5}{9}$

24. Which is smaller? $\frac{3}{10}, \quad \frac{5}{10}$

25. You are serving pizza and you give $\frac{1}{4}$ of it to each of 3 adults. You divide the remaining piece between two children. What portion of the whole pizza is each child's slice? (Think carefully. HINT: Draw yourself a picture.) _____

26. If 1 medicine bottle contains 12 doses, how many bottles must be purchased to supply 18 doses? _____

27. A nursing school class consists of 3 men and 57 women. What fraction of the students in the class are men? (Express your answer as a fraction in lowest terms.) _____

28. A nursing student answers 18 out of 20 questions correctly on a test. Write a proper fraction (reduced to lowest terms) to represent the student's score.

       _____

29. A typical dose of Children's Tylenol contains 160 milligrams of Tylenol per teaspoonful. Each 80 milligrams is what part of a typical dose?

       _____

30. In number 29, how many teaspoons of Children's Tylenol would you need to give 80 milligrams?

       _____

After completing these problems, see page 288 to check your answers.

NOTE: If you answered question 30 correctly, you can already calculate dosages!

Addition and Subtraction of Fractions

To add or subtract fractions all the denominators must be the same.

> **▶ rule** To add or subtract fractions,
> 1. convert all fractions to equivalent fractions with the least common denominators,
> 2. add or subtract the numerators, and
> 3. Reduce the result to lowest terms.

NOTE: The denominators must be the same. You do not perform any calculations on the denominators in addition or subtraction of fractions.

EXAMPLE 1: $\frac{3}{4} + \frac{1}{4} + \frac{2}{4}$

  1. Find the least common denominator: This step is not necessary because they already have the same denominator.

  2. Add the numerators: $\frac{3+1+2}{4} = \frac{6}{4}$

  3. Reduce to lowest terms: $\frac{6}{4} = 1\frac{2}{4} = 1\frac{1}{2}$

EXAMPLE 2: $\frac{1}{3} + \frac{3}{4} + \frac{1}{6}$

  1. Find the least common denominator: 12.
Convert to equivalent fractions in twelfths. This is the same as enlarging the fractions.

$$\frac{1}{3} = \frac{4}{12}$$

$$\frac{3}{4} = \frac{9}{12}$$

$$\frac{1}{6} = \frac{2}{12}$$

  2. Add the numerators: $\frac{4+9+2}{12} = \frac{15}{12}$

  3. Reduce to lowest terms: $\frac{15}{12} = 1\frac{3}{12} = 1\frac{1}{4}$

EXAMPLE 3: $1\frac{1}{10} - \frac{3}{5}$

1. Find the least common denominator: 10
   Convert to equivalent fractions in tenths.

   $$1\frac{1}{10} = \frac{11}{10}$$

   $$\frac{3}{5} = \frac{6}{10}$$

2. Subtract the numerators: $\frac{11-6}{10} = \frac{5}{10}$

3. Reduce to lowest terms: $\frac{5}{10} = \frac{1}{2}$

Multiplication of Fractions

To multiply fractions, multiply numerators and multiply denominators.

When possible, *cancellation of terms* shortens the process of both multiplication and division. Cancellation (like "reducing to lowest terms") is based on the fact that the division of both the numerator and denominator by the same whole number does not change the value of the number.

EXAMPLE: $\frac{250}{500} = \frac{\overset{1}{\cancel{250}}}{\underset{2}{\cancel{500}}} = \frac{1}{2}$ The numerator and the denominator are both divided by 250.

Also, the numerators and denominators of any of the fractions involved in the multiplication may be cancelled. This is called "cross-cancellation."

EXAMPLE: $\frac{1}{8} \times \frac{8}{9} = \frac{1}{\cancel{8}} \times \frac{\overset{1}{\cancel{8}}}{9} = \frac{1}{1} \times \frac{1}{9} = \frac{1}{9}$

▶ ***rule***   To multiply fractions,

1. cancel terms, if possible,
2. multiply numerators, multiply denominators, and
3. reduce the result (product) to lowest terms.

EXAMPLE 1: $\frac{3}{4} \times \frac{2}{6}$

1. Cancel terms: Divide 2 and 6 by 2

   $$\frac{3}{4} \times \frac{\overset{1}{\cancel{2}}}{\underset{3}{\cancel{6}}} = \frac{3}{4} \times \frac{1}{3}$$

   Divide 3 and 3 by 3

   $$\frac{\overset{1}{\cancel{3}}}{4} \times \frac{1}{\underset{1}{\cancel{3}}} = \frac{1}{4} \times \frac{1}{1}$$

2. Multiply numerators and denominators:

   $$\frac{1}{4} \times \frac{1}{1} = \frac{1}{4}$$

3. Reduce to lowest terms: This step is not necessary because the product is already in lowest terms.

EXAMPLE 2: $\frac{15}{30} \times \frac{2}{5}$

1. Cancel terms: Divide 15 and 30 by 15

$$\frac{\overset{1}{\cancel{15}}}{\underset{2}{\cancel{30}}} \times \frac{2}{5} = \frac{1}{2} \times \frac{2}{5}$$

Divide 2 and 2 by 2

$$\frac{1}{\underset{1}{\cancel{2}}} \times \frac{\overset{1}{\cancel{2}}}{5} = \frac{1}{1} \times \frac{1}{5}$$

2. Multiply numerators and denominators:

$$\frac{1}{1} \times \frac{1}{5} = \frac{1}{5}$$

3. Reduce to lowest terms: This step is not necessary because the product is already in lowest terms.

NOTE: Recall that when multiplying a fraction by a whole number, the same rule applies. The whole number becomes a fraction with a denominator of 1.

EXAMPLE 3: $\frac{2}{3} \times 4 = \frac{2}{3} \times \frac{4}{1}$

1. No terms to cancel. (You cannot cancel 2 and 4 since both are numerators. To do so would change the value.)
2. Multiply numerators and denominators:

$$\frac{2}{3} \times \frac{4}{1} = \frac{2 \times 4}{3 \times 1} = \frac{8}{3}$$

3. Reduce to lowest terms.

$$\frac{8}{3} = 8 \div 3 = 2\frac{2}{3}$$

NOTE: To multiply mixed fractions, first convert the mixed fraction(s) to an improper fraction(s) and then multiply.

EXAMPLE 4: $3\frac{1}{2} \times 4\frac{1}{3}$

1. Convert: $3\frac{1}{2} = \frac{7}{2}$

$$4\frac{1}{3} = \frac{13}{3}$$

Therefore, $\frac{7}{2} \times \frac{13}{3}$

2. Cancel: No number can be cancelled in this problem.

3. Multiply: $\frac{7 \times 13}{2 \times 3} = \frac{91}{6}$

4. Reduce: $\frac{91}{6} = 15\frac{1}{6}$

Division of Fractions

In division of fractions, the divisor is inverted and then the calculation is the same as for multiplication of fractions.

> **rule** To divide fractions,
>
> 1. invert the terms of the divisor,
> 2. cancel terms, if possible,
> 3. multiply the resulting fractions, and
> 4. reduce to lowest terms.

EXAMPLE 1: $\frac{3}{4} \div \frac{1}{3}$

1. Invert: $\frac{3}{4} \div \frac{1}{3} = \frac{3}{4} \times \frac{3}{1}$

2. Cancel: Not necessary since no numbers can be cancelled.

3. Multiply: $\frac{3}{4} \times \frac{3}{1} = \frac{9}{4}$

4. Reduce: $\frac{9}{4} = 2\frac{1}{4}$

EXAMPLE 2: $\frac{2}{3} \div 4$

1. Invert: $\frac{2}{3} \div \frac{4}{1} = \frac{2}{3} \times \frac{1}{4}$

2. Cancel terms: $\frac{\overset{1}{\cancel{2}}}{3} \times \frac{1}{\underset{2}{\cancel{4}}} = \frac{1}{3} \times \frac{1}{2}$

3. Multiply: $\frac{1 \times 1}{3 \times 2} = \frac{1}{6}$

4. Reduce: Not necessary.

NOTE: To divide mixed fractions, first convert the mixed fraction(s) to an improper fraction(s).

EXAMPLE 3: $1\frac{1}{2} \div \frac{3}{4}$

1. Convert: $\frac{3}{2} \div \frac{3}{4}$

2. Invert: $\frac{3}{2} \times \frac{4}{3}$

3. Cancel: $\frac{\overset{1}{\cancel{3}}}{\underset{1}{\cancel{2}}} = \frac{\overset{2}{\cancel{4}}}{\underset{1}{\cancel{3}}} = \frac{1}{1} \times \frac{2}{1}$

4. Multiply: $\frac{1 \times 2}{1 \times 1} = \frac{2}{1}$

5. Reduce: $\frac{2}{1} = 2$

NOTE: To *multiply* complex fractions also involves the division of fractions. Study this carefully.

EXAMPLE 4: $\dfrac{\frac{1}{150}}{\frac{1}{100}} \times 2$

1. Convert: Express 2 as a fraction. $\dfrac{\frac{1}{150}}{\frac{1}{100}} \times \frac{2}{1}$

2. Invert: $\frac{1}{150} \times \frac{100}{1} \times \frac{2}{1}$

3. Cancel: $\frac{1}{\overset{}{\underset{3}{150}}} \times \frac{\overset{2}{100}}{1} \times \frac{2}{1} = \frac{1}{3} \times \frac{2}{1} \times \frac{2}{1}$

4. Multiply: $\frac{1}{3} \times \frac{2}{1} \times \frac{2}{1} = \frac{4}{3}$

5. Reduce: $\frac{4}{3} = 1\frac{1}{3}$

This example appears very difficult at first, but when solved logically, one step at a time, it is just like the others.

quick review

- *To add or subtract fractions*, convert to equivalent fractions with like denominators, then add or subtract the numerators.
- *To multiply fractions*, multiply numerators and multiply denominators.
- *To divide fractions*, invert the divisor and multiply.
- Reduce results to lowest terms.

review set 3

Multiply and reduce the answers to lowest terms.

1. $\frac{3}{10} \times \frac{1}{12} =$ _____

2. $\frac{12}{25} \times \frac{3}{5} =$ _____

3. $\frac{5}{8} \times 1\frac{1}{6} =$ _____

4. $\frac{1}{100} \times 3 =$ _____

5. $\dfrac{\frac{1}{6}}{\frac{1}{4}} \times \dfrac{\frac{3}{2}}{\frac{2}{3}} =$ _____

6. $\dfrac{\frac{1}{150}}{\frac{1}{100}} \times 2\frac{1}{2} =$ _____

7. $\frac{30}{75} \times 2 =$ _____

Add and reduce the answers to lowest terms.

8. $7\frac{4}{5} + \frac{2}{3} =$ _____

9. $\frac{3}{4} + \frac{2}{3} =$ _____

10. $4\frac{2}{3} + 5\frac{1}{24} + 7\frac{1}{2} =$ _____

11. $\frac{3}{4} + \frac{1}{8} + \frac{1}{6} =$ _____

12. $12\frac{1}{2} + 20\frac{1}{3} =$ _____

Subtract and reduce the answers to lowest terms.

13. $\frac{3}{4} - \frac{1}{4} =$ _____

14. $8\frac{1}{12} - 3\frac{1}{4} =$ _____

15. $\frac{1}{8} - \frac{1}{12} =$ _____

16. $100\frac{1}{33} - 33\frac{1}{3} =$ _____

17. $355\frac{1}{5} - 55\frac{2}{5} =$ _____

Divide and reduce the answers to lowest terms.

18. $\frac{1}{60} \div \frac{1}{2} =$ _____

19. $2\frac{1}{2} \div \frac{3}{4} =$ _____

20. $\dfrac{\frac{1}{20}}{\frac{1}{3}} =$ _____

21. $\frac{1}{150} \div \frac{1}{50} =$ _____

22. $\dfrac{\frac{3}{4}}{\frac{7}{8}} \div \dfrac{1\frac{1}{2}}{2\frac{1}{3}} =$ _____

23. $\dfrac{\frac{3}{5}}{\frac{3}{4}} \div \dfrac{\frac{4}{5}}{1\frac{1}{9}} =$ _____

24. One large apple contains 80 calories. How many calories do you consume if you eat $\frac{3}{4}$ of an apple? _____

25. How many seconds are there in $9\frac{1}{3}$ minutes? _____

26. A circle is divided into 12 equal parts with 4 parts shaded. Write a fraction reduced to lowest terms to express the unshaded parts. _____

27. A bottle of Children's Tylenol contains 20 teaspoons of liquid. If each dose for a 2-year-old child is $\frac{1}{2}$ teaspoon, how many doses are available in this bottle? _____

28. You need to take $1\frac{1}{2}$ tablets of medication 3 times per day for 7 days. Over the 7 days, how many tablets will you take? _____

After completing these problems, see pages 288 and 289 to check your answers.

Decimals

Decimals or *decimal fractions* are fractions with a denominator of 10, 100, 1000, or any multiple or power of 10. The position of the number in relation to the decimal point indicates its value.

EXAMPLE: Look carefully at the decimal fraction 0.125.

$$0 \,.\, \underset{\text{Tenths}}{1} \quad \underset{\text{Hundredths}}{2} \quad \underset{\text{Thousandths}}{5}$$

$0.125 = \frac{125}{1000}$ or one hundred twenty-five thousandths

0.125 is less than 0.25 (twenty-five hundredths) but greater than 0.0125 (one hundred twenty-five ten thousandths)

Zeros added after the last digit of a decimal fraction *do not* change its value: 0.25 = 0.250. Zeros added between the decimal point and the first digit of a decimal fraction *do* change its value: 0.125 ("is *not* equal to") 0.0125.

To eliminate possible confusion by overlooking a decimal as a whole number, *always* place a zero to the left of the decimal point to emphasize it: 0.125, 0.01, 0.005.

Read decimals by naming the value of the place: $0.1 = \frac{1}{10}$ is read "one-tenth." In the case of mixed decimals, read the *decimal point* as "and": $1.01 = 1\frac{1}{100}$ is read "one *and* one-hundredth."

For dosage calculations you may need to convert decimals to fractions and vice versa.

▶ **rule** To convert a fraction to a decimal, divide the numerator by the denominator.

EXAMPLE: Convert $\frac{1}{4}$ to a decimal.

$$\frac{1}{4} = 4\overline{)1.00} = 0.25$$

$$\begin{array}{r} .25 \\ 4\overline{)1.00} \\ \underline{8} \\ 20 \\ \underline{20} \end{array}$$

▶ **rule** To convert a decimal to a fraction,

1. express the decimal number as a whole number in the numerator of the fraction,
2. express the denominator of the fraction as the number 1 followed by as many zeros as there are places to the right of the decimal point, and
3. reduce the resultant fraction to lowest terms.

EXAMPLE: Convert 0.125 to a fraction.
1. Numerator: 125
2. Denominator: 1 + 3 zeros = 1000
3. Reduce: $\frac{125}{1000} = \frac{1}{8}$

review set 4 _____

Complete the following table of equivalent fractions and decimals. Reduce fractions to lowest terms.

	Fraction	Decimal	The *decimal* is read as:
1.	$\frac{1}{5}$	_____	_____
2.	_____	_____	eighty-five hundredths
3.	_____	1.05	_____
4.	_____	0.006	_____
5.	$10\frac{3}{200}$	_____	_____
6.	_____	1.9	_____
7.	_____	_____	five and one-tenth
8.	$\frac{4}{5}$	_____	_____
9.	_____	250.5	_____

	Fraction	Decimal	The *decimal* is read as:
10.	$33\frac{3}{100}$	_____	_____
11.	_____	0.95	_____
12.	$2\frac{3}{4}$	_____	_____
13.	_____	_____	seven and five-thousandths
14.	$\frac{21}{250}$	_____	_____
15.	_____	12.125	_____
16.	_____	20.09	_____
17.	_____	_____	twenty-two and twenty-two thousandths
18.	_____	0.15	_____
19.	$1000\frac{1}{200}$	_____	_____
20.	_____	_____	four thousand eighty-five and seventy-five thousandths

After completing these problems, see page 289 to check your answers.

Addition and Subtraction of Decimals

The addition and subtraction of decimals is very similar to addition and subtraction of whole numbers. There are only two simple rules that are different.

> ▶ **rule**   To add and subtract decimal fractions, line up the decimal points.

EXAMPLE 1: $1.25 + 1.75 = $
$$\begin{array}{r} 1.25 \\ +\ 1.75 \\ \hline 3.00 = 3 \end{array}$$

EXAMPLE 2: $1.25 - 0.13 = $
$$\begin{array}{r} 1.25 \\ -\ 0.13 \\ \hline 1.12 \end{array}$$

> ▶ **rule**   To add and subtract decimal fractions, add zeros to the right of the decimal point, making all decimal numbers of equal length.

EXAMPLE 1: $3.75 - 2.1 = $
$$\begin{array}{r} 3.75 \\ -\ 2.10 \\ \hline 1.65 \end{array}$$

EXAMPLE 2:   Add 0.9, 0.65, 0.27, 4.712
$$\begin{array}{r} 0.900 \\ 0.650 \\ 0.270 \\ +\ 4.712 \\ \hline 6.532 \end{array}$$

review set 5

Find the result of the following problems.

1. 0.16 + 5.375 + 1.05 + 16 = _____

2. 7.517 + 3.2 + 0.16 + 33.3 = _____

3. 13.009 − 0.7 = _____

4. 5.125 + 6.025 + 0.15 = _____

5. 175.1 + 0.099 = _____

6. 25.2 − 0.193 = _____

7. 0.58 − 0.062 = _____

8. $10.10 − $0.62 = _____

9. $19 − $0.09 = _____

10. $5.05 + $0.17 + $17.49 = _____

11. 4 + 1.98 + 0.42 + 0.003 = _____

12. 0.3 − 0.03 = _____

13. 16.3 − 12.15 = _____

14. 2.5 − 0.99 = _____

15. 5 + 2.5 + 0.05 + 0.15 + 2.55 = _____

16. 0.03 + 0.16 + 2.327 = _____

17. 700 − 325.65 = _____

18. 645.32 − 40.9 = _____

19. 18 + 2.35 + 7.006 + 0.093 = _____

20. 13.529 + 10.09 = _____

After completing these problems, see page 289 to check your answers.

Multiplying Decimals

The procedure in multiplication of decimals is the same as for whole numbers. The only difference is in the expression of the product or answer. Use the following simple rule:

> **▶ rule** To multiply decimals,
> 1. multiply the decimals without concern for decimal placement,
> 2. count off the number of decimal places in the decimals multiplied, and
> 3. place the decimal point in the product to the left of the total number of places counted.

EXAMPLE 1: $1.5 \times 0.5 =$

$$
\begin{array}{r}
1.5 \\
\times \ 0.5 \\
\hline
0.75
\end{array}
$$

(1 decimal place)
(1 decimal place)
(The decimal point is located 2 places to the left, because *2* decimal places are counted.)

EXAMPLE 2: $1.72 \times 0.9 =$

$$
\begin{array}{r}
1.72 \\
\times\ \ 0.9 \\
\hline
1.548
\end{array}
$$

(2 decimal places)
(1 decimal place)
(The decimal point is located 3 places to the left, because *3* decimal places are counted.)

EXAMPLE 3: $5.06 \times 1.3 =$

$$
\begin{array}{r}
5.06 \\
\times\ \ 1.3 \\
\hline
1\,518 \\
+\ 5\,06\ \ \\
\hline
6.578
\end{array}
$$

(2 decimal places)
(1 decimal place)

(The decimal point is located 3 places to the left, because *3* decimal places are counted.)

> ▶ **rule** When multiplying a decimal by a power of ten, move the decimal point as many places to the right as there are zeros in the multiplier.

EXAMPLE 1: Multiply 1.25 by 10

The multiplier 10 has 1 zero; move the decimal point 1 place to the right.

$1.25 \times 10 = 1.2.5 = 12.5$

EXAMPLE 2: Multiply 2.3 by 100

The multiplier 100 has 2 zeros; move the decimal point 2 places to the right. (Note: add zeros as necessary to complete the operation.)

$2.3 \times 100 = 2.30. = 230$

EXAMPLE 3: Multiply 0.001 by 1000

The multiplier 1000 has 3 zeros; move the decimal point 3 places to the right.

$0.001 \times 1000 = 0.001. = 1$

Dividing Decimals

When dividing decimals, set up the problem the same as for the division of whole numbers. Follow the same procedure for dividing whole numbers, after you apply the following rule.

> ▶ **rule** To divide decimals,
> 1. move the decimal in the divisor (number divided by) and the dividend (number divided), the number of places needed to make the *divisor* a *whole number;*
> 2. place the decimal point in the quotient (answer) above the new decimal place in the dividend.

NOTE: Moving the decimal point to the right is the same as multiplying by 10, 100, 1000, etc. Recall the rule: multiplying or dividing both the numerator and the denominator by the same nonzero number does not change the value.

EXAMPLE 1:

$$100.75 \div 2.5 = 2.5. \overline{\smash{\big)}\ 100.7\,5} = 40.3$$

with quotient 40.3, dividend 100.75, divisor 2.5

$$
\begin{array}{r}
4\ 0.3 \text{ (quotient)} \\
2.5. \overline{\smash{\big)}\ 100.7\,5} = 40.3 \\
\underline{100} \\
75 \\
\underline{75}
\end{array}
$$

100.75 ÷ 2.5 = 2.5. (dividend) (divisor)

EXAMPLE 2:

$$56.5 \div 0.02 = 0.02. \overline{\smash{\big)}\ 56.50} = 2825$$

$$
\begin{array}{r}
28\ 25. \\
0.02. \overline{\smash{\big)}\ 56.50} = 2825 \\
\underline{4} \\
16 \\
\underline{16} \\
5 \\
\underline{4} \\
10 \\
\underline{10}
\end{array}
$$

NOTE: Recall that adding a zero after a decimal does not change its value ($56.5 = 56.50$).

> **rule** When dividing a decimal by a power of ten, move the decimal point to the left as many places as there are zeros in the divisor.

EXAMPLE 1:   Divide 0.65 by 10
The divisor 10 has 1 zero; move the decimal point 1 place to the left.
$$0.65 \div 10 = .0.65 = 0.065$$
(Note: place the zero to the left of the decimal point to avoid confusion and to emphasize that this is a decimal.)

EXAMPLE 2:   Divide 7.3 by 100
The divisor 100 has 2 zeros; move the decimal point 2 places to the left.
$$7.3 \div 100 = .07.3 = 0.073$$
(Note: add zeros as necessary to complete the operation.)

EXAMPLE 3:   Divide 0.5 by 1000
The divisor 1000 has 3 zeros; move the decimal point 3 places to the left.
$$0.5 \div 1000 = .000.5 = 0.0005$$

Rounding Decimal Fractions

For most dosage calculations, it will only be necessary to carry decimals to thousandths (*three* decimal places) and round back to hundredths (*two* places) for the final answer. (You will also need to round to tenths.)

> **rule** To round a decimal to hundredths,
>
> 1. do not change the number in hundredths place, if the number in thousandths place is 4 or less;
> 2. increase the number in hundredths place by 1, if the number in thousandths place is 5 or more.

EXAMPLES: 0.123 = 0.12   Rounded to hundredths (two places)
1.744 = 1.74
5.325 = 5.33
0.666 = 0.67

> **rule** To round a decimal to tenths,
>
> 1. do not change the number in tenths place, if the number in hundredths place is 4 or less;
> 2. increase the number in tenths place by 1, if the number in hundredths place is 5 or more.

EXAMPLES: 0.13 = 0.1   Rounded to tenths (one place)
5.64 = 5.6
0.75 = 0.8
1.66 = 1.7

quick review

- To multiply decimals, place the decimal point in the product to the *left* as many decimal places as there are in the two decimals multiplied. Example: $0.25 \times 0.2 = 0.050 = 0.05$
- To divide decimals, move the decimal point in the divisor and dividend the number of decimal places that will make the divisor a whole number. Example:

$$1.2\overline{)24.0} \to 20.$$

- To multiply or divide decimals by powers of 10, move the decimal to the *right* (to *multiply*) or to the *left* (to *divide*) the number of decimal places as there are zeros in the multiple of 10. Examples: $5.06 \times 10 = 5.06 = 50.6$; $2.1 \div 100 = .02.1 = 0.021$
- When rounding decimals, add 1 to the place value considered if the next decimal place is 5 or greater. Examples: (rounded to hundredths) 3.054 = 3.05; 0.566 = 0.57; (rounded to tenths) 3.05 = 3.1; 0.54 = 0.5

review set 6

Multiply and round your answers to two decimal places.

1. $1.16 \times 5.03 =$ _____   6. $75.1 \times 1000.01 =$ _____

2. $0.314 \times 7 =$ _____   7. $16.03 \times 2.05 =$ _____

3. $1.71 \times 25 =$ _____   8. $55.50 \times 0.05 =$ _____

4. $3.002 \times 0.05 =$ _____   9. $23.2 \times 15.025 =$ _____

5. $16.1 \times 25.04 =$ _____   10. $1.14 \times 0.014 =$ _____

Divide and round your answers to two decimal places.

11. $16 \div 0.04 =$ _____   16. $73 \div 13.40 =$ _____

12. $25.3 \div 6.76 =$ _____   17. $16.36 \div 0.06 =$ _____

13. $0.02 \div 0.004 =$ _____   18. $0.375 \div 0.25 =$ _____

14. $45.5 \div 15.25 =$ _____   19. $100.04 \div 0.002 =$ _____

15. $515 \div 0.125 =$ _____   20. $45 \div 0.15 =$ _____

Multiply or divide by the power of 10 indicated. Draw an arrow to demonstrate movement of the decimal point.

21. $562.5 \times 100 =$ _____   26. $23.25 \times 10 =$ _____

22. $16 \times 10 =$ _____   27. $717.717 \div 10 =$ _____

23. $25 \div 1000 =$ _____   28. $83.16 \times 10 =$ _____

24. $32.005 \div 1000 =$ _____   29. $0.33 \times 100 =$ _____

25. $0.125 \div 100 =$ _____   30. $14.106 \times 1000 =$ _____

After completing these problems, see page 290 to check your answers.

Ratio and Percent

Other expressions equivalent to fractions ($\frac{1}{2}$) and decimals (0.5) are ratios (1:2) and percents (50%).

A *ratio* is used to indicate the relationship of one quantity to another. When written, the two quantities are separated by a colon (:).

In drug solutions, the ratio is used occasionally to indicate the amount of drug to the amount of solution.

EXAMPLE: Adrenalin 1:1000 solution = 1 part Adrenalin to 1000 parts solution.

Actually a ratio is the same as a fraction; 1:1000 is the same as $\frac{1}{1000}$.

Percent means per hundred parts or hundredth part. Percent is a fraction or a ratio with the denominator always being 100. The symbol for percent is %.

EXAMPLE: $25\% = \frac{25}{100} = 25{:}100 = 25$ parts per 100 parts

Since the denominator of a percent is always 100, it is easy to find the equivalent decimal. Recall, to divide by 100 move the decimal point to the left the number of places equal to the number of zeros in the denominator.

EXAMPLE: $25\% = \frac{25}{100} = 25 \div 100 = .25. = 0.25$

quick review

- To change a percent to a decimal fraction, move the decimal point two places to the left. Example: 4% = .04. = 0.04
- To change a decimal fraction to a percent, move the decimal point two places to the right. Example: 0.04 = 0.04. = 4%.

review set 7

Find the equivalent decimal, fraction, percent, and ratio forms. Reduce fractions and ratios to lowest terms; round decimals to two places.

	Decimal	Fraction	Percent	Ratio
1.	_____	$\frac{2}{5}$	_____	_____
2.	0.05	_____	_____	_____
3.	_____	_____	17%	_____
4.	_____	_____	_____	1:4
5.	_____	_____	6%	_____
6.	_____	$\frac{1}{6}$	_____	_____
7.	_____	_____	50%	_____
8.	_____	_____	_____	1:100
9.	0.09	_____	_____	_____
10.	_____	$\frac{3}{8}$	_____	_____
11.	_____	_____	_____	2:3
12.	_____	$\frac{1}{3}$	_____	_____
13.	0.52	_____	_____	_____
14.	_____	_____	_____	9:20
15.	_____	$\frac{6}{7}$	_____	_____
16.	_____	_____	_____	3:10
17.	_____	$\frac{1}{50}$	_____	_____
18.	0.6	_____	_____	_____
19.	0.04	_____	_____	_____
20.	_____	_____	10%	_____

After completing these problems, see page 290 to check your answers.

Solving Simple Equations for X

Common formulas used in clinical calculations involve solving a simple equation for an unknown value X. Having completed your math review to this point, you have mastered the skills necessary to perfect this operation. The following examples demonstrate various forms of this equation you will encounter. *Learn to express your answers in decimal form* since decimals will be used most often in dosage calculations and administration. Round decimals to hundredths or to two places.

EXAMPLE 1: $\frac{100}{200} \times 1 = X$

HINT: You can drop the 1 since a number multiplied by 1 is the same number.

Therefore, $\frac{100}{200} = X$

1. Reduce to lowest terms: $\frac{100}{200} = \frac{\overset{1}{\cancel{100}}}{\underset{2}{\cancel{200}}} = \frac{1}{2} = X$

2. Convert to decimal form: $\frac{1}{2} = 0.5 = X$

3. You have your answer. $X = 0.5$

EXAMPLE 2: $\frac{3}{5} \times 2 = X$

1. Convert: Express 2 as a fraction. $\frac{3}{5} \times \frac{2}{1} = X$

2. Multiply fractions: $\frac{3}{5} \times \frac{2}{1} = \frac{6}{5} = X$

3. Reduce to lowest terms: $\frac{6}{5} = 1\frac{1}{5} = X$

4. Convert to decimal form: $1\frac{1}{5} = 1.2 = X$

5. You have your answer. $X = 1.2$

EXAMPLE 3: $\frac{\frac{1}{6}}{\frac{1}{4}} \times 5 = X$

1. Convert: Express 5 as a fraction. $\frac{\frac{1}{6}}{\frac{1}{4}} \times \frac{5}{1} = X$

2. Divide fractions: Invert the divisor and multiply. $\frac{1}{6} \times \frac{4}{1} \times \frac{5}{1} = X$

3. Cancel terms: $\frac{1}{\cancel{6}} \times \frac{\overset{2}{\cancel{4}}}{1} \times \frac{5}{1} = \frac{1}{3} \times \frac{2}{1} \times \frac{5}{1} = \frac{10}{3} = X$

4. Reduce to lowest terms: $\frac{10}{3} = 3\frac{1}{3} = X$

5. Convert to decimal form: $3\frac{1}{3} = 3.333 = X$

6. Round to hundredths place: $3.333 = 3.33 = X$

7. Easy, when you take it one step at a time. $X = 3.33$

EXAMPLE 4: $\frac{\frac{1}{100}}{\frac{1}{150}} \times 2.2 = X$

1. Convert: Express 2.2 in fraction form. $\frac{\frac{1}{100}}{\frac{1}{150}} \times \frac{2.2}{1} = X$

2. Divide fractions: Invert the divisor and multiply. $\frac{1}{100} \times \frac{150}{1} \times \frac{2.2}{1} = X$

3. Cancel terms: $\dfrac{1}{\overset{\,}{\underset{2}{\cancel{100}}}} \times \dfrac{\overset{3}{\cancel{150}}}{1} \times \dfrac{2.2}{1} =$

$$\frac{1}{2} \times \frac{3}{1} \times \frac{2.2}{1} = X$$

4. Multiply: $\dfrac{1}{2} \times \dfrac{3}{1} \times \dfrac{2.2}{1} = \dfrac{6.6}{2} = X$

5. Divide: $\dfrac{6.6}{2} = 3.3 = X$

6. That's it! $X = 3.3$

EXAMPLE 5: $\dfrac{0.125}{0.25} \times 1.5 = X$

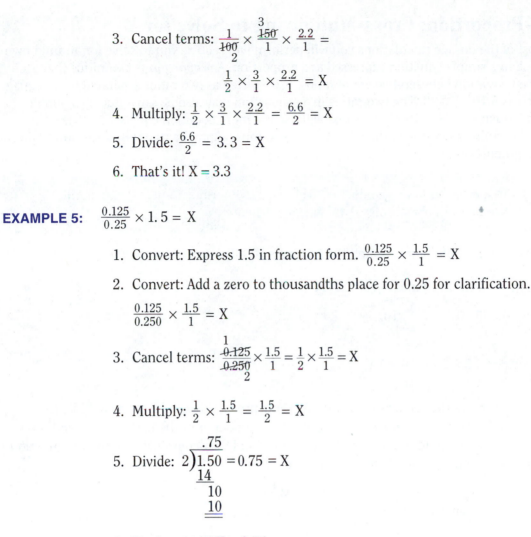

1. Convert: Express 1.5 in fraction form. $\dfrac{0.125}{0.25} \times \dfrac{1.5}{1} = X$

2. Convert: Add a zero to thousandths place for 0.25 for clarification.

$$\frac{0.125}{0.250} \times \frac{1.5}{1} = X$$

3. Cancel terms: $\dfrac{\overset{1}{\cancel{0.125}}}{\underset{2}{\cancel{0.250}}} \times \dfrac{1.5}{1} = \dfrac{1}{2} \times \dfrac{1.5}{1} = X$

4. Multiply: $\dfrac{1}{2} \times \dfrac{1.5}{1} = \dfrac{1.5}{2} = X$

5. Divide:
$$
\begin{array}{r}
.75 \\
2\overline{)1.50} \\
\underline{14} \\
10 \\
\underline{10} \\
\end{array}
= 0.75 = X
$$

6. You've got it! $X = 0.75$

HINT: Example 5 can also be solved by canceling both terms and working in common fractions instead of decimal fractions.

Try this: $\dfrac{0.125}{0.25} \times 1.5 = X$

1. Convert: Express 1.5 in fraction form. $\dfrac{0.125}{0.25} \times \dfrac{1.5}{1} = X$

2. Convert: Add zeros, making *both* decimal fractions of equal length.

$$\frac{0.125}{0.250} \times \frac{1.5}{1.0} = X$$

3. Cancel terms: $\dfrac{\overset{1}{\cancel{0.125}}}{\underset{2}{\cancel{0.250}}} \times \dfrac{3}{2} = \dfrac{1}{2} \times \dfrac{3}{2} = X$

4. Multiply: $\dfrac{1}{2} \times \dfrac{3}{2} = \dfrac{3}{4} = X$

5. Convert: $\dfrac{3}{4} = 0.75 = X$

6. You've got it again! $X = 0.75$

Which way do you find easier?

Ratio-Proportion: Cross-Multiplying to Solve for X

Most of the dosage calculations you will perform will require you to solve for an unknown quantity X in a simple equation expressed as a proportion. A *proportion* is two ratios that are equal or an equation between two equal ratios. It is written as two ratios separated by an equals sign, such as 5:10 = 10:20. The two ratios in a proportion may also be separated by a double colon sign, such as 5:10 :: 10:20. This text will use the more common equals sign (=).

To determine the value of the unknown X, you must apply the rule for cross-multiplying used in a proportion.

> **rule**   In a proportion the product of the means (two inside numbers) equals the product of the extremes (two outside numbers).

Finding the product of the means and the extremes is called *cross-multiplying*.

EXAMPLE:
$$\text{Extremes}$$
$$5{:}10 \quad = \quad 10{:}20$$
$$\text{Means}$$
$$5 \times 20 = 10 \times 10$$
$$100 = 100$$

Since ratios are the same as fractions, the same proportion can be expressed like this: $\frac{5}{10} = \frac{10}{20}$. The fractions are *equivalent* or equal. The numerator of the first fraction and the denominator of the second fraction are the extremes, and the denominator of the first fraction and the numerator of the second fraction are the means.

EXAMPLE: Extreme $\frac{5}{10} \quad \times \quad \frac{10}{20}$ Mean
                 Mean   Extreme

Cross-multiply to find the equal products of the means and extremes.

> **rule**   If two fractions are *equivalent* or equal, their cross-products are also equal.

EXAMPLE: $\frac{5}{10} \quad \times \quad \frac{10}{20}$
$$5 \times 20 = 10 \times 10$$
$$100 = 100$$

When one of the quantities in a proportion is unknown, a letter, such as X, may be substituted for this unknown quantity. You would solve the equation to find the value of X. In addition to cross-multiplying, there is one more rule you need to know to solve for X in a proportion.

> **rule**   Dividing or multiplying each side (member) of an equation by the same non-zero number produces an equivalent equation.

Dividing each side of an equation by the same nonzero number is the same as *reducing* or simplifying the equation. Multiplying each side by the same nonzero number *enlarges* the equation. Let's examine how to simplify an equation.

EXAMPLE: $25X = 100$

$$\frac{25X}{25} = \frac{100}{25}$$ Simplify the equation to find X.
Divide both sides by 25.

$$X = 4$$

Replace X with its value of 4 in the same equation and you can prove that the calculations are correct.

$$25 \times 4 = 100$$

$$\frac{25 \times 4}{25} = \frac{100}{25}$$

$$4 = 4$$

Now you are ready to apply the concepts of *cross-multiplying* and *simplifying an equation* to solve for X in a proportion. Let's look at some examples.

EXAMPLE 1: $\dfrac{90}{2} = \dfrac{45}{X}$

You have a proportion with an unknown quantity X in the denominator of the second fraction. Find the value of X.

1. Cross-multiply: $\dfrac{90}{2} \diagdown\!\!\!\!\diagup \dfrac{45}{X}$

2. Multiply terms: $90 \times X = 2 \times 45$

$$90X = 90$$

3. Simplify the equation: Divide both sides of the equation by the number before the unknown X. You are equally reducing the terms on both sides of the equation.

$$\frac{90X}{90} = \frac{90}{90}$$

$$X = 1$$

Try another one. The unknown X is a different term.

EXAMPLE 2: $\dfrac{80}{X} \times 60 = 20$

1. Convert: Express "60" as a fraction.

$$\frac{80}{X} \times \frac{60}{1} = 20$$

2. Multiply fractions: $\dfrac{80}{X} \times \dfrac{60}{1} = 20$

$$\frac{4800}{X} = 20$$

3. Convert: Express "20" as a fraction.

$$\frac{4800}{X} = \frac{20}{1}$$

You now have a proportion.

4. Cross-multiply: $\dfrac{4800}{X} \diagdown\!\!\!\!\diagup \dfrac{20}{1}$

$$20X = 4800$$

5. Simplify: Divide both sides of the equation by the number before the unknown X.

$$\frac{20X}{20} = \frac{4800}{20}$$

$$X = 240$$

EXAMPLE 3: $\frac{160}{X} = \frac{80}{2.5}$

1. Cross-multiply: $\frac{160}{X} \diagtimes \frac{80}{2.5}$

   $80 \times X = 2.5 \times 160$

   $80X = 400$

2. Simplify: $\frac{80X}{80} = \frac{400}{80}$

   $X = 5$

EXAMPLE 4: $\frac{\frac{1}{4}}{3} = \frac{\frac{1}{2}}{X}$

1. Cross-multiply: $\frac{\frac{1}{4}}{3} \diagtimes \frac{\frac{1}{2}}{X}$

   $\frac{1}{4} X = 3 \times \frac{1}{2}$

   $\frac{1}{4} X = \frac{3}{1} \times \frac{1}{2}$

   $\frac{1}{4} X = \frac{3}{2}$

2. Simplify: $\frac{\frac{1}{4}X}{\frac{1}{4}} = \frac{\frac{3}{2}}{\frac{1}{4}}$

   $X = \dfrac{\frac{3}{2}}{\frac{1}{4}}$

3. Divide fractions; invert and multiply: $X = \frac{3}{2} \times \frac{4}{1}$

4. Cancel: $X = \frac{3}{\cancel{2}_1} \times \frac{\cancel{4}^2}{1} = \frac{3}{1} \times \frac{2}{1}$

5. Multiply: $X = \frac{3}{1} \times \frac{2}{1} = \frac{6}{1}$

   $X = 6$

When the value of X includes a fraction, *learn to express your answer in a decimal form.* Round decimals to hundredths or to two decimal places.

EXAMPLE 5: $\frac{288}{73} = \frac{14}{X}$

1. Cross-multiply: $\frac{288}{73} \diagtimes \frac{14}{X}$

   $288X = 73 \times 14$

   $288X = 1022$

2. Simplify: $\frac{288X}{288} = \frac{1022}{288}$

   $X = 3.549$

3. Round to two decimal places: $X = 3.55$

review set 8

Find the value of X. Express answers as decimals rounded to two places.

1. $\frac{1000}{2} = \frac{125}{X}$ _____

2. $\frac{500}{1.8} = \frac{250}{X}$ _____

3. $\frac{500}{1} = \frac{280}{X}$ _____

4. $\frac{0.5}{2} = \frac{250}{X}$ _____

5. $\frac{75}{1.5} = \frac{35}{X}$ _____

6. $\frac{X}{12} = \frac{1200}{28}$ _____

7. $\frac{X}{60} = \frac{1000}{28}$ _____

8. $\frac{2000}{X} = \frac{2}{0.5}$ _____

9. $\frac{500}{X} = \frac{15}{6}$ _____

10. $\frac{\frac{1}{4}}{500} = \frac{\frac{2.5}{100}}{X}$ _____

11. $\frac{250}{1} = \frac{750}{X}$ _____

12. $\frac{80}{5} = \frac{10}{X}$ _____

13. $\frac{5}{20} = \frac{X}{40}$ _____

14. $\frac{\frac{1}{100}}{1} = \frac{\frac{1}{150}}{X}$ _____

15. $\frac{2.2}{X} = \frac{8.8}{5}$ _____

16. $\frac{125}{60} \times 15 = X$ _____

17. $\frac{100}{60} \times 10 = X$ _____

18. $\frac{80}{X} \times 60 = 20$ _____

19. $\frac{6}{X} \times 0.5 = 4$ _____

20. $\frac{X}{5} \times 2.2 = 1$ _____

21. $\frac{X}{\frac{1}{4}} \times 15 = 60$ _____

22. $\frac{5}{25\%} \times 30\% = X$ _____

After completing these problems, see pages 290 and 291 to check your answers.

practice problems—chapter 1

Directions:
1. Carry answers to three decimal places and round to two places.
2. Express fractions in lowest terms.

Time Limit: 90 minutes

Convert to Roman numerals:

1. 14 _____   2. 25 _____   3. 8 _____   4. 20 _____

Convert to Arabic numbers:

5. VII _____   6. XXIV _____   7. XIX _____   8. XXX _____

Complete the operations indicated:

9. $\frac{1}{4} + \frac{2}{3} =$ _____

10. $\frac{6}{7} - \frac{1}{9} =$ _____

11. $1\frac{3}{5} \times \frac{5}{8} =$ _____

12. $\frac{3}{8} \div \frac{3}{4} =$ _____

13. $13.2 + 32.55 + 0.029 =$ _____

14. $80.3 - 21.06 =$ _____

15. $0.3 \times 0.3 =$ _____

16. $1.5 \div 0.125 =$ _____

17. $\frac{1}{150} \div \frac{1}{100} =$ _____

18. $\frac{\frac{1}{120}}{\frac{1}{60}} =$ _____

19. $20\% \times 0.09 =$ _____

20. $\frac{16\%}{\frac{1}{4}} =$ _____

Arrange in order from smallest to largest:

21. $\frac{1}{3}, \frac{1}{2}, \frac{1}{6}, \frac{1}{10}, \frac{1}{5}$ _____

22. $\frac{3}{4}, \frac{7}{8}, \frac{5}{6}, \frac{2}{3}, \frac{9}{10}$ _____

23. 0.25, 0.125, 0.3, 0.009, 0.1909   _____

24. 0.9%, $\frac{1}{2}$%, 50%, 500%, 100%   _____

Convert as indicated:

25. 1:100 to a decimal   _____   31. $\frac{1}{2}$% to a ratio   _____

26. $\frac{6}{150}$ to a decimal   _____   32. 2:3 to a fraction   _____

27. 0.009 to a percent   _____   33. 3:4 to a percent   _____

28. $33\frac{1}{3}$% to a fraction   _____   34. $\frac{2}{5}$ to a percent   _____

29. $\frac{5}{9}$ to a ratio   _____   35. $\frac{1}{6}$ to a decimal   _____

30. 0.05 to a fraction   _____

Find the value of X in the following equations. Express your answers as decimals rounded to the nearest hundredth.

36. $\frac{0.35}{1.3} \times 4.5 = X$ _____   41. $\frac{0.125}{2} = \frac{0.25}{X}$ _____

37. $\frac{0.3}{2.6} = \frac{0.15}{X}$ _____   42. $\frac{\frac{1}{2}\%}{1000} = \frac{10\%}{X}$ _____

38. $\frac{1,500,000}{500,000} \times X = 7.5$ _____   43. $\frac{\frac{1}{100}}{\frac{1}{150}} \times 2.2 = X$ _____

39. $\frac{\frac{1}{4}}{1} = \frac{\frac{1}{6}}{X}$ _____   44. $\frac{X}{15} = \frac{150}{7.5}$ _____

40. $\frac{1:4}{2500} = \frac{1:100}{X}$ _____   45. $\frac{1,000,000}{600,000} \times 5 = X$ _____

46. Each nurse can care for 6 patients. How many nurses will be needed to care for 30 patients?   _____

47. If you have a roll of dimes and you must pay $1.10, how many dimes will you use?   _____

48. If 1 pound of apples costs $0.69, how much do $3\frac{1}{2}$ pounds cost?   _____

49. To prepare orange juice from frozen concentrate, you mix 3 cans of water to every 1 can of juice concentrate. How many cans of water will you need to prepare 4 cans of juice concentrate?   _____

50. If 1 centimeter equals $\frac{3}{8}$ inch, how many centimeters are there in 3 inches?   _____

After completing these problems, see pages 318 and 319 to check your answers. Give yourself two points for each correct answer.

Perfect score = 100   My score = _____
Passing score = 86 or higher

For more practice, go back to the beginning of this chapter and repeat the Mathematics Diagnostic Test.

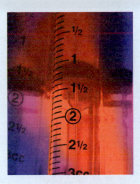

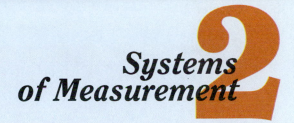

objectives

Upon mastery of Chapter 2, you will be able to recognize and express the basic systems of measurement used to calculate dosages. To accomplish this you will also be able to:

- Interpret and properly express metric, apothecaries', and household notation.
- Memorize and recall metric, apothecaries', and household equivalents.
- Explain the use of *mEq* and *U* in dosage calculation.

In order to administer the correct amount of the prescribed medication to the patient, you must be familiar with dosage calculations. A thorough knowledge of weights and measures used in the prescription and administration of medications is essential. The systems of weights and measures used by health professionals are the metric, apothecaries', and household systems. It is necessary for you to understand these systems and how to interchange from one system to another.

Most prescriptions are written using the metric system and all U. S. drug labels today give metric measurement. There are still a *few* prescriptions for older drugs written in the apothecaries' system, usually by physicians trained in this system. Until the metric system completely replaces the apothecaries' system, it is necessary for nurses to be familiar with both systems.

You are probably most familiar with the English system of measurement in your everyday experiences. In the English system,

- *length* is measured in inches, feet, yards, miles, etc.
- *weight* is measured in ounces, pounds, tons, etc.
- *volume* is measured in pints, quarts, gallons, etc.

Dosage calculations are most concerned with measurement of weight and volume. (*Volume*, or how much a container holds, is also called *capacity*.) However, linear measure (length) is also important in health care. For example, linear measure is used to measure the height of an individual to determine the person's growth patterns. Other examples include measurement of the circumference of a newborn baby's head and chest to assess the newborn's size in relation to birth weight, and to describe the size of incisions, lacerations, or tumors. In this text, you will learn about the measurement of body surface area to determine drug dosage. Body surface area is measured in the metric linear measure of meters–based on a comparison of weight and height.

The Metric System

The metric system is the most widely used system of measurement in the world today. It is the system most commonly used for prescribing and administering medications.

The metric system is a decimal system, which means it is based on multiples of ten. The base units of the metric systems are *gram* used for weight, *liter* used for volume, and *meter* used for length. In this system, prefixes are used to show which portion of the base unit is being considered. It is important that you learn the most commonly used prefixes.

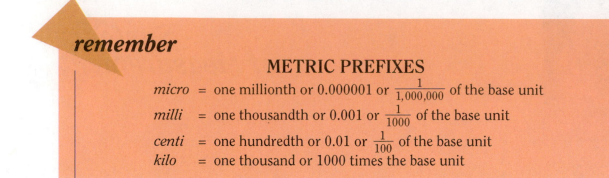

remember

METRIC PREFIXES

micro = one millionth or 0.000001 or $\frac{1}{1,000,000}$ of the base unit

milli = one thousandth or 0.001 or $\frac{1}{1000}$ of the base unit

centi = one hundredth or 0.01 or $\frac{1}{100}$ of the base unit

kilo = one thousand or 1000 times the base unit

The international standardization of metric units was adopted in 1960 with the *International System of Units* or *"SI."* The abbreviations of this system of metric notation are the most widely accepted.

The metric units of measure and their SI abbreviations that are most often used for dosage calculations and measurement of health status are given in the following units of volume, weight, and length. Other acceptable abbreviations are given in parentheses. This text will use the first or standardized abbreviation throughout; you should do the same.

remember

METRIC UNITS AND ABBREVIATIONS

weight: gram–g	**volume:** liter–L (ℓ)	**length:** meter–m
milligram–mg	milliliter–mL (mℓ)	centimeter–cm
microgram–mcg (μg)		millimeter–mm
kilogram–kg		

NOTE: Cubic centimeter (cc) is another common way of expressing milliliter. A cubic centimeter is the amount of space occupied by one milliliter of liquid. You may also see gram abbreviated as Gm or gm, and milliliter abbreviated as ml, but you should use the standardized abbreviations listed previously.

In addition to learning the metric units, their values, and their abbreviations, it is important to use the following rules of metric notation.

► *rules of metric notation*

1. The unit or abbreviation always follows the amount. Example: 5 g, NOT g 5.
2. Decimals are used to designate fractional metric units. Example: 1.5 mL, not $1\frac{1}{2}$ mL.
3. Use a zero to emphasize the decimal point for fractional metric units of less than 1. Example: 0.5 mg, NOT .5 mg. This is a critical rule as it will prevent confusion and potential dosage error. Consider for a moment if you overlooked the decimal point and misinterpreted the medication order as 5 mg instead of 0.5 mg. The patient would be overdosed 10 times.
4. Omit unnecessary zeros. Example: 1.5 g, NOT 1.50 g. This is another critical rule.
5. When in doubt, double check, and ask the writer for clarification.

The following table represents the basic metric units, abbreviations, and equivalents that are important for you to know. Learn the prefixes and you will find the metric system easy to understand and use. Notice that most calculations of equivalents you will use are derived

remember

M E T R I C

UNIT	ABBREVIATION	EQUIVALENTS
Weight		
gram	g	1 g = 1000 mg
milligram	mg	1 mg = 1000 mcg, or 0.001 g
microgram	mcg (μg)	1 mcg = 0.001 mg = 0.000001 g
kilogram	kg	1 kg = 1000 g
Volume		
liter	L (or ℓ)	1 L = 1000 mL
milliliter	mL (or m ℓ)	1 mL = 0.001 L, or 1 cc
cubic centimeter	cc	1 cc = 1 mL, or 0.001 L
Length		
meter	m	1 m = 100 cm, or 1000 mm
centimeter	cm	1 cm = 0.01 m, or 10 mm
millimeter	mm	1 mm = 0.001 m, or 0.1 cm

simply by multiplying or dividing by 1000. See Chapter 1 to review the rules for multiplying and dividing decimals by a power of ten.

The metric system is the common system of measurement in health care. Therefore, body weight is more often expressed in kilograms than in pounds. It is important for you to know the equivalent of pounds in kilograms since some drug dosages are now computed per kilogram of body weight (rather than pound). You can easily convert from pounds to kilograms if you know that 1 kilogram = 2.2 pounds (lb).

quick review

In the metric system:

- The metric base units are gram, liter, and meter.
- Subunits are designated by the appropriate prefix and the base unit, such as *milli*gram.
- The unit or abbreviation always follows the amount.
- Decimals are used to designate fractional amounts.
- Use a zero to emphasize the decimal point for fractional amounts of less than 1.
- Omit unnecessary zeros.
- Multiply or divide by 1000 to derive most equivalents needed for dosage calculations. 1 cc = 1 mL.
- When in doubt about the exact amount or the abbreviation used, do not guess. Ask the writer to clarify.

review set 9

1. The system of measurement most commonly used for prescribing and administering medications is the _____ system.

2. Liter and milliliter are metric units that measure _____.

3. Gram and milligram are metric units that measure _____.

4. Meter and millimeter are metric units that measure _____.

5. 1 mg is _____ of a g.

6. There are _____ mL in a liter.

7. 10 mL = _____ cc

8. Which is largest, kilogram, gram, or milligram? _____

9. Which is smallest, kilogram, gram, or milligram? _____

10. 1 liter = _____ cc

11. 1000 mcg = _____ mg

12. 1 kg = _____ lb

13. 1 cm = _____ mm

Select the *correct* metric notation.

14. .3 g, 0.3 Gm, 0.3 g, .3 Gm, 0.30 g   _____

15. $1\frac{1}{3}$ ml, 1.33 mL, 1.33 ML, $1\frac{1}{3}$ ML, 1.330 mL   _____

16. 5 Kg, 5.0 kg, kg 05, 5 kg, 5 kG   _____

17. 1.5 mm, $1\frac{1}{2}$ mm, 1.5 Mm, 1.50 MM, $1\frac{1}{2}$ MM   _____

18. mg 10, 10 mG, 10.0 mg, 10 mg, 10 MG   _____

Interpret these metric abbreviations.

19. mcg	_____	23. mm	_____
20. mL	_____	24. kg	_____
21. cc	_____	25. cm	_____
22. g	_____		

After completing these problems, see page 291 to check your answers.

Apothecaries' System

It seems likely that within a few years the metric system will be used exclusively in the measurement of medicines. However, as long as prescriptions are being written with apothecaries' and household notation, it is necessary that health care workers be knowledgeable about both of these systems.

In the apothecaries' system, Roman numerals are used more often than Arabic numbers to express whole numbers. Fractions are used to express amounts of less than one, except the fraction $\frac{1}{2}$ which is represented by the symbol "ss." (You will recall that in the metric system, amounts of less than one are expressed in decimals.)

Express apothecaries' amounts of ten or less in lowercase Roman numerals. Amounts greater than ten may be expressed in Arabic numbers except 20 and 30, which usually are expressed xx and xxx, respectively. For example, three grains = gr iii; twelve ounces = ℥ 12; and twenty grains = gr xx.

The common apothecaries' units still in use for medicines are the grain (gr) and ounce (℥). The most common unit of weight in the apothecaries' system is the *grain (gr)*. Aspirin is a familiar medicine dispensed in grains. There are no essential equivalents of length to learn in the apothecaries' system. The units of measurement and essential equivalents for volume in the apothecaries' system are given in the following table.

remember

APOTHECARY

UNIT	ABBREVIATION	EQUIVALENTS
quart	qt	qt i = pt ii
pint	pt	qt i = ℥ 32
fluidounce	℥	pt i = ℥ 16
dram	ℨ	
minim	♏	

NOTE: The minim (♏) and dram (ℨ) are given only so that you will be able to recognize them. Many syringes still have the minim scale identified and the medicine cup continues to show the dram scale. Both have become obsolete as a unit of measure, so there are no equivalents that you need to learn.

In the apothecaries' system, abbreviations or symbols are correctly written before the quantity. An example of this is gr iii, which is read "three grains." (Recall that this is different from the metric system wherein the number precedes the unit, such as 3 g or 3 mg.) Notice that the abbreviation for grain (gr) and gram (g) can be confusing. The system of indicating the abbreviation or symbol before the quantity in apothecaries' measurement further distinguishes it from the metric. But, if you are ever doubtful about the meaning that is intended, be sure to ask the writer for clarification.

Following are some examples of apothecaries' notations and their interpretations.

NOTATION	INTERPRETATION
gr i	one grain
gr vi	six grains
gr ss	one-half grain
gr iss	one and one-half grains
gr $\frac{1}{8}$	one-eighth grain
℥ ii	two ounces
ℨ iiss	two and one-half drams

HINT: The ounce (℥) is a larger unit and its symbol has one more loop on top than the dram (ℨ).

quick review

In the apothecaries' system:

- The common units for dosage calculations are grain and ounce.
- The quantity is best expressed in lowercase Roman numerals. Amounts greater than ten may be expressed in Arabic numbers, *except* 20 (xx) and 30 (xxx).
- Quantities of less than one are expressed as fractions, *except* $\frac{1}{2}$.
- One-half ($\frac{1}{2}$) is expressed by the symbol *ss*.
- The abbreviation or symbol is clearly written before the quantity.
- If you are unsure about the exact meaning of any medical notation, do not guess or assume; ask the writer for clarification.

review set 10 _____

Interpret the following apothecaries' symbols.

1. ℥ _____   3. **m** _____   5. gr _____

2. ℥ _____   4. ss _____

Correctly write the following quantities in the apothecaries system.

6. one-half ounce _____   12. eight and one-half ounces _____

7. one-sixth grain _____   13. two grains _____

8. four ounces _____   14. sixteen pints _____

9. two pints _____   15. three grains _____

10. one and one-fourth quarts _____   16. thirty-two ounces _____

11. ten grains _____   17. seven and one-half grains _____

Give the equivalent units.

18. qt i = ℥ _____   20. qt i = pt _____

19. ℥ 16 = pt _____

After completing these problems, see page 291 to check your answers.

Household System

Household units are likely to be used by the patient at home where hospital measuring devices are not available. You should be familiar with the household system of measurement so that you can explain take-home prescriptions to your patient at the time of discharge. These units are the least accurate and should not be relied upon in the hospital administration of medicines. The common household units and equivalents are given in the following table. There is no standardized system of notation for household measure; but, generally, the quantity is expressed in Arabic numbers with the abbreviation following.

remember

HOUSEHOLD

UNIT	ABBREVIATION	EQUIVALENT
drop	gtt	
teaspoon	tsp (or t)	1 T = 3 t
tablespoon	tbs (or T)	

NOTE: Like the minim (**m**) and dram (℥), the drop (**gtt**) unit is given only for the purpose of recognition. There are no standard equivalents to learn. The amount of each drop varies according to the diameter of the utensil used for measurement. (See Figure 4–2: Calibrated Dropper and Figure 11–9: Intravenous Drip Chambers.)

Other Common Drug Measures: Units and Milliequivalents

Two other measures may be used to indicate the quantity of medicine prescribed: the milliequivalent (mEq) and the unit (U). The *milliequivalent* is one-thousandth ($\frac{1}{1000}$) of an equivalent weight of a chemical. The *unit* (U) is a standardized amount needed to produce a desired effect. The meaning of the term *unit* varies for each drug measured in this way. Medications such as penicillin, heparin, and insulin are measured in standardized units. One-thousandth ($\frac{1}{1000}$) of a unit (U) is the *milliunit* (mU); equivalent : 1 U = 1000 mU. Pitocin is a drug prescribed in mU.

The quantity is expressed in Arabic numbers with the symbol following the amount.

EXAMPLE 1: Heparin 7500 U is ordered and Heparin 10,000 units per 1 mL is the stock drug.

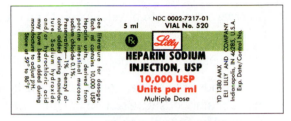

EXAMPLE 2: Potassium chloride 10 mEq is ordered and Potassium chloride 20 mEq per 15 mL is the stock drug.

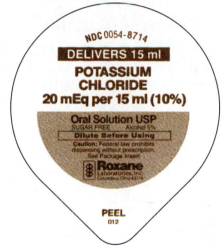

review set 11

Interpret the following notations.

1. 20 gtt   _____
2. 1000 U   _____
3. 10 mEq   _____
4. 4t   _____
5. 10 T   _____

Express the following using correct notation.

6. four drops   _____
7. 30 milliequivalents   _____
8. 5 tablespoons   _____
9. 1500 units   _____
10. 10 teaspoons   _____

11. The household system of measurement is commonly used in hospital dosage calculations.
    (True)   (False)

12. Drugs such as heparin and insulin are commonly measured in _____, abbreviated _____.

13. 1 T = _____ t   14. 3 T = _____ t   15. 1 U = _____ mU

After completing these problems, see page 291 to check your answers.

The importance of the placement of the decimal point cannot be overemphasized. Let's look at some examples of potential medication errors related to the placement of the decimal point.

■ *error 1*

Not placing a zero before a decimal point on medication orders.

possible scenario

An emergency room physician wrote an order for the bronchodilator terbutaline for a patient with asthma. The order was written as follows:

Terbutaline .5 mg subcutaneously now, repeat dose in 30 minutes if no improvement

Suppose the nurse, not noticing the faint decimal point, administered terbutaline 5 mg subcutaneously instead of 0.5 mg. The patient would receive ten times the dose intended by the physician.

potential outcome

Within minutes of receiving the injection the patient would likely complain of headache, and develop tachycardia, nausea, and vomiting. The patient's hospital stay would have been lengthened due to the need to recover from the overdose.

prevention

This type of medication error is avoided by remembering the rule to place a 0 in front of a decimal to avoid confusion regarding the dosage: 0.5 mg. Further, remember to question orders that are unclear or seem unreasonable.

■ *error 2*

Using decimal points and zero on medication orders when they serve no purpose.

possible scenario

Suppose a physician ordered oral Coumadin (an anticoagulant) for a patient with a history of phlebitis. The physician wrote an order for 1 mg, but while writing the order placed a decimal point after the 1 and added a 0:

Coumadin 1.0 mg orally once per day

Coumadin 1.0 mg could easily be transcribed on the medication record by the unit clerk as Coumadin 10 mg. Should this occur, the patient would receive ten times the correct dose.

potential outcome

The patient would likely begin hemorrhaging. An antidote, such as vitamin K, would be necessary to reverse the effects of the overdose. However, it is important to remember that not all drugs have antidotes.

prevention

This type of error can be avoided by not using a decimal point or extra zero when not necessary. In this instance the decimal point serves no purpose and can easily be misinterpreted, especially if the decimal point is difficult to see. Question any order that is unclear or unreasonable.

critical thinking skills

Many medication errors occur by confusing mg's and mL's. Remember that mg is the weight of the medication, and mL is the volume of the medication preparation.

■ error 3

Confusing mg and mL.

possible scenario

Suppose a physician ordered Prelone (prednisolone, a steroid) 15 mg by mouth twice a day for a patient with cancer. Prelone syrup is supplied in a concentration of 15 mg in 5 mL. The pharmacist supplied a bottle of Prelone containing a total volume of 240 mL with 15 mg of Prelone in every 5 mL. The nurse, in a rush to give her medications on time, misread the order as 15 mL and gave the patient Prelone 15 mL instead of 5 mL. Therefore, the patient received 45 mg of Prelone, or three times the correct dosage.

potential outcome

The patient could develop a number of complications related to a high dosage of steroids: gastrointestinal bleeding, headaches, seizures, and hypertension, to name a few.

prevention

Mg is the weight of medication, and mL is the volume you prepare. Do not allow yourself to get rushed or distracted so that you would confuse milligrams with milliliters. When you know you are distracted or stressed, have another nurse double check your dose.

practice problems—chapter 2

Give the metric prefix for the following amounts.

1. 0.001 _____
2. 0.000001 _____
3. 0.01 _____
4. 1000 _____

Identify the metric base unit for the following.

5. length _____
6. weight _____
7. volume _____

Interpret the following notations.

8. gtt _____
9. ℥ _____
10. m _____
11. gr _____
12. mg _____
13. mcg _____
14. U _____
15. mEq _____
16. t _____
17. ℨ _____
18. mL _____
19. cc _____
20. pt _____
21. T _____
22. mm _____
23. g _____

24. cm _____   26. m   _____

25. L _____   27. kg   _____

Express the following amounts in proper notation.

28. one-half grain

29. two teaspoons

30. one-third ounce

31. five hundred milliunits

32. one-half liter

33. one-fourth grain

34. one two-hundredths of a grain

35. five-hundredths of a milligram

After completing these problems, see page 319 to check your answers.

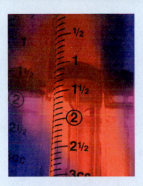

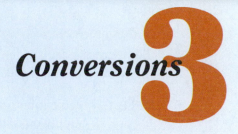

objectives

Upon mastery of Chapter 3, you will be able to complete step 1, conversions, in the three-step process of dosage calculations. To accomplish this, you will also be able to:

- Convert from one unit to another within the same system of measurement.
- Recall from memory the metric, apothecaries', and household approximate equivalents.
- Convert units of measure from one system of measurement to another system of measurement.

Also upon mastery of Chapter 3, you will be able to convert between Celsius and Fahrenheit temperature, and from traditional to 24-hour time.

Medications are usually prescribed or ordered in a unit of weight measure such as grams or grains. The nurse must interpret this order and administer the correct number of tablets, capsules, teaspoons, milliliters or some other unit of volume or capacity measure.

EXAMPLE 1: A prescription notation may read:
Tenormin 200 mg to be given orally

The nurse has on hand unit dose blister packets labeled *100 mg of Tenormin in each tablet*. In order to administer the correct amount of the drug, the nurse must convert the prescribed weight of 100 mg to the correct number of tablets. In this case, the nurse gives the patient two of the 100-mg tablets, which equals 200 mg of *Tenormin*. In order to give the prescribed dosage, the nurse must be able to calculate the order in weight to the correct amount in volume or capacity of the drug on hand or in stock. (If one tablet equals 100 mg, then two tablets equal 200 mg.)

EXAMPLE 2: A prescription notation may read:
Versed 2.5 mg by intramuscular injection

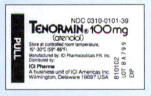

The nurse has on hand a vial of *Versed* labeled *5 mg/mL*. In order to adminis-ter the correct amount of the drug, the

(Courtesy of Roche Laboratories)

nurse must be able to fill the injection syringe with the correct number of milliliters. As the nurse, how many milliliters would you give? (If 5 mg = 1 mL, then 2.5 mg = 0.5 mL. Therefore, 0.5 mL should be administered.)

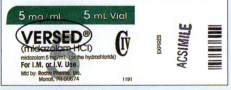

Sometimes a drug order may be written in a unit of measure that is different from the supply of drugs the nurse has on hand.

EXAMPLE 1:   Medication order: *Keflex 0.5 g orally*
Supply on hand: *Keflex 250 mg capsules*

The drug order is written in grams, but the drug is supplied in milligrams.

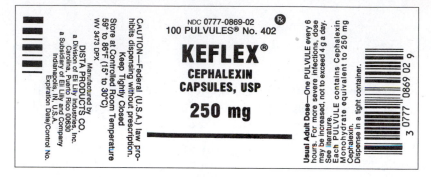

EXAMPLE 2:   Medication order: *Codeine gr ss orally*
Supply on hand: *Codeine 30 mg tablets*

The drug order is written in grains (apothecaries' measure), but the drug is supplied in milligrams (metric measure).

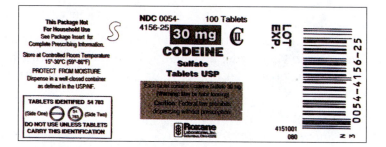

In such cases, the prescribed quantities must be converted into the units as supplied. The nurse can then calculate the correct dosage to prepare and administer to the patient. Thus, conversion is the first step in the calculation of dosages.

In this chapter you will learn two methods to do conversions: the *ratio-proportion* method and the *conversion factor* method. Study them both and then choose to use whichever one is easier and more logical to you.

Converting from One Unit to Another Using the Ratio-Proportion Method

After learning the systems of measurement common for dosage calculation and their equivalents (Chapter 2), the next step is to learn how to use them. First, you must be able to convert or change from one unit to another. To accomplish this simple operation you need to:

- recall the equivalents,
- set up a proportion of two equivalent ratios, and
- cross-multiply to solve for X.

rule   Ratio for known equivalent equals ratio for unknown equivalent.

EXAMPLE 1:   Let's start with units already familiar to you.

How many cups are in 3 quarts?

In units of household measure, 1 quart (qt) = 4 cups (c).

The first ratio of the proportion contains the *known equivalent,* for example 1 quart : 4 cups. The second ratio contains the *desired unit of measure* and the *unknown equivalent* expressed as X, for example 3 quarts : X cups.

This proportion in fractional form looks like this:

$$\frac{1 \text{ qt}}{4 \text{ c}} = \frac{3 \text{ qt}}{X \text{ c}}$$

Notice that the ratios follow the same sequence. The units in the numerators match (qt) and the units in the denominators match (c).

Be sure to label the units in each ratio. Cross-multiply to solve the proportion for X. Refer to Chapter 1 to review this skill if needed.

Step 1. $\frac{1 \text{ qt}}{4 \text{ c}} \diagdown\!\!\!\diagup \frac{3 \text{ qt}}{X \text{ c}}$ (Cross multiply.)

Step 2. $1X = 12$

Step 3. $\frac{1X}{1} = \frac{12}{1}$ (Simplify.)

Step 4. $X = 12$ cups

Note: You can eliminate steps 2 and 3, because any number multiplied or divided by one is the same number. Look at how this simplified the calculation in the next example.

EXAMPLE 2:   Let's look at another conversion of units already familiar to you.

How many inches (in) are in 2 feet (ft)?

Known equivalent: 1 ft = 12 in

$\frac{1 \text{ ft}}{12 \text{ in}} \diagdown\!\!\!\diagup \frac{2 \text{ ft}}{X \text{ in}}$ (Cross multiply.)

$X = 24$ inches   (It is not necessary to simplify; you have the answer.)

EXAMPLE 3:   Let's examine how to convert from cups to quarts.

How many quarts do 24 cups make?

Known equivalent: 1 qt = 4 cups

The sequence of units is still the same, but now the unknown X is quarts.

$\frac{1 \text{ qt}}{4 \text{ c}} \diagdown\!\!\!\diagup \frac{X \text{ qt}}{24 \text{ c}}$ (Cross multiply.)

$4X = 24$

$\frac{4X}{4} = \frac{24}{4}$ (Simplify.)

$X = 6$ quarts

EXAMPLE 4:   Let's also examine converting inches to feet.

How many feet do 48 inches make?

Known equivalent: 1 ft = 12 in

$$\frac{1\text{ ft}}{12\text{ in}} \diagdown \frac{X\text{ ft}}{48\text{ in}} \quad \text{(Cross multiply.)}$$

$$12X = 48$$

$$\frac{12X}{12} = \frac{48}{12} \quad \text{(Simplify.)}$$

$$X = 4 \text{ feet}$$

Converting Within the Metric System Using Ratio-Proportion

The most common conversions in dosage calculations are within the metric system. As you recall, most metric conversions are simply derived by multiplying or dividing by 1000. Recall from Chapter 1 that multiplying by 1000 is the same as moving the decimal point three places to the right. Also recall that dividing by 1000 is the same as moving the decimal point three places to the left.

To convert 2 grams to the equivalent number of milligrams, you would first recall the *known equivalent*: 1 g = 1000 mg. Then set up a proportion of the *known equivalent* to the *unknown equivalent* and cross-multiply to solve for the unknown X.

$$\frac{1\text{ g}}{1000\text{ mg}} \diagdown \frac{2\text{ g}}{X\text{ mg}}$$

$$X = 2 \times 1000 = 2.000. = 2000 \text{ mg}$$

Remember, to multiply a number by 1000, you move the decimal point three places to the right.

EXAMPLE 1:   0.3 g = X mg

Known equivalent: 1 g = 1000 mg

$$\frac{1\text{ g}}{1000\text{ mg}} \diagdown \frac{0.3\text{ g}}{X\text{ mg}}$$

$$X = 0.3 \times 1000 = 0.300. = 300 \text{ mg} \quad \text{(Move decimal point 3 places to the right.)}$$

0.3 g = 300 mg

EXAMPLE 2:   2.5 L = X mL

Known equivalent: 1 L = 1000 mL

$$\frac{1\text{ L}}{1000\text{ mL}} \diagdown \frac{2.5\text{ L}}{X\text{ mL}}$$

$$X = 2.5 \times 1000 = 2.500. = 2500 \text{ mL} \quad \text{(Move decimal point 3 places to the right.)}$$

2.5 L = 2500 mL

EXAMPLE 3:   0.15 g = X mg

Known equivalent: 1 g = 1000 mg

$$\frac{1\text{ g}}{1000\text{ mg}} \diagdown \frac{0.15\text{ g}}{X\text{ mg}}$$

$$X = 0.15 \times 1000 = 0.150. = 150 \text{ mg} \quad \text{(Move decimal point 3 places to the right.)}$$

0.15 g = 150 mg

EXAMPLE 4:   0.04 mg = X mcg

Known equivalent: 1 mg = 1000 mcg

$$\frac{1 \text{ mg}}{1000 \text{ mcg}} \diagup\!\!\!\!\!\diagdown \frac{0.04 \text{ mg}}{X \text{ mcg}}$$

X = 0.04 × 1000 = 0.040. = 40 mcg   (Move decimal point 3 places to the right.)

0.04 mg = 40 mcg

Now, let's convert in the other direction: mg to g, mL to L, and mcg to mg. Remember that to divide by 1000, you move the decimal point 3 places to the left.

EXAMPLE 1:   5000 mg = X g

Known equivalent: 1 g = 1000 mg

$$\frac{1 \text{ g}}{1000 \text{ mg}} \diagup\!\!\!\!\!\diagdown \frac{X \text{ g}}{5000 \text{ mg}}$$

1000X = 5000

$$\frac{1000X}{1000} = \frac{5000}{1000}$$

X = 5.000. = 5 g   (Move decimal point 3 places to the left.)

5000 mg = 5 g

EXAMPLE 2:   500 mL = X L

Known equivalent: 1 L = 1000 mL

$$\frac{1 \text{ L}}{1000 \text{ mL}} \diagup\!\!\!\!\!\diagdown \frac{X \text{ L}}{500 \text{ mL}}$$

1000X = 500

$$\frac{1000X}{1000} = \frac{500}{1000}$$

X = .500. = 0.5 L   (Move decimal point 3 places to the left.)

500 mL = 0.5 L

EXAMPLE 3:   50 mL = X L

Known equivalent: 1 L = 1000 mL

$$\frac{1 \text{ L}}{1000 \text{ mL}} \diagup\!\!\!\!\!\diagdown \frac{X \text{ L}}{50 \text{ mL}}$$

1000X = 50

$$\frac{1000X}{1000} = \frac{50}{1000}$$

X = .050. = 0.05 L   (Move decimal point 3 places to the left.)

50 mL = 0.05 L

EXAMPLE 4:   5 mcg = X mg

Known equivalent: 1 mg = 1000 mcg

$$\frac{1 \text{ mg}}{1000 \text{ mcg}} \times \frac{X \text{ mg}}{5 \text{ mcg}}$$

$$1000X = 5$$

$$\frac{1000X}{1000} = \frac{5}{1000}$$

$X = 0.005. = 0.005 \text{ mg}$ (Move decimal point 3 places to the left.)

$5 \text{ mcg} = 0.005 \text{ mg}$

quick review

To convert between metric units:

- Recall the metric equivalents.
- Follow the rule: Ratio for known equivalent equals ratio for unknown equivalent.
- Label the units and match the units in the numerators and denominators.
- Cross-multiply to find the value of the unknown X.

You can probably do most of these calculations in your head with little difficulty. If you feel you do not understand the concept of conversions within the metric system, review the decimal and ratio-proportion sections in Chapter 1 and get help from your instructor before proceeding further.

review set 12

Convert each of the following to the equivalent unit indicated.

1. 500 cc = _____ L
2. 0.015 g = _____ mg
3. 8 mg = _____ g
4. 10 mg = _____ g
5. 60 mg = _____ g
6. 300 mg = _____ g
7. 0.2 mg = _____ g
8. 1.2 g = _____ mg
9. 0.0025 kg = _____ g
10. 0.065 g = _____ mg
11. 0.005 L = _____ mL
12. 1.5 L = _____ cc
13. 2 mL = _____ cc
14. 250 cc = _____ L
15. 2 kg = _____ g
16. 56.08 cc = _____ mL
17. 79,200 mL = _____ L
18. 1 L = _____ mL
19. 1 g = _____ mg
20. 1 mL = _____ L
21. 0.23 mcg = _____ mg
22. 1.05 g = _____ kg
23. 0.01 mcg = _____ mg
24. 0.4 mg = _____ mcg
25. 25 g = _____ kg
26. 50 cm = _____ m
27. 10 L = _____ mL
28. 450 cc = _____ L
29. 5 mL = _____ L
30. 30 mg = _____ mcg

After completing these problems, see page 291 to check your answers.

Approximate Equivalents

Fortunately, the use of the apothecaries' and household systems is becoming less and less frequent. But until they are obsolete, the nurse must be familiar with conversions between the metric, apothecaries', and household systems of measurement.

Approximate equivalents are used for conversions from one system to another. Exact equivalents are usually not practical for dosage calculations by nurses. The exact equivalent of one gram as measured in grains is: 1 gram = 15.432 grains. This is rounded off to give the approximate equivalent of 1 g = gr 15.

Learn the approximate equivalents listed here so that you can change from one system to another quickly and accurately. The equivalents should be committed to memory. Review them often. When you learn these essential equivalents in addition to the other equivalents you learned in Chapter 2, you are on your way to mastering the skill of dosage calculations.

remember

APPROXIMATE EQUIVALENTS

1 g = gr 15	1 L = qt i = pt ii = ʒ 32 = 4 cups
gr i = 60 mg	pt i = 500 mL = ʒ 16 = 2 cups
1 t = 5 mL	1 cup = 250 mL = ʒ viii
1 T = 3 t = 15 mL = ʒ ss	1 kg = 2.2 lb
ʒ i = 30 mL = 6 t	1 in = 2.5 cm

Figures 3–1 and 3–2 are visual aids of most of the equivalents. You may find these diagrams easier to remember than the tables.

Look at the first triangle of *weight equivalents* (Figure 3–1). Beginning at the top of the triangle, use your finger to trace the arrow from *g* (gram) down to *gr* (grain). The arrow indicates that *1 g = gr 15*. On the other side, trace down from *g* (gram) to *mg* (milligram). This arrow indicates that *1 g = 1000 mg*. Likewise, the bottom arrow goes from *gr* to *mg* to remind you that *gr i = 60 mg*. In summary, the triangle simply says:

1 g = gr 15, 1 g = 1000 mg, and gr i = 60 mg.

Look at the second triangle of *volume equivalents* (Figure 3–2). Beginning at the top of the triangle, use your finger to trace the arrow from ʒ (ounce) down to *t* (teaspoon). The arrow indicates that *ʒ i = 6 t*. On the other side, trace down from ʒ (ounce) to *mL* (milliliter). This arrow reminds you that *ʒ i = 30 mL*. Likewise, the bottom arrow goes from *t* (teaspoon) to *mL* (milliliter). This arrow reminds you that *1 t = 5 mL*. (Remember that 1 cc = 1 mL.) In summary, this triangle simply says:

ʒ i = 6 t, ʒ i = 30 mL, and 1 t = 5 mL.

WEIGHT EQUIVALENTS

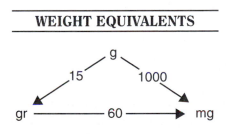

Fig. 3–1 Weight Equivalents

VOLUME EQUIVALENTS

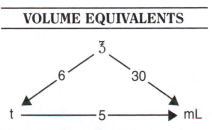

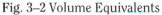

Fig. 3–2 Volume Equivalents

Converting Between Systems of Measurement Using the Ratio-Proportion Method

Now let's convert units between systems of measurement using approximate equivalents. Recall that to convert between units, you must apply the rule: *ratio for known equivalent equals ratio for unknown equivalent*. The first three examples demonstrate converting from a larger to a smaller unit of measure.

Note: Although arabic numbers may be used for calculations, final answers should be reported in proper apothecaries' notation.

EXAMPLE 1:   Convert 0.5 gram to grains.

Approximate equivalent: 1 g = gr 15

$$\frac{1\ g}{gr\ 15} \quad \overset{\longrightarrow}{\longleftarrow} \quad \frac{0.5\ g}{gr\ X}$$

$X = 0.5 \times 15$

$X = gr\ 7.5 = gr\ viiss$

Note: As is customary, the capital letter X is consistently used in this text to denote the unknown quantity. It is important that you do not confuse the unknown X with the value of "gr x," which designates "ten grains."

EXAMPLE 2:   Convert 2 ounces to milliliters.

Approximate equivalent: ℥ i = 30 mL

$$\frac{℥\ i}{30\ mL} = \frac{℥\ ii}{X\ mL}$$

$$\frac{℥\ 1}{30\ mL} \quad \overset{\longrightarrow}{\longleftarrow} \quad \frac{℥\ 2}{X\ mL} \qquad \text{(Cross multiply and solve for X.)}$$

$X = 2 \times 30$

$X = 60\ mL$

EXAMPLE 3:   Convert 40 kilograms to pounds.

Approximate equivalent: 1 kg = 2.2 lb

$$\frac{1\ kg}{2.2\ lb} \quad \overset{\longrightarrow}{\longleftarrow} \quad \frac{40\ kg}{X\ lb} \qquad \text{(Cross multiply and solve for X.)}$$

$X = 40 \times 2.2$

$X = 88\ lb$

Now let's convert from a smaller to a larger unit of measure. The unknown X is in a different place in the proportion, but the sequence of the units must still match, such as:

$$\frac{gr}{mg} = \frac{gr}{mg}.$$

EXAMPLE 1:   Convert 120 milligrams to grains.

Approximate equivalent: gr i = 60 mg

$$\frac{gr\ 1}{60\ mg} \quad \overset{\longrightarrow}{\longleftarrow} \quad \frac{gr\ X}{120\ mg} \qquad \text{(Cross multiply and solve for X.)}$$

$6X = 120$

$$\frac{60X}{60} = \frac{120}{60}$$

$X = gr\ 2 = gr\ ii$

EXAMPLE 2: Convert 45 milliliters to teaspoons.

Approximate equivalent: 1 t = 5 mL

$$\frac{1\ t}{5\ mL} \quad\bowtie\quad \frac{X\ t}{45\ mL}$$ (Cross multiply and solve for X.)

$$5X = 45$$

$$\frac{5X}{5} = \frac{45}{5}$$

$$X = 9\ t$$

EXAMPLE 3: Convert 66 pounds to kilograms.

Approximate equivalent: 1 kg = 2.2 lb

$$\frac{1\ kg}{2.2\ lb} \quad\bowtie\quad \frac{X\ kg}{66\ lb}$$ (Cross multiply and solve for X.)

$$2.2X = 66$$

$$\frac{22X}{2.2} = \frac{66}{2.2}$$

$$X = 30\ kg$$

Try this: Convert your weight in pounds to kilograms rounded to hundredths or two decimal places.

quick review

To use the ratio and proportion method to convert between systems of measurement:

- Recall the approximate equivalents.
- Follow the rule: Ratio for known equivalent equals ratio for unknown equivalent.
- Label and match units in the numerators and denominators.
- Cross-multiply to solve for the unknown X.

review set 13

Use ratio and proportion to convert each of the following amounts to the unit indicated. Indicate the approximate equivalent used in the conversion.

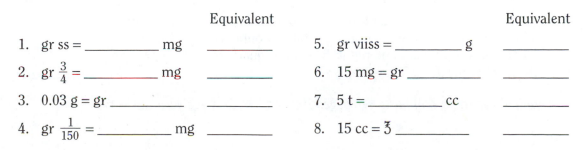

		Equivalent			Equivalent
1.	gr ss = _____ mg	_____	5.	gr viiss = _____ g	_____
2.	gr $\frac{3}{4}$ = _____ mg	_____	6.	15 mg = gr _____	_____
3.	0.03 g = gr _____	_____	7.	5 t = _____ cc	_____
4.	gr $\frac{1}{150}$ = _____ mg	_____	8.	15 cc = ℥ _____	_____

	Equivalent		Equivalent
9. ℥ iiss = _____ mL	_____	20. 99 lb = _____ kg	_____
10. 750 mL = pt _____	_____	21. 0.4 mg = gr _____	_____
11. 60 mL = _____ t	_____	22. 0.6 mg = gr _____	_____
12. 4 T = _____ cc	_____	23. pt i = _____ mL	_____
13. 9 kg = _____ lb	_____	24. gr x = _____ mg	_____
14. 110 lb = _____ kg	_____	25. 300 mg = gr _____	_____
15. 3 L = ℥ _____	_____	26. 30 cm = _____ in	_____
16. 3.5 kg = _____ lb	_____	27. 90 mg = gr _____	_____
17. 12 in = _____ cm	_____	28. 60 mL = ℥ _____	_____
18. qt ii = _____ L	_____	29. gr $\frac{1}{6}$ = _____ mg	_____
19. 3 t = _____ mL	_____	30. 30 mg = gr _____	_____

31. Calculate the total fluid intake in mL for 24 hours.

Breakfast	8 ounces milk
	6 ounces orange juice
	4 ounces water with medication
Lunch	8 ounces iced tea
Snack	10 ounces coffee
	4 ounces gelatin dessert
Dinner	8 ounces water
	6 ounces tomato juice
	6 ounces beef broth
Snack	5 ounces pudding
	12 ounces diet soda
	4 ounces water with medication Total = _____ mL

32. A child who weighs 55 lb is to receive 0.05 mg of a drug per kg of body weight. How much of the drug should the child receive for each dose?   _____

33. The doctor prescribes 60 mL of Epsom Salts crystals in 1000 mL of warm water as a soak for a sprained ankle. Using measures commonly found in the home, how would you instruct the patient to prepare the solution?   _____

34. The patient is to receive 10 mL of a drug. How many teaspoonsful should the patient take?   _____

35. An infant is taking a "ready-to-feed" formula. The formula comes in quart containers. If the infant usually takes 4 ounces of formula every 3 hours during the day and night, how many quarts of formula should the mother buy for a 3-day supply?   _____

After completing these problems, see pages 292 and 293 to check your answers.

Converting Using the Conversion Factor Method

An alternate method of converting between units and systems of measurement is the conversion factor method. To use this method you need to:

- recall the equivalents, and
- multiply or divide.

The following information will help you to remember when to multiply and when to divide. The *conversion factor* is a number used with either multiplication or division to change a measurement from one unit of measure to its equivalent in another unit of measure.

 rule To convert from a larger to smaller unit of measure, multiply by the conversion factor. Larger → Smaller: (×)

This is true because it takes *more* parts of a *smaller* unit to make an equivalent amount of a larger unit. In order to get more parts, *multiply*.

Let's examine units already familiar to you.

EXAMPLE 1: How many cups are in two quarts? In units of measure, 1 quart = 4 cups. It takes 4 of the cup units to equal 1 of the quart units; cups are *smaller* than quarts, larger → smaller: multiply. The conversion factor for the cup and quart units is 4. Multiply by the conversion factor. Therefore, 2 quarts = 2 × 4 = 8 cups.

EXAMPLE 2: How many inches are in 4 feet?

To convert 4 feet to the equivalent number of inches, multiply by the conversion factor of 12, because 1 foot = 12 inches. Multiplication is used because it takes *more* inches to represent the same amount in feet; because inches are smaller units than feet. Therefore, 4 feet = 4 × 12 = 48 inches.

rule To convert from a smaller to a larger unit of measure, divide by the conversion factor. Smaller → Larger: (÷)

This is true because it takes *fewer* parts of the *larger* unit to make an equivalent amount of a smaller unit. In order to get fewer parts, *divide*.

EXAMPLE 1: How many feet are in 36 inches?

1 foot = 12 inches. Inches are smaller units than feet.

To convert 36 inches to the equivalent number of feet, divide by the conversion factor of 12. Division is used because it takes *fewer* feet to represent the same amount in inches; smaller → larger: divide.

Therefore, 36 inches = 36 ÷ 12 = 3 feet.

EXAMPLE 2: How many quarts are in 16 cups?

You know that 1 quart = 4 cups. The conversion factor is 4. A quart is *larger* than a cup.

Divide by the conversion factor because it takes *fewer* of the quart units to equal the same amount in the cup units; smaller → larger: divide.

Therefore, 16 cups = 16 ÷ 4 = 4 quarts.

Apply the conversion factor method to convert between metric, apothecary, and household units of measure.

EXAMPLE 1:   How many grams are equivalent to 3.5 kg?

Equivalent: 1 kg = 1000g. Larger → smaller: multiply by the conversion factor of 1000.

$$3.5 \text{ kg} = 3.5 \times 1000 = 3.500. = 3500 \text{ g}$$

EXAMPLE 2:   Convert 45 milligrams to grains.

Approximate equivalent: gr i = 60 mg. Smaller → larger: divide by the conversion factor of 60.

$$45 \text{ mg} = \frac{45}{60} = \text{gr} \frac{3}{4}$$

EXAMPLE 3:   Convert 10 milliliters to teaspoons.

Approximate equivalent: 1 t = 5 mL. Smaller → larger: divide by the conversion factor of 5.

$$10 \text{ mL} = \frac{10}{5} = 2 \text{ t}$$

EXAMPLE 4:   Convert 50 kilograms to pounds.

Approximate equivalent: 1 kg = 2.2 lb. Larger → smaller: multiply by the conversion factor of 2.2.

$$50 \text{ kg} = 50 \times 2.2 = 110 \text{ lb}$$

quick review

To use the conversion factor method to convert from one unit of measure to another:

- Recall the equivalents.
- Identify the conversion factor.
- MULTIPLY by the conversion factor to convert to a smaller unit.
  Larger → Smaller: (×)
- DIVIDE by the conversion factor to convert to a larger unit.
  Smaller → Larger: (÷)

review set 14

Use the conversion factor method to convert each of the following amounts to the unit indicated. Indicate the equivalent used in the conversion.

		Equivalent			Equivalent
1.	0.5 mL = _____ L	_____	3.	84 lb = _____ kg	_____
2.	3 g = gr _____	_____	4.	gr xx = _____ g	_____

Equivalent   Equivalent

5. gr $\frac{1}{8}$ = _____ mg   _____   13. 7.5 mg = gr _____   _____

6. 75 mL = ℥ _____   _____   14. 0.6 mg = gr _____   _____

7. 750 mL = pt _____   _____   15. 7.5 cm = _____ in   _____

8. ℥ iss = _____ mL   _____   16. 16 g = _____ mg   _____

9. 15 mg = gr _____   _____   17. 15 mL = ℥ _____   _____

10. 0.625 mcg = _____ mg _____   18. ℥ 16 = qt _____   _____

11. 2.5 mL = _____ t   _____   19. qt ii = _____ L   _____

12. gr ss = _____ mg   _____   20. pt i = qt _____   _____

21. The medicine order states to administer a potassium chloride supplement to the patient in at least 150 mL of juice. How many ounces of juice should you pour? _____

22. The child should have 5 mL of liquid Children's Tylenol (acetaminophen) every 4 hours as needed for fever above 100° F. To relate these instructions to the child's mother, you should advise her to give her child _____ teaspoon(s) of Tylenol.

23. The doctor advises his patient to drink at least 2000 mL of fluid per day. The patient should have at least _____ 8-ounce glasses of water per day.

24. A child weighs 50 pounds. What is the child's weight in kilograms? _____

25. The doctor orders codeine gr $\frac{1}{4}$. How many milligrams is this equivalent to? _____

After completing these problems, see page 293 to check your answers.

For more practice rework Review Sets 12 and 13 using the conversion factor method.

Converting between Traditional and 24-Hour Time

It is becoming increasingly popular in the health care setting to measure time using the 24-hour clock. Look at the 24-hour clock (Figure 3–3).

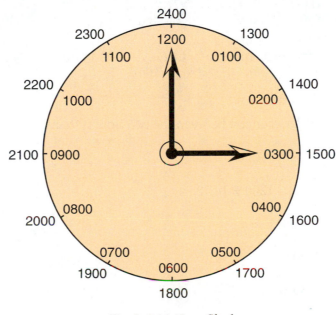

Fig. 3–3 24-Hour Clock

The inside numbers represent the hours for AM time and the outside numbers represent the hours for PM time. The *minutes* between 2400 (12 midnight) and 0100 (1 AM) are represented as 0001, 0002, 0003. . .0058, 0059, 0100.

Hours on the 24-hour clock after 0059 ("zero zero fifty nine") minutes are stated in 100s.

EXAMPLE 1:   2400 is stated as "twenty-four hundred."

EXAMPLE 2:   0100 is stated as "zero one hundred."

Use of the 24-hour clock decreases the chance for error in administering medications and documenting time because no two times are expressed by the same number. For example, 8 AM – 8 PM on the traditional clock is 0800 – 2000 on the 24-hour clock. Figure 3–4 lists the comparison of traditional time to international time (24-hour time).

AM	INT'L. TIME	PM	INT'L. TIME
12 midnight	2400	12 Noon	1200
1	0100	1	1300
2	0200	2	1400
3	0300	3	1500
4	0400	4	1600
5	0500	5	1700
6	0600	6	1800
7	0700	7	1900
8	0800	8	2000
9	0900	9	2100
10	1000	10	2200
11	1100	11	2300

Fig. 3–4 Comparison of Traditional and International Time (24-Hour Clock)

rules   1. Traditional time and 24-hour time are the same hours starting with 1:00 AM (0100) through 12:59 PM (1259).
2. Hours after 12:00 AM (midnight) and before 1:00 AM are 0001–0059 in 24-hour time.
3. Hours starting with 1:00 PM through 12:00 AM (midnight) are 12:00 hours greater in 24-hour time (1300–2400).

Let's apply these rules to convert between the two time systems.

EXAMPLE 1:   3:00 PM = 3:00 + 12:00 = 1500

EXAMPLE 2:   2212 = 2212 – 1200 = 10:12 PM

EXAMPLE 3:   12:45 AM = 0045

EXAMPLE 4:   0004 = 12:04 AM

EXAMPLE 5:   0130 = 1:30 AM

EXAMPLE 6:   11:00 AM = 1100

review set 15

Convert 24-hour time to traditional AM/PM time.

1. 0032 = _____   6. 1215 = _____

2. 0730 = _____   7. 0220 = _____

3. 1640 = _____   8. 1010 = _____

4. 2121 = _____   9. 1315 = _____

5. 2359 = _____   10. 1825 = _____

Convert traditional to 24-hour time.

11. 1:30 PM = _____   16. 3:45 AM = _____

12. 12:04 AM = _____   17. 12:00 midnight = _____

13. 9:45 PM = _____   18. 3:30 PM = _____

14. 12:00 noon = _____   19. 6:20 AM = _____

15. 11:15 PM = _____   20. 5:45 PM = _____

After completing these problems, see page 294 to check your answers.

Converting between Celsius and Fahrenheit Temperature

Another important conversion in health care involves Celsius and Fahrenheit temperature. Simple formulas are used for converting between the two temperature scales. It is easier to remember the formulas when you understand how they have been developed.

The Fahrenheit (F) scale establishes the freezing point for pure water at 32° and the boiling point for pure water at 212°. The Celsius (C) scale establishes the freezing point of pure water at 0° and the boiling point of pure water at 100°.

Look at Figure 3–5. Note that there is 180° difference between the boiling and freezing points on the Fahrenheit thermometer, and 100° between the boiling and freezing points on the Celsius thermometer. Therefore, each Celsius degree is $\frac{180}{100}$ or 1.8 the size of a Fahrenheit degree. Taken the other way, each Fahrenheit degree is $\frac{100}{180}$ the size of a Celsius degree. Every one degree Celsius is equivalent to 1.8 degrees Fahrenheit.

To convert between Fahrenheit and Celsius temperature, formulas have been developed based on the differences between the freezing and boiling points on each scale.

> **rule** To convert a given Fahrenheit temperature to Celsius, first subtract 32 and then divide the result by 1.8. The formula is:
>
> $$°C = \frac{°F - 32}{1.8}$$

EXAMPLE: Convert 98.6°F to °C

$$°C = \frac{98.6 - 32}{1.8}$$

$$°C = \frac{66.6}{1.8}$$

$$°C = 37°$$

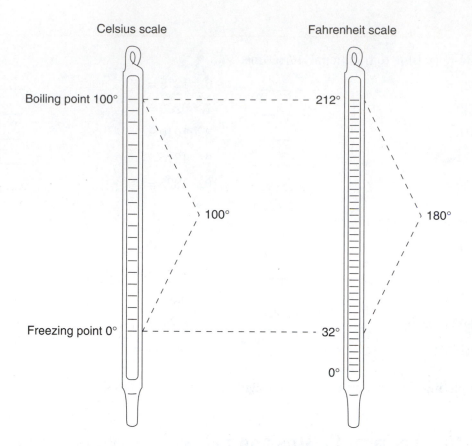

Fig. 3–5 Comparison of Celsius and Fahrenheit Scales

Note: Glass thermometers pictured here are for demonstration purposes. Electronic digital temperature devices are more commonly used in health care settings. However, the nurse's ability to convert temperature scales of these devices between Celsius and Fahrenheit remains an important skill.

rule   To convert Celsius temperature to Fahrenheit, multiply by 1.8 and add 32. The formula is:

$$°F = 1.8\,°C + 32$$

EXAMPLE: Convert 35°C to °F

°F = 1.8 × 35 + 32

°F = 63 + 32

°F = 95°

quick review

Use these formulas to convert between Fahrenheit and Celsius temperatures:

■ $°C = \dfrac{°F - 32}{1.8}$

■ $°F = 1.8\,°C + 32$

review set 16

Convert these temperatures as indicated. Round your answer to tenths.

1.	0°F =	_____ °C	9.	80°C =	_____ °F
2.	85°C =	_____ °F	10.	36.4°C =	_____ °F
3.	100°C =	_____ °F	11.	100°F =	_____ °C
4.	32°C =	_____ °F	12.	19°C =	_____ °F
5.	72°F =	_____ °C	13.	4°C =	_____ °F
6.	99°F =	_____ °C	14.	94.2°F =	_____ °C
7.	103.6°F =	_____ °C	15.	102.8°F =	_____ °C
8.	40°C =	_____ °F			

After completing these problems, see page 294 to check your answers.

critical thinking skills

The ability to convert from one unit or system of measure to another is used often in nursing practice. Let's look at an example in which the conversion was performed incorrectly.

■ error

Incorrectly converting pounds (lbs) to kilograms (kg).

possible scenario

An attending physician ordered Ceclor (an antibiotic) for a 22 pound child with severe otitis media (ear infection). The doctor prescribed a dosage of Ceclor 40 mg per day for every kilogram of the child's body weight. To administer the correct dosage, the nurse had to first convert the child's weight in pounds to the equivalent weight in kilograms. The nurse, in a rush to start the medication, converted the child's weight and calculated the daily dosage this way:

1 is to 2.2 as 22 is to X

Based on this scenario, the nurse set up a proportion and calculated the child's weight in kg in this manner:

$$\frac{1}{2.2} = \frac{22}{X}$$
$$X = 22 \times 2.2$$
$$X = 48.4 \text{ kg}$$

The nurse concluded that the child would require 48.4 x 40 or 1,936 mg of Ceclor per day, almost 2000 mg (2 g) per day. The nurse concluded 2 g would be the correct dosage.

As you noticed, the nurse didn't correctly use the ratio and proportion rules for conversions. Look again at the correct conversion method using ratio and proportion.

$$\frac{1 \text{ kg}}{2.2 \text{ lb}} = \frac{X \text{ kg}}{22 \text{ lb}}$$

$$2.2 \, X = 22$$

$$\frac{2.2 \, X}{2.2} = \frac{22}{2.2}$$

$$X = 10 \text{ kg}$$

The correct daily dosage should have been $10 \times 40 = 400$ mg, not 2000 mg.

potential outcome

The child would have received 5 times the correct daily dosage. The patient would have developed serious complications from overdosage with a high potential for a fatal outcome.

prevention

Remember to set up proportions to convert between equivalent ratios that follow the same sequence and label the units. The units in the numerators should match and the units in the denominators should match. If the units had been properly labeled in the calculation, the nurse would have more likely discovered the error.

Summary

At this point, you should be quite familiar with the equivalents for converting within the metric, apothecaries', and household systems, and from one system to another. From memory, you should be able to recall quickly and accurately the equivalents for conversions. If you are having difficulty understanding the concept of converting from one unit of measurement to another, review this chapter and seek additional help from your instructor.

You have also learned the formulas for converting between Celsius and Fahrenheit temperature scales, and for converting between the traditional and 24-hour clock.

Work the practice problems for Chapter 3. Concentrate on accuracy. One error can be a serious mistake when calculating the dosages of medicines or performing critical measurements of health status.

practice problems—chapter 3

Give the following equivalents without consulting conversion tables.

1. 0.5 g = _____ mg
2. 0.01 g = _____ mg
3. 7.5 cc = _____ mL
4. qt iii = _____ L
5. 4 mg = _____ g
6. 500 mL = _____ L
7. 250 mL = pt _____
8. 300 g = _____ kg
9. 28 in = _____ cm
10. 68 kg = _____ lb
11. gr iii = _____ mg
12. ℥ iiiss = _____ mL
13. gr $\frac{1}{200}$ = _____ mg
14. gr $\frac{1}{4}$ = _____ mg
15. gr $\frac{1}{10}$ = _____ mg
16. gr iss = _____ mg
17. 70 $\frac{1}{2}$ lb = _____ kg
18. 3634 g = _____ lb
19. 8 mL = _____ L
20. gr xxx = _____ g

21. 237.5 cm = _____ in

22. 0.5 g = gr _____

23. 0.6 mg = gr _____

24. gr x = _____ g

25. 150 lb = _____ kg

26. 60 mg = gr _____

27. gr 15 = _____ g

28. 2 cups = _____ cc

29. 6 t = _____ T

30. 90 mL = ℥ _____

31. 1 ft = _____ cm

32. 2 T = _____ cc

33. 2.2 lb = _____ kg

34. 5 cc = _____ t

35. 1000 mL = _____ L

36. 1.5 g = _____ mg

37. ℥ iss = _____ cc

38. 1500 mL = qt _____

39. 10 mg = gr _____

40. 25 mg = _____ g

41. 4.3 kg = _____ g

42. 60 mg = _____ g

43. 0.015 g = _____ mg

44. 45 cc = _____ mL

45. gr 12 = _____ g

46. 3.6 g = _____ mg

47. 3.6 mg = _____ g

48. 10 mL = _____ L

49. 2 t = _____ mL

50. 170 mg = _____ g

51. 1730 = _____ AM/PM

52. 8:30 PM = _____ hours

53. 0915 = _____ AM/PM

54. 98°F = _____ °C

55. 110°C = _____ °F

56. 30°C = _____ °F

57. 2°F = _____ °C

58. 2001 = _____ AM/PM

59. 7:30 PM = _____ hours

60. 6:45 AM = _____ hours

61. 12 midnight = _____ hours

62. As a camp nurse for 9- to 12-year-old children, you are administering $2\frac{1}{2}$ teaspoonsful of oral liquid Tylenol to 6 feverish campers every 4 hours for oral temperatures above 100°F. You have on hand a 4-ounce bottle of liquid Tylenol. How many complete doses are available from this bottle? _____

63. At this same camp, the standard dosage of Pepto-Bismol for 9- to 12-year-olds is 1 tablespoonful. How many complete doses are available in a 120-mL bottle? _____

64. Calculate the total fluid intake in mL of this clear liquid lunch:

    apple juice   4 ounces
    chicken broth   8 ounces
    gelatin dessert   6 ounces
    hot tea   10 ounces

    TOTAL = _____ mL

65. An ampule contains 10 mg of morphine. The doctor orders morphine gr $\frac{1}{6}$. What percentage of the solution in the ampule should the patient receive? _____

After completing these problems, see page 319 to check your answers.

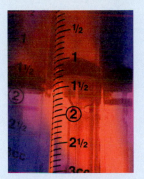

Equipment Used in Dosage Measurement 4

objectives

Upon mastery of Chapter 4, you will be able to correctly measure the prescribed dosages that you calculate. To accomplish this, you will also be able to:

- Recognize and select the appropriate equipment for the medication, dosage, and method of administration ordered.
- Read and interpret the calibrations of each utensil presented.

Now that you are familiar with the systems of measurement used in the calculation of dosages, let's take a look at the common utensils used to measure the correct dosage. In this section you will learn to recognize and read the calibrations of a medicine cup, a calibrated dropper, a regular 3-cc syringe, a prefilled syringe, a standard U-100 insulin syringe, a Lo-Dose® U-100 insulin syringe, and a tuberculin syringe.

Oral Administration

Medicine Cup

Figure 4–1 shows the 30-milliliter or 1-ounce medicine cup that is used to measure most liquids for oral administration. Two views are presented to show all of the scales. Notice that the approximate equivalents of the metric, apothecaries', and household systems of measurement are indicated on the cup. You can see that 30 milliliters equal 1 ounce, 5 milliliters equal 1 teaspoon, and so forth. Look at the calibrations. Milliliters are marked in 5 unit increments (plus 2.5 and 7.5 mL), teaspoons and tablespoons are marked in 2 unit increments after $\frac{1}{2}$ t, drams are marked in 2 unit increments after 1 dram, and ounces are marked in $\frac{1}{4}$ unit increments after $\frac{1}{8}$ oz. For volumes less than 2.5 mL, a smaller, more accurate container should be used (see Figures 4–2, 4–3, and 4–4).

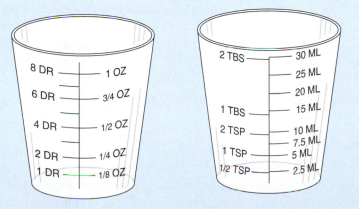

Fig. 4–1 Medicine Cup with Approximate Equivalent Measures

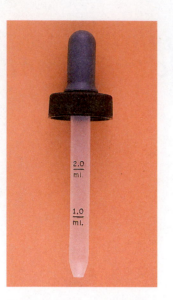

Fig. 4–2 Calibrated Dropper

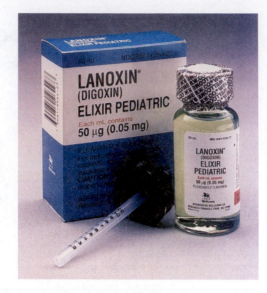

Fig. 4–3 Digoxin Dropper *(Reproduced with permission of Burroughs Wellcome Co.)*

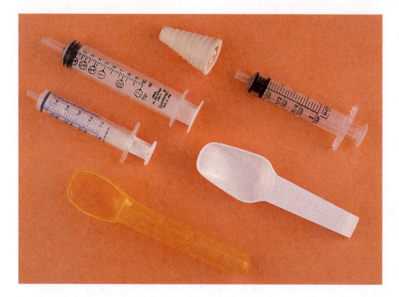

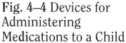

Fig. 4–4 Devices for Administering Medications to a Child

Calibrated Dropper

Figure 4–2 shows the calibrated dropper which is used to administer some small quantities. A dropper is used when giving medicine to children and when adding small amounts of liquid to water or juice. Eye and ear medications are also dispensed from a squeeze-drop bottle. The amount of the drop varies according to the diameter or the hole at the end of the dropper. For this reason, the dropper usually accompanies the medicine and is calibrated according to the way the drug is ordered, as pictured in Figure 4–3. The calibrations are usually given in milliliters, cubic centimeters, or drops. To be safe, do not interchange droppers from other medications.

Note: The inside diameter affects the scale of milliliters on it, if given; the *hole* will affect the volume of the *drop*, if drops are counted.

Pediatric Oral Devices

Various types of calibrated equipment are available to administer oral medications to children. Several devices intended for oral use only are shown in Figure 4–4. To be safe, do not use syringes intended for injections in the administration of oral medications. Confusion about the route of administration may occur.

Parenteral Administration

The term *parenteral* is used to designate routes of administration other than gastrointestinal. However, in this text, parenteral always means injection routes.

3-cc Syringe

Figure 4-5 shows a 3-cc syringe assembled with needle unit. The black rubber tip of the suction plunger is visible. The plunger withdraws the medicine from the storage container. The calibrations are read from the top black ring, NOT the raised middle section and NOT the bottom ring. Look closely at the metric scale which is calibrated in cubic centimeters (cc) for each tenth (0.1) of a cubic centimeter. Each $\frac{1}{2}$ cubic centimeter is marked up to 3 cubic centimeters.

The apothecaries' scale is calibrated in minims. You may disregard this scale, since it is becoming obsolete. It will not be used for the measurement of dosages.

Standard drug dosages are to be rounded to the nearest tenth (0.1) of a cc or mL and measured on the cc scale.

EXAMPLE: 1.45 cc is rounded to 1.5 cc. Notice that the colored liquid in Figure 4-5 identifies 1.5 cc.

Figure 4-6 shows another 3-cc syringe assembled with needle unit. Notice that the plunger in both the photo and the drawing measure 2 cc.

Prefilled Syringe

Figure 4–7 is an example of a prefilled, single-dose syringe. Such syringes contain the usual single dose of a medication and are to be used once and discarded.

If you are to give **less than the full single dose** of a drug provided in a prefilled, single-dose syringe, you should discard the extra amount **before** injecting the patient.

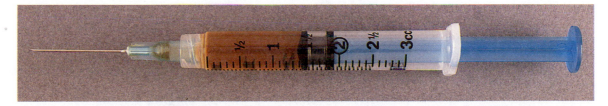

Fig. 4–5 3-cc Syringe with Needle Unit Measuring 1.5 cc

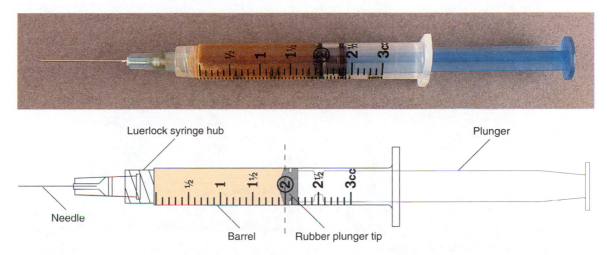

Fig. 4–6 3-cc Syringe with Needle Unit Measuring 2 cc

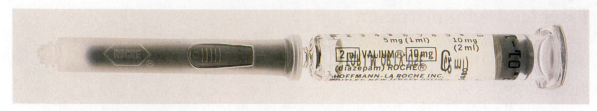

Fig. 4–7 Prefilled, Single-Dose Syringe *(Courtesy of Roche Laboratories, Inc.)*

EXAMPLE: The drug order prescribes 7.5 mg of Valium to be administered to a patient. You have a prefilled, single-dose syringe of Valium containing 10 mg per 2 mL of solution (as in Figure 4–7). You would discard 2.5 mg (0.5 mL) of the drug solution; then, 7.5 mg would be remaining in the syringe. You will learn more about calculating drug dosages beginning in Chapter 7.

Figure 4–8 is an example of the Carpuject® brand injection syringe system. The disposable system contains a single-dose cartridge-needle unit. The cartridge-needle unit is to be used only once and discarded. The medication contained in the cartridge is measured and supplied in the usual single dose. However, if the medication order is for **less than the full single dose**, you should discard the extra amount **before** injecting the patient.

NOTE: Most syringes are marked in cubic centimeters (cc), whereas most drugs are prepared and labeled with the strength given per milliliter (mL). Remember that the cubic centimeter and milliliter are equivalent measurements in dosage calculations (1 cc = 1 mL).

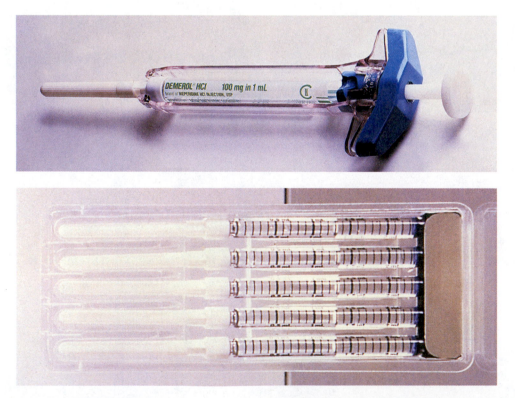

Fig. 4–8 Carpuject® Sterile Cartridge-Needle Unit and a Package of Prefilled Cartridges. *(Courtesy Sanofi Winthrop Pharmaceuticals)*

Insulin Syringe

Figure 4–9(a), shows a standard U-100 insulin syringe. This syringe is to be used for the measurement and administration of U-100 insulin **only**. It must not be used to measure other medications that are measured in units. Insulin should not be measured in any other type of syringe. (See Chapter 8 on insulin dosage.) Notice that Figure 4–9(a) pictures both sides of the same 100-unit dual-scale insulin syringe. One side is calibrated in odd unit increments and the opposite side is calibrated in even unit increments. The plunger in Figure 4–10(a) on page 66 simulates the measurement of 70 units of U-100 insulin. (NOTE: For U-100 insulin, 100 U = 1 cc or mL.)

Figure 4–9(b) shows U-100 Lo-Dose® insulin syringes. The enlarged scales are easier to read. The top syringe is calibrated for each 1 unit (U) up to 50 units per 0.5 cc. Every 5 units are labeled. Figure 4–9(b) also shows a smaller U-100 Lo-Dose® syringe (bottom) calibrated for each unit up to 30 units (0.3 cc). This syringe is commonly used for pediatric administration of insulin. The plunger in Figure 4–10(b) on page 66 simulates the measurement of 19 units for U-100 insulin.

Tuberculin Syringe

Figure 4–11(a) on page 66 shows the 1 cc tuberculin syringe. Figure 4–11(b) shows the 0.5 mL tuberculin syringe. This syringe should be used when a small dose of a drug must be measured, such as an allergen extract, vaccine, or child's medication. Notice that the tuberculin

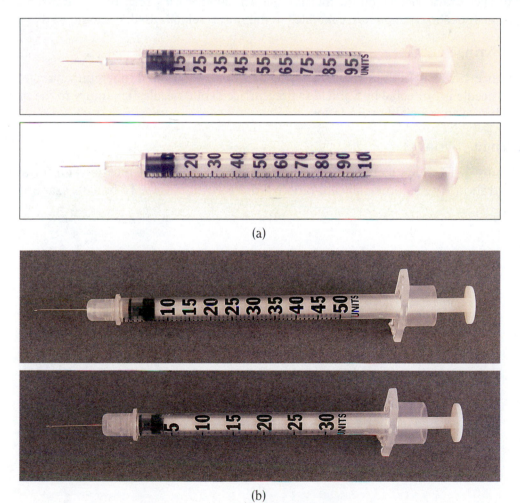

(a)

(b)

Fig. 4–9 (a) Standard 100-Unit Dual-Scale U-100 Insulin Syringe and (b) Lo-Dose® Insulin Syringes, 50 and 30 Units *(Courtesy Becton Dickinson and Company)*

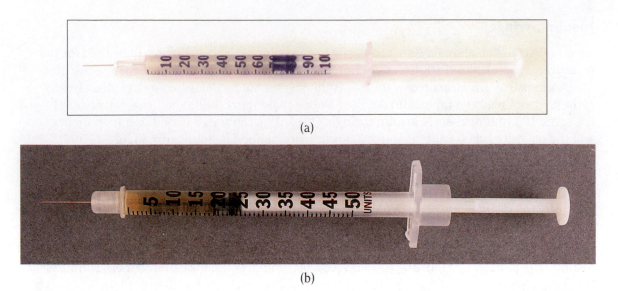

(a)

(b)

Fig. 4–10 (a) Standard U-100 Insulin Syringe Measuring 70 U of U-100 Insulin and **(b)** U-100 Lo-Dose® Insulin Syringe Measuring 19 Units of U-100 Insulin

syringe is calibrated in hundredths (0.01) of one cubic centimeter or milliliter with each one-tenth (0.1) cc or mL labeled on the metric scale. The apothecaries' scale on the reverse side of the syringe (not shown in photo), calibrated in minims, is seldom used. It should be disregarded.

Safety Syringe

Figure 4–12 shows the safety 3-cc syringe, insulin syringe, and tuberculin syringe. Notice that the needle is protected by a shield to prevent accidental needlestick injury to the nurse administering an injectable medication.

Intravenous Syringes

Figure 4–13 shows common large syringes used to prepare medications for intravenous administration. The volume and calibration of these syringes vary. To be safe, examine

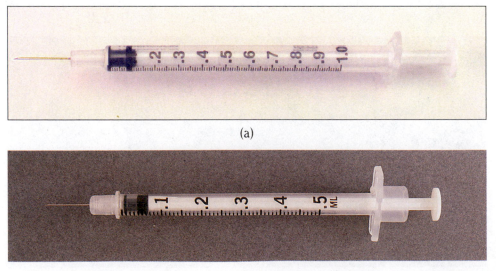

(a)

(b)

Fig. 4–11 (a) 1-cc Tuberculin Syringe and **(b)** 0.5-mL Tuberculin Syringe *(Courtesy Becton Dickinson and Company)*

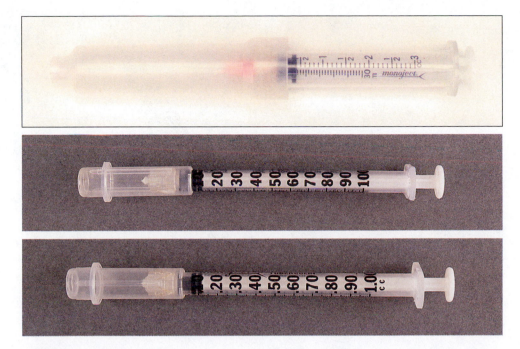

Fig. 4–12 Safety Syringes

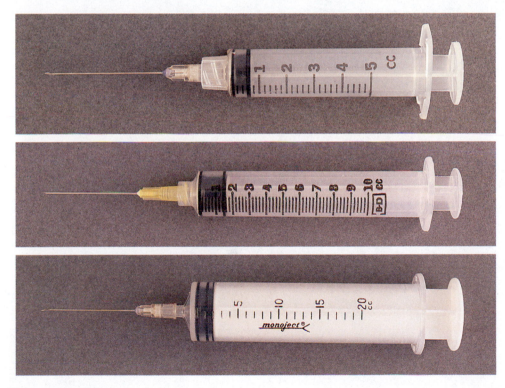

Fig. 4–13 Intravenous Syringes

the calibrations of the syringes, and select the one that is best suited for the volume to be administered.

Needleless Syringes

Figure 4–14 pictures a needleless syringe system designed to prevent accidental needlesticks during intravenous administration.

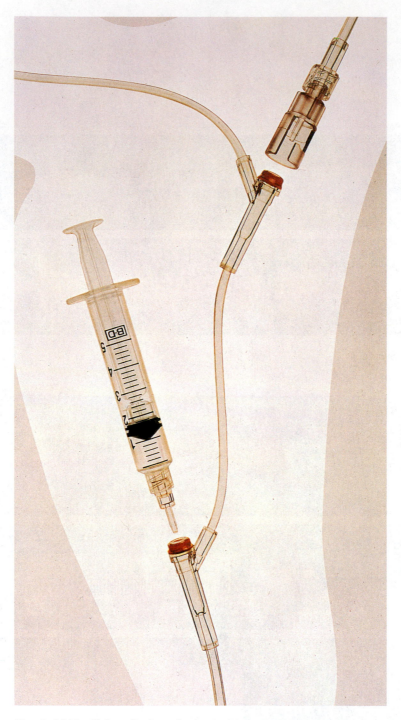

Fig. 4–14 Needleless Syringe System *(Courtesy Becton Dickinson and Company)*

quick review

■ The medicine cup has a 1-ounce or 30-milliliter capacity for oral liquids. It is also calibrated to measure teaspoons, tablespoons, and drams. Amounts less than 2.5 milliliters should be measured in a smaller device, such as an oral syringe.

■ The calibrated dropper measures small amounts of oral liquids. The size of the drop varies according to the diameter of the dropper.

■ The standard 3-cc syringe is used to measure most injectable drugs. It is calibrated in tenths of a cc.

■ The prefilled, single-dose syringe is to be used once and discarded.

■ The standard U-100 insulin syringe is used to measure U-100 insulin only. It is calibrated for a total of 100 units or 1 cc.

■ The Lo-Dose® U-100 insulin syringe is used for measuring small amounts of U-100 insulin. It is calibrated for a total of 50 units or 0.5 cc. A smaller Lo-Dose® U-100 insulin syringe is calibrated for 30 units or 0.3 cc. This syringe is commonly used for administering insulin to children.

■ The tuberculin syringe is used to measure small or critical amounts of injectable drugs. It is calibrated in hundredths of a mL for a total of 0.5 mL or 1 mL.

■ Do not use syringes intended for injections in the administration of oral medications.

review set 17

1. In which syringe should 0.25 mL of a drug solution be measured? _____

2. a. Can 1.25 mL be measured in the regular 3-cc syringe? _____

   b. How? _____

3. Should insulin be measured in a tuberculin syringe? _____

4. Fifty (50) units of U-100 insulin equals how many cubic centimeters? _____

5. a. The gtt is considered a consistent quantity for comparisons between different droppers. (True) (False)

   b. Why? _____

6. Can you measure 3 mL in a medicine cup? _____

7. How would you measure 3 mL of oral liquid to be administered to a child? _____

8. The medicine cup indicates that each teaspoon is the equivalent of _____ mL.

9. Describe your action if you are to administer less than the full amount of a drug supplied in a prefilled, single-dose syringe. _____

10. What is the primary purpose of the safety and needleless syringes? _____

   _____

note to learner

The drawings on subsequent pages of the 3-cc, 1-mL tuberculin, and 50-unit and 100-unit insulin syringes, represent actual sizes.

Draw an arrow to indicate the calibration that corresponds to the dose to be administered.

11. Administer 0.75 cc

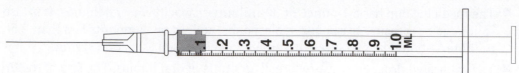

12. Administer 1.33 cc

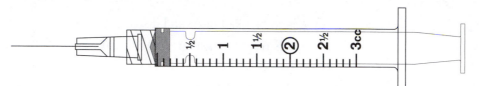

13. Administer 2.2 cc

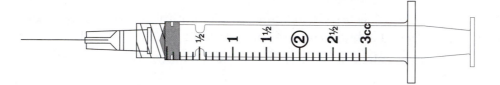

14. Administer 1.3 cc

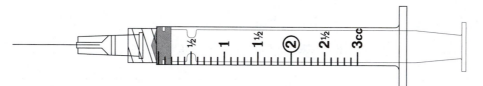

15. Administer 0.33 cc

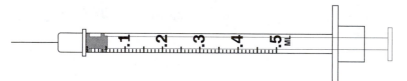

16. Administer 66 U of U-100 insulin

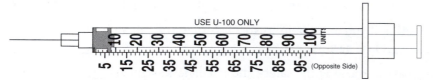

17. Administer 27 U of U-100 insulin

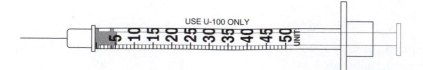

18. Administer 75 U of U-100 insulin

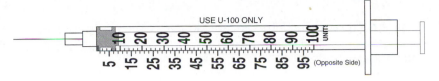

19. Administer 4.4 cc

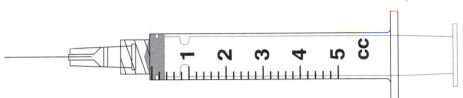

20. Administer 16 cc

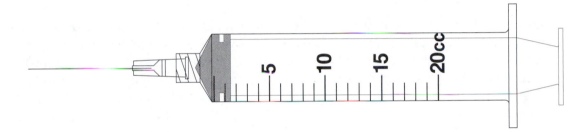

After completing these problems, see pages 294 and 295 to check your answers.

critical thinking skills

Select correct equipment to prepare medications. In the following examples the correct dosage was not given because incorrect measuring devices were used.

■ error 1

Using inaccurate measuring devices for oral medications.

possible scenario

Suppose a pediatrician ordered Amoxil suspension (250 mg/5 mL), 1 teaspoon, every 8 hours, to be given to a child seen in the pediatric clinic. The child should receive the medication for 10 days for otitis media, an ear infection. The pharmacy dispensed the medication in a bottle containing 150 mL, or a 10-day supply. The nurse did not clarify for the mother how to measure and administer the medication. The child returned to the clinic in ten days for routine follow-up. The nurse asked whether the child had taken all the prescribed Amoxil. The child's mother stated, "No, we have almost half of the bottle left." When the nurse asked how the medication had been given, the mother described the bright pink plastic teaspoon she had obtained from the local ice cream parlor. The nurse measured the spoon's capacity and found it to be less than 3 mL. (Remember, 1 tsp = 5 mL.) The child would have received only 3/5, or 60%, of the correct dose.

potential outcome

The child would not have been receiving a therapeutic dosage of the medication and was actually underdosed. The child could develop a super infection, which could lead to a more severe illness like meningitis.

prevention

Use calibrated measuring spoons or specially designed oral syringes to measure the correct dosage of medication. The volumes of spoons may vary considerably as they did in this situation.

■ error 2

Using unorthodox containers for measurement of medications.

possible scenario

Suppose a client with cancer is ordered Compazine liquid orally for nausea. Because the patient has had difficulty taking the medication, the nurse decided to draw up the medication in a syringe without a needle to facilitate giving the medication. The nurse found this to be quite helpful and prepared several doses in syringes without the needle. A nurse from another unit covered for the nurse during lunch, and when the patient complained of nausea, assumed the Compazine prepared in an injection syringe was to be given via injection. The nurse attached a needle and injected the oral medication.

potential outcome

The medication would be absorbed systemically, and the patient could develop an abscess at the site of injection.

prevention

This error could have been avoided by following the principle of not putting oral drugs in syringes intended for injection. Instead, place the medication in an oral syringe to which a needle cannot be attached. In addition, the medication should have been labeled for oral use only. The medication was ordered orally, not by injection. The alert nurse would have noticed the discrepancy. Last, and even more important, a medication should be administered only by the nurse who prepared it.

practice problems—chapter 4 _____

1. In the U-100 insulin syringe, 100 U = _____ cc.

2. The tuberculin syringe is calibrated in _____ of cc.

3. Can you measure 1.25 cc in a single tuberculin syringe? Explain. _____
    _____
    _____

4. How would you measure 1.33 mL in a 3-cc syringe? _____

5. The medicine cup has a _____ mL or _____ ounce capacity.

6. To administer 0.52 cc to a child, select a _____ syringe.

7. 75 U of U-100 insulin equals _____ cc.

8. All droppers are calibrated to deliver a standardized drop of equal amounts, regardless of the dropper used. (True) (False)

9. The prefilled syringe is a multiple-dose system. (True) (False)

10. Insulin should be measured in an insulin syringe **only**. (True) (False)

Draw an arrow to indicate the calibration that corresponds to the dose to be administered.

11. Administer 0.45 cc

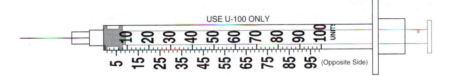

12. Administer 80 U of U-100 insulin

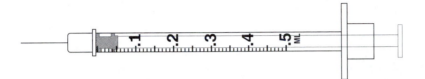

13. Administer 2t

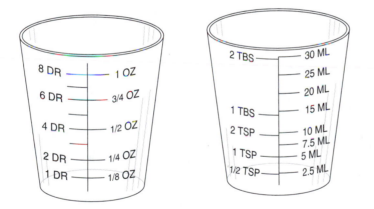

14. Administer 2.4 cc

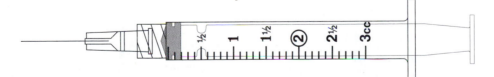

15. Administer 1.1 cc

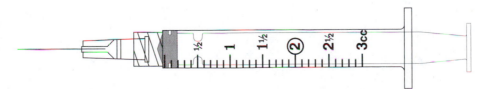

16. Administer 6.2 cc

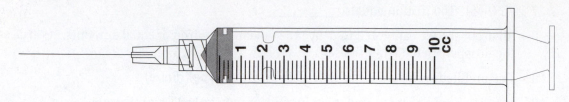

After completing these problems, see pages 319 and 320 to check your answers.

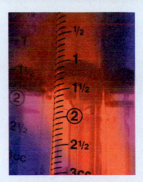

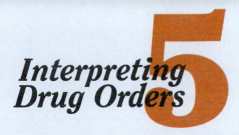
objectives

Upon mastery of Chapter 5, you will be able to interpret the medication (drug) order. To accomplish this you will also be able to:

- Read and write proper medical notation.
- Write the standard medical abbreviation from a list of common terminology.
- Classify the notation that specifies the dosage, route, and frequency of the medication to be administered.

The prescription or medication order conveys the therapeutic drug plan for the patient. It is the responsibility of the nurse to:

- interpret the order,
- prepare the exact dosage of the prescribed drug,
- identify the patient,
- administer the proper dosage at the prescribed time intervals, by the prescribed route,
- record the administration of the prescribed drug, and
- monitor the patient's response for desired (therapeutic) or adverse effects.

Before you can prepare the proper dosage of the prescribed drug, you must learn to interpret or read the written drug order. For brevity and speed, the health professions have adopted certain standards and common abbreviations for use in notation. You should learn to recognize and interpret the abbreviations from memory. As you practice reading drug orders, you will find that this skill becomes second nature to you.

An example of a typical written drug order is:

Amoxil 500 mg p.o. q.i.d. (p.c. & h.s.)

This order means the patient should receive 500 milligrams of an antibiotic named Amoxil (or amoxicillin) orally four times a day (after meals and at bedtime). You can see that the medical notation considerably shortens the written order.

Hospitals have a special form for recording drug orders (Figure 5–1). The drug orders from this form are transcribed to a medication administration record. Figure 5–2 shows a sample medication administration record. The nurse uses this record as a guide to prepare the correct drug dosages and to record the drugs administered.

			ENTERED	FILLED	CHECKED	VERIFIED
						—

NOTE: A NON-PROPRIETARY DRUG OF EQUAL QUALITY MAY BE DISPENSED - IF THIS COLUMN IS NOT CHECKED!

DATE	TIME WRITTEN	PLEASE USE BALL POINT - PRESS FIRMLY	✓	TIME NOTED	NURSES SIGNATURE
11/3/xx	0815	Keflex 250 mg p.o. q.6h.	✓		
		Human NPH Insulin 40 U SC ā breakfast	✓	0830	
		Demerol 75 mg IM q. 3–4 h p.r.n. severe pain	✓		
		Codeine 30 mg p.o. q.4h p.r.n. mild–mod pain	✓		G. Pickar, R.N.
		Tylenol 650 mg p.o. q.4h p.r.n., fever > 101° F	✓		
		Lasix 40 mg p.o. q.d.	✓		
		Slow-K 8 mEq p.o. b.i.d.	✓		
		J. Physician, M.D.			
11/3/xx	2200	Lasix 80 mg IV stat			
		J. Physician, M.D.	✓	2210	M. Smith, R.N.

AUTO STOP ORDERS: UNLESS REORDERED, FOLLOWING WILL BE D/C'D AT 0800 ON:

DATE	ORDER		
		☐ CONT	PHYSICIAN SIGNATURE
		☐ D/C	
		☐ CONT	PHYSICIAN SIGNATURE
		☐ D/C	
		☐ CONT	PHYSICIAN SIGNATURE
		☐ D/C	

CHECK WHEN ANTIBIOTICS ORDERED ☐ Prophylactic ☐ Empiric ☐ Therapeutic

Allergies: None Known

PATIENT DIAGNOSIS: Diabetes

HEIGHT 5' 5"   WEIGHT 130 lb.

FORM 959-708 (8-90)   **PHYSICIANS ORDER**   Reynolds + Reynolds LITHO IN U.S.A. K41814 (7-90) D339360

Patient, Mary Q.
#3-11316-7

Fig. 5–1 Physician's Order

PAGE _____ of _____

MEDICATION ADMINISTRATION RECORD

ORIGINAL ORDER DATE	DATE STARTED / RENEWED	MEDICATION - DOSAGE	ROUTE	SCHEDULE 11-7	7-3	3-11	DATE 11-3-xx 11-7	7-3	3-11	DATE 11-4-xx 11-7	7-3	3-11	DATE 11-5-xx 11-7	7-3	3-11	DATE 11-6-xx 11-7	7-3	3-11
11-3	11-3	Keflex 250 mg q. 6 h	PO	12/6	12	6		GP 12	MS 6	12JJ 6JJ	GP 12	MS 6						
11-3	11-4	Human NPH Insulin 40 U ā breakfast	SC		7³⁰						GP 7³⁰ Ⓡ							
11-3	11-3	Lasix 40 mg q.d.	PO		9			GP 9			GP 9							
11-3	11-3	Slow-K 8 mEq b.i.d.	PO		9	9			MS 9		GP 9	MS 9						

PRN

11-3	11-3	Demerol 75 mg q. 3-4 h	IM	severe pain				GP 12 Ⓛ	MS 6 Ⓜ-10 Ⓙ									
11-3	11-4	Codeine 30 mg q. 4 h	PO	mild–mod pain						JJ 6	GP 2							
11-3	11-3	Tylenol 650 mg q. 4 h	PO	fever >101°F				GP 12	MS 4–8	JJ 12–4	GP 8–12							

INJECTION SITES

B - RIGHT ARM	D - RIGHT ANTERIOR THIGH	H - LEFT ABDOMEN	L - LEFT BUTTOCKS
C - RIGHT ABDOMEN	G - LEFT ARM	J - LEFT ANTERIOR THIGH	M - RIGHT BUTTOCKS

DATE GIVEN	TIME	INT.	ONE-TIME MEDICATION - DOSAGE	RT.	SCHEDULE 11-7	7-3	3-11	DATE 11-7	7-3	3-11	DATE 11-7	7-3	3-11	DATE 11-7	7-3	3-11	DATE 11-7	7-3	3-11
11-3	2200		Lasix 80 mg stat	IV															

SIGNATURE OF NURSE ADMINISTERING MEDICATIONS

SCHEDULE	DATE	DATE	DATE	DATE
11-7		JJ J. Jones, LPN		
7-3	GP G. Pickar, RN	GP G. Pickar, RN		
3-11	MS M. Smith, RN	MS M. Smith, RN		

DATE GIVEN	TIME	INT.	MEDICATION-DOSAGE-CONT.	RT.

LITHO IN U.S.A. K8508 (7-92) D095538

RECOPIED BY:

CHECKED BY:

Patient, Mary Q.

#3-11316-7

ALLERGIES: None Known

602-31 (7-92) (MPC# 1355)

① ORIGINAL COPY

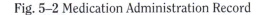

Fig. 5–2 Medication Administration Record

Computerized Medication Administration Records

Many hospitals now use computers for processing drug orders. The drug order is entered in the computer from the order form (Figure 5–3). The computer can process the order much more rapidly than people can. It can transmit the order within seconds to the pharmacy for filling the order, and to the business office for posting charges. It can even scan information previously entered, such as drug incompatibilities, drug allergies, safe dosage ranges, or recommended administration times. The health care staff can be readily alerted to potential problems or inconsistencies. The medication administration record may also be printed directly from the computer (Figure 5–4 on page 79). The nurse may even document the administration of the medication at the computer terminal.

			ENTERED	FILLED	CHECKED	VERIFIED
						—

NOTE: A NON-PROPRIETARY DRUG OF EQUAL QUALITY MAY BE DISPENSED - IF THIS COLUMN IS NOT CHECKED!

DATE	TIME WRITTEN	PLEASE USE BALL POINT - PRESS FIRMLY	✓	TIME NOTED	NURSES SIGNATURE
8/31/XX	1500	Procan SR 500 mg p.o. q 6 h	✓		
		J. Physician, M.D.		1515	MS
9/3/XX	0830	Digoxin 0.125 mg p.o. q.o.d.	✓		
		Lasix 40 mg p.o. q.d	✓		
		Reglan 10 mg p.o. stat & a.c. & h.s.	✓		
		K-Lyte 25 mEq p.o. b.i.d.-start 9/4/XX	✓		
		Nitroglycerin gr $^1/_{150}$ SL p.r.n. chest pain	✓	0845	GP
		Darvocet-N 100 tab. 1 p.o. q. 4-6 h p.r.n. mild-moderate pain	✓		
		Demerol 50 mg IM q. 4 h c̄	✓		
		Phenergan 50 mg IM q. 4h } p.r.n. severe pain	✓		
		J. Physician, M.D.			

AUTO STOP ORDERS: UNLESS REORDERED, FOLLOWING WILL BE D/C'ᴰ AT 0800 ON:

DATE	ORDER		
		☐ CONT	PHYSICIAN SIGNATURE
		☐ D/C	
		☐ CONT	PHYSICIAN SIGNATURE
		☐ D/C	
		☐ CONT	PHYSICIAN SIGNATURE
		☐ D/C	

CHECK WHEN ANTIBIOTICS ORDERED   ☐ Prophylactic   ☐ Empiric   ☐ Therapeutic

Allergies:
No Known allergies

PATIENT DIAGNOSIS
congestive heart failure

HEIGHT   5' 10"   WEIGHT   165 lb.

FORM 959-708 (8-90)   **PHYSICIANS ORDER**   Reynolds + Reynolds LITHO IN U.S.A. K41814 (7-90) D339060

Patient, John D.
#3-81512-3

①

Fig. 5–3 Physician's Order

PHARMACY MAR

START	STOP	MEDICATION	SCHEDULED TIMES	OK'D BY	0001 HRS. TO 1200 HRS.	1201 HRS. TO 2400 HRS.
08/31/xx 1800 SCH		PROCAN SR 500 MG TAB-SR [500 MG] Q6H [PO]	0600 1200 1800 2400	JD	0600GP 1200 GP	1800 MS 2400 JD
09/03/xx 0900 SCH		DIGOXIN (LANOXIN) 0.125 MG TAB [1 TAB] QOD [PO] ODD DAYS-SEPT	0900	JD	0900 GP	
09/03/xx 0900 SCH		FUROSEMIDE (LASIX) 40 MG TAB [1 TAB] QD [PO]	0900	JD	0900 GP	
09/03/xx 0845 SCH		REGLAN 10 MG TAB [10 MG] AC&HS [PO] GIVE ONE NOW!!	0730 1130 1630 2100	JD	0730 GP 1130 GP	1630 MS 2100 MS
09/04/xx 0900 SCH		K-LYTE 25 MEQ EFFERVESCENT TAB [1 EFF. TAB] BID [PO] DISSOLVE AS DIR START 9-4	0900 1700	JD	0900 GP	1700 GP
09/03/xx 1507 PRN		NITROGLYCERIN 1/50 GR 0.4 MG TAB-SL [1 TABLET] PRN* [SL] PRN CHEST PAIN		JD		
09/03/xx 1700 PRN		DARVOCET-N 100* [1 TAB] Q4-6H [PO] PRN MILD–MODERATE PAIN		JD		
09/03/xx 2100 PRN		MEPERIDINE* (DEMEROL) INJ [50 MG] Q4H [IM] PRN SEVERE PAIN W PHENERGAN		JD		2200 Ⓗ MS
09/03/xx 2100 PRN		PROMETHAZINE (PHENERGAN) INJ [50 MG] Q4H [IM] PRN SEVERE PAIN W DEMEROL		JD		2200 Ⓗ MS

Gluteus	Thigh	NURSE'S SIGNATURE	INITIAL		
A. Right	H. Right			ALLERGIES: NKA	Patient: Patient, John D.
B. Left	I. Left	7–3 G. Pickar, R.N.	GP		Patient # 3-81512-3
Ventro Gluteal		3–11 M. Smith, R.N.	MS		Admitted: 08/31/xx
C. Right	J. Right				Physician: J. Physician, MD
D. Left	K. Left	11–7 J. Doe, R.N.	JD	DIAGNOSIS: CHF	Room: PCU-14 PCU
E. Abdomen 1|2 3|4					

730-13 (12/83)

Fig. 5–4 Computerized Medication Administration Record

review set 18

Refer to the **Computerized Pharmacy MAR** (Figure 5–4) to answer items 1–10.

Convert the scheduled 24-hour time to traditional AM/PM time.

1. Scheduled times for administering Procan SR. _____

2. Scheduled times for administering Lanoxin and Lasix. _____

3. Scheduled times for administering Reglan. _____

4. Scheduled times for administering K-Lyte. _____

5. How often can the Demerol be given? _____

6. If the Lanoxin was last given on 9/5/xx at 0900, when is the next time and date it will be given? _____

7. What is the ordered route of administration for the nitroglycerin? _____

8. How many times a day is furosemide ordered? _____

9. The equivalent dosage of Lanoxin measured in micrograms is _____ .

10. Which drugs are ordered to be administered "as necessary?" _____

Refer to the **Medication Administration Record** (Figure 5–2) on page 77 to answer items 11–20.

11. What is the route of administration for the insulin? _____

12. How many times in a 24-hour period will Lasix be administered? _____

13. The only medication ordered to be given routinely at noon is _____ .

14. What time of day is the insulin to be administered? _____

15. A dosage of 8 mEq of Slow-K is ordered. What does mEq mean? _____

16. You work 3-11 on November 5. Which routine medications will you administer to Mary Q. Patient during your shift? _____

17. Mary Q. Patient has a fever of 101.4° F. What medication should you administer? _____

    _____

18. How many times in a 24-hour period will Slow-K be administered? _____

19. The equivalent of the scheduled administration time(s) for the Slow-K as converted to 24-hour time is _____ .

20. The equivalent of the scheduled administration time(s) for the Keflex as converted to 24-hour time is _____ .

21. Identify the place on the MAR where the stat IV Lasix was charted. _____

    _____

After completing these problems, see page 295 to check your answers.

The Drug Order

The drug order consists of seven parts:

1. Name of the patient

2. Name of the drug to be administered

3. Dosage of the drug

4. Route by which the drug is to be administered

5. Time and/or frequency of administration

6. Date and time when the order was written

7. Signature of the person writing the order

Parts 1–5 are known as "THE FIVE RIGHTS" of medication administration and are essential for safe medication administration. The *right patient* must receive the *right drug* in the *right amount* (or dosage) by the *right route* at the *right time*. If the nurse has difficulty interpreting the order or any of the above information is not complete, the nurse MUST clarify the order with the writer. Usually this person is the physician or nurse practitioner.

remember

COMMON MEDICAL ABBREVIATIONS

ABBREVIATION	INTERPRETATION	ABBREVIATION	INTERPRETATION
Route:		**Frequency:**	
IM	intramuscular	b.i.d.	twice a day
IV	intravenous	t.i.d.	three times a day
IV PB	intravenous piggyback	q.i.d.	four times a day
SC	subcutaneous	min.	minute
SL	sublingual, under the tongue	h	hour
ID	intradermal	q.h	every hour
GT	gastrostomy tube	q.2h	every two hours
NG	nasogastric tube	q.3h	every three hours
NJ	nasojejunal tube	q.4h	every four hours
p.o.	by mouth, orally	q.6h	every six hours
p.r.	per rectum	q.8h	every eight hours
O.D.	right eye	q.12h	every twelve hours
O.S.	left eye		
O.U.	both eyes	**General:**	
A.D.	right ear	$\bar{a}$	before
A.S.	left ear	$\bar{p}$	after
A.U.	both ears	$\bar{c}$	with
		$\bar{s}$	without
Frequency:		q	every
a.c.	before meals	aq	water
p.c.	after meals	NPO	nothing by mouth
ad. lib.	as desired, freely	ss	one-half
p.r.n.	when necessary	gtt	drop
h.s.	hour of sleep, at bed time	tab	tablet
		cap	capsule
stat	immediately, at once	et	and
q.d.	once a day, every day	noct	night
q.o.d.	every other day		

For the purposes of learning dosage calculations, you will be concerned with parts 2–5 of the medication order. The dosage of the drug is expressed in the standard abbreviations or symbols given in Chapter 2. For instance, you recall that milliliter is abbreviated mL and the symbol for ounce is ℥, etc. Other common abbreviations used in writing drug orders are listed here. The abbreviations are grouped according to those which refer to the route (method) of administration, the frequency (time interval), and other general terms. Commit these abbreviations to memory along with the others you have already learned.

For the drug order, the name of the drug is written first, followed by the dosage, route, and frequency. When correctly written, the brand name of the drug begins with a capital letter, while the generic (nonproprietary) name begins with a lowercase letter. Also drug labels and published literature use the ® sign following the brandname, indicating the name is registered. For instance, meperidine hydrochloride is the generic name of Demerol®, a brand of the same drug; acetominophen is the generic name of Tylenol®, a brand.

EXAMPLES: Interpreting drug orders.

1. Dilantin 100 mg p.o. t.i.d.
   Reads: "Give 100 milligrams of Dilantin orally three times a day."
2. procaine penicillin G 400,000 U IM q.6h
   Reads: "Give 400,000 units of procaine penicillin G intramuscularly every 6 hours."
3. Demerol 75 mg IM q.4h p.r.n., pain
   Reads: "Give 75 milligrams of Demerol intramuscularly every 4 hours when necessary for pain."
4. Humulin R insulin 5 U SC stat
   Reads: "Give 5 units of Humulin R insulin subcutaneously immediately."
5. Ancef 1 g IV PB q.6h
   Reads: "Give one gram of Ancef intravenous piggyback every six hours."

The administration times are designated by hospital policy; such as t.i.d. administration times may be 0900 or 9 AM, 1300 or 1 PM, and 1700 or 5 PM.

quick review

■ All parts of the drug order must be stated clearly, for accurate, exact interpretation. If you are ever in doubt as to the meaning or any part of a drug order, ask the writer to clarify.

review set 19

Interpret the following physician's medication (drug) orders:

1. naproxen 250 mg p.o. b.i.d. _____

   _____

2. Humulin N U-100 insulin 30 U SC q.d. 30 min. ā breakfast _____

   _____

3. Ceclor 500 mg p.o. stat, then 250 mg q.8h _____

   _____

4. Synthroid 25 mcg p.o. q.d. _____

   _____

5. Ativan 10 mg IM q.4h p.r.n., agitation _____

   _____

6. furosemide 20 mg IV stat (slowly) _____

   _____

7. Gelusil 10 cc p.o. h.s. _____

   _____

8. atropine sulfate ophthalmic 1% 2 gtt O.D. q. 15 min × 4 _____

   _____

9. morphine sulfate gr $\frac{1}{4}$ IM q.3–4h p.r.n., pain _____

    _____

10. Lanoxin 0.25 mg p.o. q.d. _____

    _____

11. tetracycline 250 mg p.o q.i.d. _____

    _____

12. nitroglycerin gr $\frac{1}{400}$ SL stat _____

    _____

13. Cortisporin Otic 2 gtt A.U. t.i.d. et h.s. _____

    _____

14. Of the preceding medication orders, which are given in the generic name? (Write the numbers of the drug order, e.g.,#1, etc.) _____

    _____

15. Describe your action if no method of administration is written. _____

    _____

16. Do q.i.d. and q.4h have the same meaning? Explain. _____

    _____

17. Who determines the medication administration times? _____

    _____

18. Name the seven parts of a written medication prescription. _____

    _____

19. Which parts of the written medication prescription/order represent the "Five Rights" of medication administration? _____

    _____

20. Interpret (state) the "Five Rights." _____

    _____

After completing these problems, see pages 295 and 296 to check your answers.

critical thinking skills

It is the responsibility of the nurse to clarify any order that is incomplete; that is, an order that does not contain the seven parts discussed on page 80. It is also the responsibility of the nurse to clarify any discrepancies in the written order. Let's look at some examples in which these errors occurred.

■ error 1

Failing to clarify incomplete orders.

possible scenario

Suppose a physician ordered Pepcid one tablet p.o. at h.s. for a patient with an active duodenal ulcer. You will note that there is no dosage listed.

The nurse thought the dosage came in only one strength, added 20 mg to the order, and sent it to the pharmacy. The pharmacist prepared the dosage written on the physician order sheet. Two days later, during rounds, the physician noted that the patient had not responded well to the Pepcid. When asked about the Pepcid, the nurse explained that the patient had received 20 mg at bedtime. The physician informed the nurse that the patient should have received the 40 mg tablet.

potential outcome

Potentially, the delay in correct dose could result in gastrointestinal bleeding or delayed healing of the ulcer.

prevention

This medication error could have been avoided simply by the physician writing the strength of the medication. When this was omitted, the nurse should have checked the dosage before sending the order to the pharmacy. When you fill in an incomplete order, you are essentially practicing medicine without a license, which is illegal.

■ *error 2*

Not checking for discrepancies.

possible scenario

Suppose a physician wrote an order for Gentamicin 100 mg to be given IV q.8h to a patient hospitalized with meningitis. The unit secretary transcribed the order as:

Gentamicin 100 mg IV q.8h
(12 AM–6 AM–12 PM–6 PM)

The medication nurse checked the order without noticing the discrepancy in the administration times. Suppose the patient received the medication every six hours for three days before the error was noticed.

potential outcome

The patient would have received one extra dose each day, which is equivalent to one-third more medication daily. Most likely, the physician would be notified of the error, and the medication would be discontinued with serum gentamicin levels drawn. The levels would likely be in the toxic range, and the patient's gentamicin levels would be monitored until the levels returned to normal. This patient would be at risk of developing ototoxicity or nephrotoxicity from the overdose of Gentamicin.

prevention

This error could have been avoided by paying careful attention to the ordered frequency and if the frequency had been written on the MAR.

practice problems—chapter 5 _____

Interpret the following abbreviations and symbols without consulting another source.

1. ʒ   _____   9. q.d.   _____

2. p.r.   _____   10. O.D.   _____

3. a.c.   _____   11. stat   _____

4. p̄   _____   12. ad.lib.   _____

5. t.i.d.   _____   13. h.s.   _____

6. q.4h   _____   14. IM   _____

7. p.r.n.   _____   15. s̄   _____

8. p.o.   _____

Give the abbreviation or symbol for the following terms without consulting another source.

16. one-half   _____   24. subcutaneous   _____

17. drop   _____   25. teaspoon   _____

18. milliliter   _____   26. twice daily   _____

19. grain   _____   27. every 3 hours   _____

20. gram   _____   28. after meals   _____

21. with   _____   29. before   _____

22. four times a day   _____   30. kilogram   _____

23. both eyes   _____

Interpret the following physician's drug orders without consulting another source.

31. Toradol 60 mg IM stat and q.6h _____

32. procaine penicillin G 300,000 U IM q.i.d. _____

33. Mylanta 5 mL p.o. 1 h a.c., 1 h p.c., h.s., et q.2h p.r.n. @ noc. _____

34. Librium 25 mg p.o. q.6h p.r.n., agitation _____

35. heparin 5,000 U SC stat _____

36. Demerol 50 mg IM q.3–4h p.r.n., pain _____

37. digoxin 0.25 mg p.o. q.d. _____

38. Neosynephrine ophthalmic 10% 2 gtt O.S. q. 30 min × 2 _____

39. Lasix 40 mg IM stat _____

40. Decadron 4 mg IV b.i.d. _____

Refer to the **Medication Administration Record** (Figure 5–5) on page 86 to answer items 41–45.

41. Convert the scheduled times for Isosorbide SR to traditional AM/PM time.

_____   _____   _____

42. How many units of heparin will the patient receive at 2200? _____

43. What route is ordered for the Humulin R insulin? _____

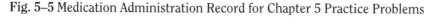

ORIGINAL ORDER DATE	DATE STARTED / RENEWED	MEDICATION - DOSAGE	ROUTE	SCHEDULE			DATE 11-3-xx			DATE 11-4-xx			DATE 11-5-xx			DATE 11-6-xx		
				11-7	7-3	3-11	11-7	7-3	3-11	11-7	7-3	3-11	11-7	7-3	3-11	11-7	7-3	3-11
11-3	11-3	Heparin lock Central line flush (10u/cc solution) 2cc bid	IV		1000	2200												
11-3	11-3	Isosorbide SR 40 mg. q 8h	PO	2400	0800	1600												
11-3	11-3	Cipro 500 mg. q. 12h	PO		1000	2200												
11-3	11-3	Humulin N insulin 15u q. am	SC	0700														
11-3	11-3	Humulin R insulin 30 min. ac and hs per sliding rule scale: Blood glucose 0-150 3U 151-250 8U 251-350 13U 351-400 18U >400 call Dr.	SC		0730 1130	1730 2200												
	11-3	PRN Tylenol tabs 2 q 3-4 h prn headache	PO															

PRN

INJECTION SITES		B - RIGHT ARM			D - RIGHT ANTERIOR THIGH			H - LEFT ABDOMEN			L - LEFT BUTTOCKS		
		C - RIGHT ABDOMEN			G - LEFT ARM			J - LEFT ANTERIOR THIGH			M - RIGHT BUTTOCKS		

DATE GIVEN	TIME	INT.	ONE - TIME MEDICATION - DOSAGE	RT.	SCHEDULE 11-7	7-3	3-11	DATE 11-7	7-3	3-11	DATE 11-7	7-3	3-11	DATE 11-7	7-3	3-11	DATE
					11-7												
					7-3												
					3-11												

SIGNATURE OF NURSE ADMINISTERING MEDICATIONS

DATE GIVEN	TIME	INT.	MEDICATION-DOSAGE-CONT.	RT.	LITHO IN U.S.A. K6508 (7-92) D395538

RECOPIED BY:

CHECKED BY:

ALLERGIES:

602-31 (7-92) (MPC# 1355)

1

ORIGINAL COPY

Fig. 5–5 Medication Administration Record for Chapter 5 Practice Problems

44. Interpret the order for Cipro. _____

45. If the administration times for the sliding scale insulin are accurate, what times will meals be served (use traditional AM/PM time)? _____

Refer to the **Computerized Pharmacy MAR** (Figure 5–6) to answer items 46–50.

46. The physician visited about 5:00 PM 8/8/xx. What order did he write? _____

PHARMACY MAR

START	STOP	MEDICATION	SCHEDULED TIMES	OK'D BY	0701 TO 1500	1501 TO 2300	2301 TO 0700
21:00 8/17/xx SCH		MEGESTROL ACETATE (MEGACE) 40 MG TAB 2 TABS PO BID	0900 2100				
12:00 8/17/xx SCH		VANCOMYCIN 250 MG CAP 1 CAPSULE PO QID	0800 1200 1800 2200				
9:00 8/13/xx SCH		FLUCONAZOLE (DIFLUCAN) 100 MG TAB 100MG PO QD	0900				
21:00 8/11/xx SCH		PERIDEX ORAL RINSE 480 ML 30 ML ORAL RINSE BID SWISH & SPIT	0900 2100				
17:00 8/10/xx SCH		RANITIDINE (ZANTAC) 150 MG TAB 1 TABLET PO BID W/BREAK.&SUPPER	0800 1700				
17:00 8/08/xx SCH		DIGOXIN (LANOXIN) 0.125MG TAB 1 TAB PO QD1700	1700				
0:01 8/27/xx PRN		LIDOCAINE 5% OINT 35 GM TUBE APPLY TOPICAL PRN* TO RECTAL AREA					
14:00 8/22/xx PRN		SODIUM CHLORIDE INJ 10 ML AS DIR IV TID DILUENT FOR ATIVAN IV					
14:00 8/22/xx PRN		LORAZEPAM (ATIVAN)*2MG INJ 1 MG IV TID PRN ANXIETY					
9:30 8/21/xx PRN		TUCKS 40 PADS APPLY APPLY TOPICAL Q4-6H TO RECTUM PRN					
9:30 8/21/xx PRN		ANUSOL SUPP 1 SUPP 1 SUPP PR Q4-6H					
16:00 8/18/xx PRN		MEPERIDINE* (DEMEROL) INJ 25 MG 10 MG IV Q1H PRN PAIN IN ADDITION TO PCA					

Gluteus	Thigh	STANDARD TIMES	NURSE'S SIGNATURE	INITIAL	ALLERGIES:	NAFCILLIN		
A. Right	H. Right	QD = 0900	0701-			BACTRIM	Patient	Smith, John
B. Left	I. Left	BID = Q12H = 0900 & 2100	1500 ___			SULFA	Patient #	3-90301-4
		TID = 0800, 1400, 2200	1501-			TRIMETHOPRIM		
Ventro Gluteal	Deltoid	Q8H = 0800, 1600, 2400	2300 ___			CIPROFLOXACIN HCL	Physician:	J. Physician, M.D.
C. Right	J. Right	QID = 0800, 1200, 1800, 2200	2301-				Room:	407-4 South
D. Left	K. Left	Q6H = 0600, 1200, 1800, 2400	0700 ___					
E. Abdomen	1 / 2	Q4H = 0400, 0800, 1200...	Ok'd					
	3 / 4	QD DIGOXIN = 1700	by ___		FROM: 08/30/xx 0701		TO: 08/31/xx 0700	
Page 1 of 2	QD	QD WARFARIN = 1600						

Fig. 5–6 Computerized Pharmacy MAR for Chapter 5 Practice Problems

47. Using the time, as a clue, interpret the symbol "w/" in the Zantac order and give the proper medical abbreviation. _____

48. Interpret the order for ranitidine. _____

49. Which of the routine meds is (are) ordered for 6:00 PM? _____

50. How many hours are between the scheduled administration times for Megace?_____

After completing these problems, see page 321 to check your answers.

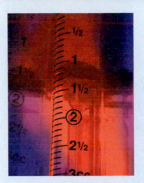

Understanding Drug Labels 6

objectives

Upon mastery of Chapter 6, you will be able to read and interpret the labels of the medications you have available. To accomplish this you will also be able to:

- Find and differentiate the brand and generic names of drugs.
- Determine the dosage strength or amount of drugs by weight.
- Determine the form in which the drug is supplied.
- Identify the total volume of the drug container.
- Differentiate the total volume of the container from the dosage strength.
- Find the directions for mixing or preparing the supply strength of drugs as needed.
- Identify the administration route.
- Recognize manufacturer's name.
- Check the drug expiration date.
- Identify the lot number.

The drug order prescribes how much of a drug the patient is to receive. The nurse must prepare the order from the drugs on hand. The drug label tells how the available drug is supplied.

Look at the following common drug labels and learn to recognize pertinent information about the drugs supplied.

Generic and brand names of the drug:

By law the generic name must be identified on all drug labels. The brand name is followed by the sign ® meaning the name is registered. Occasionally, only the generic name appears.

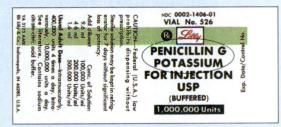

Generic Name (penicillin G potassium)

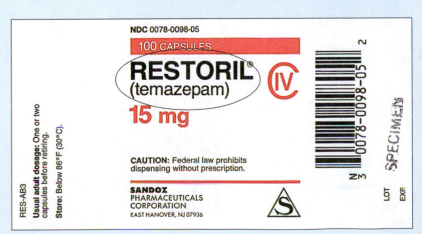

Brand Name (Restoril) and
Generic Name (temazepam)

Dosage strength: weight of the drug.

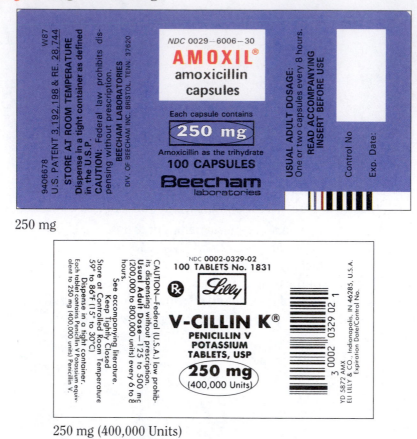

250 mg

250 mg (400,000 Units)

Form: tablets, capsules, milliliters, etc.

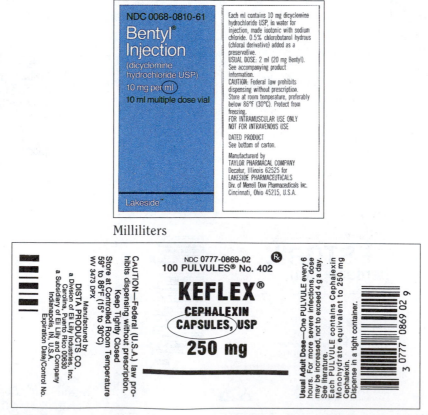

Milliliters

Capsules

Supply dosage: dosage strength and form read together.

NDC 0002-7217-01 VIAL No. 520 5 ml ℞ *Lilly* **HEPARIN SODIUM INJECTION, USP** **10,000 USP Units per ml** Multiple Dose	NDC 0590-0399-01 **NUBAIN®** (nalbuphine HCl) **20** mg/ml injection **10 ml** VIAL Each ml contains: 20 mg nalbuphine HCl, 0.94% sodium citrate hydrous, 1.26% citric acid anhydrous, 0.1% sodium metabisulfite and 0.2% of a 9:1 mixture of methyl and propylparaben, as preservatives. pH is adjusted, if neces- sary, with hydrochloric acid. **FOR IM, SC OR IV USE** **DOSAGE:** Read accompanying product information. **CAUTION:** Federal law prohibits dispen- sing without prescription. Store at controlled room temperature (59°-86°F, 15°-30°C). **PROTECT FROM EXCESSIVE LIGHT** **Du Pont Pharmaceuticals, Inc.** Subsidiary of E. I. du Pont de Nemours & Co. (Inc.) Manati, Puerto Rico 00701 XB LOT: EXP:

10,000 Units per milliliter   20 milligrams per milliliter

Total volume of liquid containers

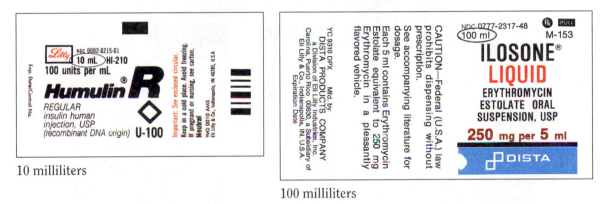

10 milliliters   100 milliliters

Administration route: such as for oral, sublingual, injection, otic, optic, rectal, vaginal, topical, IV, IM use. Unless specified otherwise, tablets, capsules, and caplets are intended for oral use.

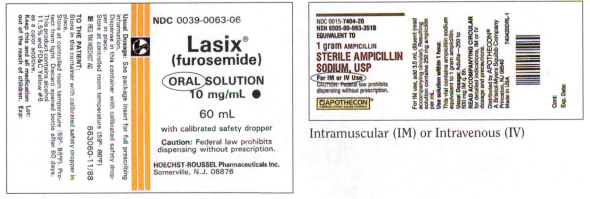

Oral   Intramuscular (IM) or Intravenous (IV)

Directions for mixing or reconstituting powdered forms of drugs.

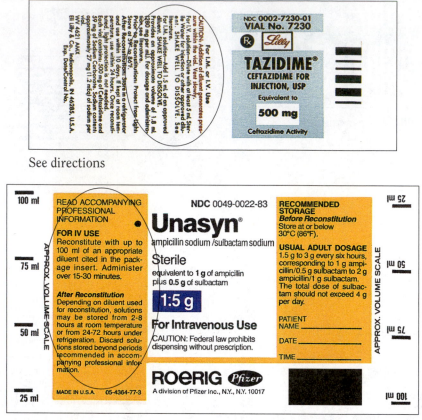

See directions

See directions

Name of the manufacturer.

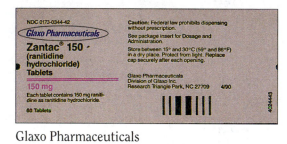

Glaxo Pharmaceuticals

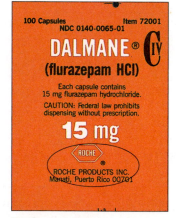

Roche

Expiration date: The medication should be used, discarded, or returned to the pharmacy by this date.

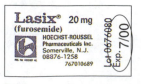

7/00

Unit dose labels: Most oral medications administered in the hospital setting are available in unit dosage, in which a single capsule or tablet is packaged separately in a typical blister pack. The pharmacy provides a 24-hour supply of each drug for the patient. Figure 6–1 shows two samples of labels from unit dose packaging. Notice that the only major difference in this form of labeling is that the total volume of the container is omitted since the volume is one tablet or capsule. Likewise, the dosage strength is understood as "per one."

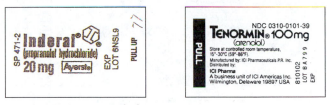

Fig. **6–1** Unit Dose Labels

Lot number: Federal law requires all medication packages to be identified with a lot or control number. This identification process is required so that if a given medication is damaged or tampered with, the lot number can be used to identify the group of medications to be removed from the shelves of hospitals or pharmacies.

Currently the lot number and expiration date of all vaccines administered in the United States are required to be documented. This information is documented on a form known as the Vaccine Adverse Event Reporting System. This is done routinely in case a given vaccine is recalled.

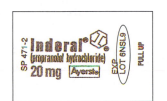

Combination drugs: Figure 6–2 shows labels of combination drugs. Read the labels for Claritin-D and Darvocet-N, and notice the different drugs that are combined. Combination drugs like Claritin-D and Darvocet-N are usually prescribed by the number of tablets or capsules to be given, rather than by the dosage strength.

quick review

Read labels carefully to:

- identify the drug and the manufacturer.
- differentiate between dosage strength, form, supply dosage, total container volume, and administration route.
- find the directions for reconstitution, as needed.
- note expiration date.
- describe lot or control number.

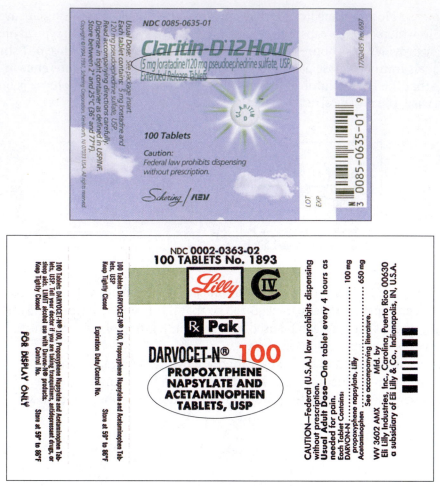

Fig. 6–2 Combination Drug Labels

review set 20

Use the labels A–G that follow to find the information requested for the review. Indicate your answer by letter (A–G).

1. The total volume of the liquid container is circled. _____

2. The dosage strength is circled. _____

3. The form of the drug is circled. _____

4. The brand name of the drug is circled. _____

5. The generic name of the drug is circled. _____

6. The expiration date is circled. _____

7. The lot number is circled. _____

8. Look at label E and determine how much of the supply drug you will administer to the patient per dose for the order *Ceclor 250 mg p.o. q.8h p.r.n.* _____

9. Look at label A and determine the route of administration. _____

After completing these problems, see page 296 to check your answers.

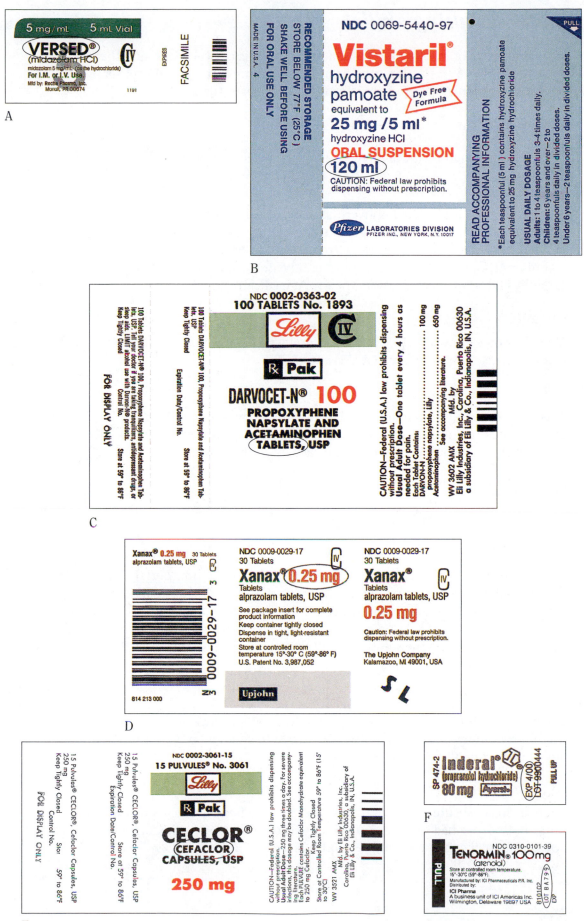

A

5 mg/mL   5 mL Vial
VERSED®
(midazolam HCl)
midazolam 5 mg/mL (as the hydrochloride)
For I.M. or I.V. Use.
Mfd by: Roche Pharma, Inc.
Manati, PR·00674
1191
EXPIRES
FACSIMILE
IV

B

MADE IN U.S.A. 4
FOR ORAL USE ONLY
SHAKE WELL BEFORE USING
STORE BELOW 77°F (25°C)
RECOMMENDED STORAGE

NDC 0069-5440-97
Vistaril®
hydroxyzine
pamoate   *Dye Free Formula*
equivalent to
25 mg /5 ml*
hydroxyzine HCl
ORAL SUSPENSION
120 ml
CAUTION: Federal law prohibits
dispensing without prescription.

Pfizer LABORATORIES DIVISION
PFIZER INC., NEW YORK, N.Y. 10017

READ ACCOMPANYING
PROFESSIONAL INFORMATION

*Each teaspoonful (5 ml) contains hydroxyzine pamoate
equivalent to 25 mg hydroxyzine hydrochloride
USUAL DAILY DOSAGE
Adults: 1 to 4 teaspoonfuls 3-4 times daily.
Children: 6 years and over—2 to
4 teaspoonfuls daily in divided doses.
Under 6 years—2 teaspoonfuls daily in divided doses.

C

NDC 0002-0363-02
100 TABLETS No. 1893
Lilly   C IV
℞ Pak
DARVOCET-N® 100
**PROPOXYPHENE
NAPSYLATE AND
ACETAMINOPHEN
TABLETS, USP**

100 Tablets DARVOCET-N® 100, Propoxyphene Napsylate and Acetaminophen Tab-
lets, USP. Tell your doctor if you are taking tranquilizers, antidepressant drugs, or
sleep aids. LIMIT alcohol use with Darvon-N® products.
Keep Tightly Closed
FOR DISPLAY ONLY
Store at 59° to 86°F

100 Tablets DARVOCET-N® 100, Propoxyphene Napsylate and Acetaminophen Tab-
lets, USP.
Keep Tightly Closed
Expiration Date/Control No.
Store at 59° to 86°F

CAUTION—Federal (U.S.A.) law prohibits dispensing
without prescription.
Usual Adult Dose—One tablet every 4 hours as
needed for pain.
Each Tablet Contains:
DARVON-N
propoxyphene napsylate, Lilly .... 100 mg
Acetaminophen .... 650 mg
See accompanying literature.
WV 3602 AMX   Mfd. by
Eli Lilly Industries, Inc., Carolina, Puerto Rico 00630
a subsidiary of Eli Lilly & Co., Indianapolis, IN, U.S.A.

D

Xanax® 0.25 mg   30 Tablets
alprazolam tablets, USP   IV

NDC 0009-0029-17
30 Tablets
Xanax® 0.25 mg
Tablets
alprazolam tablets, USP
See package insert for complete
product information
Keep container tightly closed
Dispense in tight, light-resistant
container
Store at controlled room
temperature 15°-30° C (59°-86° F)
U.S. Patent No. 3,987,052

0009-0029-17 3
ZЄM
814 213 000

NDC 0009-0029-17
30 Tablets
Xanax®
Tablets
alprazolam tablets, USP   IV
0.25 mg
Caution: Federal law prohibits
dispensing without prescription.
The Upjohn Company
Kalamazoo, MI 49001, USA
Upjohn
SL

E

15 Pulvules® CECLOR®, Cefaclor Capsules, USP
250 mg
Keep Tightly Closed
Control No.
FOR DISPLAY ONLY

15 Pulvules® CECLOR®, Cefaclor Capsules, USP
250 mg
Keep Tightly Closed
Expiration Date/Control No.

NDC 0002-3061-15
15 PULVULES® No. 3061
Lilly
℞ Pak
**CECLOR®
(CEFACLOR)
CAPSULES, USP**
250 mg

CAUTION—Federal (U.S.A.) law prohibits dispensing
without prescription.
Usual Adult Dose—250 mg three times a day. For severe
infections, this dosage may be doubled. See accompany-
ing literature.
Each PULVULE contains Cefaclor Monohydrate equivalent
to 250 mg Cefaclor.
Keep Tightly Closed
Store at Controlled Room Temperature 59° to 86°F (15°
to 30°C)
WV 3521 AMX   Mfd. by Eli Lilly Industries, Inc.,
Carolina, Puerto Rico 00630, a subsidiary of
Eli Lilly & Co., Indianapolis, IN, U.S.A.
Store at
59° to 86°F

F

SP 474-2
Inderal®
(propranolol hydrochloride)
80 mg   Ayerst
EXP 4/00
LOT 9900444
PULL UP

G

NDC 0310-0101-39
TENORMIN® 100 mg
(atenolol)
PULL
Store at controlled room temperature.
15°-30°C (59°-86°F).
Manufactured by: ICI Pharmaceuticals P.R. Inc.
Distributed by:
ICI Pharma
A business unit of ICI Americas Inc.
Wilmington, Delaware 19897 USA
810102
LOT BA79?
EXP

The importance of reading the labels of medications is critical. Make sure that the drug you want is what you have on hand before you administer it. Let's look at some examples of medication errors related to reading the label incorrectly.

■ error 1

The medication administration record and the label do not match.

possible scenario

Suppose a physician ordered Antivert (an antiemetic) 50 mg p.o. stat. The writing was not clear on the order, and Ativan (an antianxiety medication) 0.5 mg was sent up by the pharmacy. However, the order was correctly transcribed to the medication administration record (MAR). In preparing the medication, the nurse did not read the MAR or label carefully and administered Ativan, the wrong medication.

potential outcome

A medication error occurred because the wrong medication was given. In addition, the patient's nausea probably was not alleviated.

prevention

This error could have been prevented by carefully comparing the drug label and dosage to the MAR drug and dosage. In this instance both the incorrect drug and the incorrect dosage sent by the pharmacy were not picked up by the nurse.

■ error 2

Not checking the label for correct dosage.

possible scenario

A nurse flushed a triple central venous catheter (an IV with three ports). According to hospital policy, the nurse was to flush each port with 10 mL of normal saline followed by 2 mL of heparin flush solution in the concentration of 100 units/mL. The nurse mistakenly picked up a vial of heparin containing heparin 10,000 units/mL. Without checking the label, she prepared the solution for all three ports. The patient received 60,000 units of heparin instead of 600 units.

potential outcome

The patient in this case would be at great risk for hemorrhage, leading to shock and death. Protamine sulfate would likely be ordered to counteract the action of the heparin, but a successful outcome is questionable.

prevention

There is no substitute for checking the label before administering a medication. The nurse in this case had three opportunities to catch the error, having drawn three different syringes of medication for the three ports.

practice problems—chapter 6

Look at the labels A–G and identify the information requested.

Label A:

1. The supply dosage of the drug in milliequivalents is _____ .

2. The manufacturer is _____ .

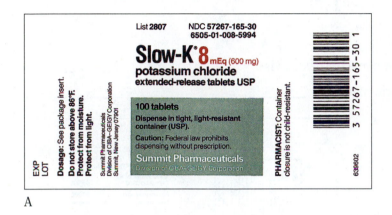

A

Label B:

3. The generic name of the drug is _____ .

4. The reconstitution instruction to mix a supply dosage of 1.5 g per 100 mL for intravenous use is _____ .

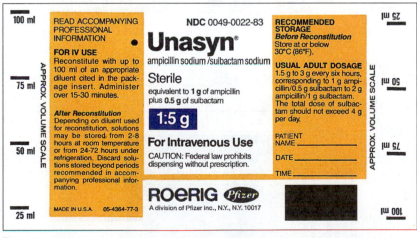

B

Label C:

5. The total volume of the medication container is _____ .

6. The supply dosage is _____ .

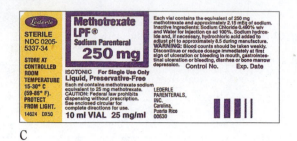

C

Label D:

7. The brand name of the drug is _____ .

8. The generic name is _____ .

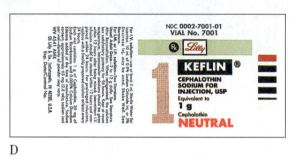

D

Label E:

9. The form of the drug is _____ .

10. The total volume of the medication container is _____ .

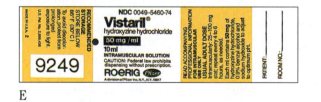

E

Label F:

11. The name of the drug manufacturer is _____ .

12. The form of the drug is _____ .

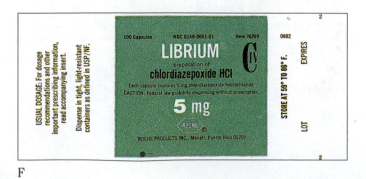

F

Label G:

13. The expiration date of the drug is _____ .

14. The dosage strength of the drug is _____ .

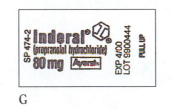

G

Match the label H or J with the correct descriptive statement. Indicate your answer by letter H or J.

15. This label represents a unit dose drug.   _____

16. This label represents a combination drug.   _____

17. This label represents a drug usually ordered by the number(s) of tablets
     or capsules to be administered rather than the dosage strength.   _____

H

J

18. The administration route for the drug labeled H is _____ .

19. The lot number for the drug labeled J is _____ .

20. The supply dosage of the drug labeled J is _____ .

After completing these problems, see page 321 to check your answers.

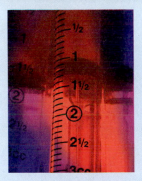

Oral Dosage of Drugs 7

objectives

Upon mastery of Chapter 7, you will be able to calculate the oral dosages of drugs.
To accomplish this you will also be able to:

- Convert all units of measurement to the same system and same size units.
- Estimate the reasonable amount of the drug to be administered.
- Set up and solve the dosage calculation ratio-proportion: ratio for the drug you have on hand equals the ratio for the desired drug.
- Calculate the number of tablets or capsules that are contained in prescribed dosages.
- Calculate the volume of liquid per dose when the prescribed dosage is in solution form.

Medications for oral administration are supplied in a variety of forms such as tablets, capsules, and liquids. Tablets, capsules, and liquids are usually ordered by mouth, or *p.o.* Many of these medications may also be ordered to be given via other routes such as nasogastric (NG) tube, nasojejunal (NJ) tube, or gastrostomy (GT) tube. A nasogastric tube is a tube placed from the nares to the stomach; a nasojejunal tube is placed from the nares to the jejunum; and a gastrostomy tube is placed directly into the stomach.

Tablets and Capsules

Medications prepared in tablet and capsule form come in the strengths or dosages in which they are commonly given (Figure 7–1). It is desirable to obtain the drug in the strength of the dosage ordered, or in multiples of that dosage. When necessary, *scored tablets* (those marked for division) can be divided in halves or quarters. Only scored tablets are intended to be divided.

When a choice is possible, the strength of the drug should be selected so that the fewest number of tablets, caplets, or capsules can be administered.

EXAMPLE: The doctor's order reads:

Tylenol (acetaminophen) 500 mg p.o. q.3-4h p.r.n. for mild pain

Tylenol comes in strengths of 325 milligrams per tablet or caplet and 500 milligrams per tablet, caplet, or gelcap. When both strengths are available, the nurse should select the 500 milligram strength and give one tablet for each dose.

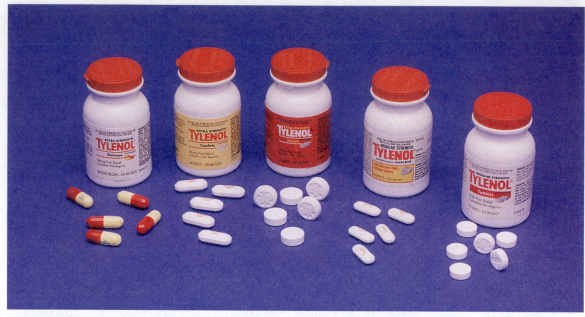

Fig. 7–1 Tablets, Caplets, and Gelcaps

> ▶ **_rule_** To calculate the correct dosage of the medication ordered, use the following three simple steps.
>
> Step 1. **Convert:** Be sure that all measures are in the same system, and all units are in the same size, converting when necessary.
>
> Step 2. **Think:** Carefully estimate what is a reasonable amount of the drug that should be administered.
>
> Step 3. **Calculate:** Compute the drug dosage using the ratio for the drug you have on hand as equivalent to the ratio for the desired drug.

Look at each of the three steps separately.

Step 1. Convert: Be sure that all measures are in the same system, and all units are in the same size, converting when necessary.

Step 1 means that medication orders written and supplied in the same system but in different size units will need to be converted to the *same size*. For instance, a drug ordered in grams but supplied in milligrams will need to be converted to the same size unit. In most cases, it is more practical to change to the smaller unit (g to mg) since this usually eliminates the decimal or fraction and keeps the calculation in whole numbers.

For example, 0.5 g = 500 mg (Equivalent: 1 g = 1000 mg).

$$\frac{1 \text{ g}}{1000 \text{ mg}} \underset{\longleftarrow}{\overset{\longleftarrow}{\bowtie}} \frac{0.5 \text{ g}}{X \text{ mg}} \qquad \text{(Cross-multiply and solve for X.)}$$

$X = 0.5 \times 1000$

$X = 0.500. = 500 \text{ mg}$

If the medication order is written in the apothecaries' system and the medication is supplied in the metric system, you must recall the approximate equivalents and convert both amounts to the *same system*.

The rule of thumb is to convert to the system of measure for the supply dosage you have available *on hand*. You will find that you will, in fact, convert apothecaries' or household systems to the metric system. This is true since the metric system is the predominant system of measure for drug preparations.

For example, the physician may order *phenobarbital gr $\frac{1}{4}$* p.o. and the drug you have available on hand is labeled *phenobarbital 15 mg per tablet*. To determine how many tablets to give the patient, you must first convert gr $\frac{1}{4}$ to the metric equivalent.

gr $\frac{1}{4}$ = 15 mg (Equivalent: gr i = 60 mg)

$$\frac{\text{gr i}}{60 \text{ mg}} \quad \rightleftharpoons \quad \frac{\text{gr } \frac{1}{4}}{X \text{ mg}} \qquad \text{(Cross-multiply and solve for X.)}$$

$$X = \frac{1}{4} \times 60$$

$$X = 15 \text{ mg}$$

Step 2. Think: Carefully consider what is the reasonable amount of the drug that should be administered.

Once you have converted all units to the same system and size, Step 2 asks you to logically conclude what amount should be given. Before you go on to Step 3, you should be able to picture in your mind the exact amount of medication to be administered. At least, you should be able to make a very close approximation, such as more or less than one tablet (capsule, milliliter, ounce). Basically, Step 2 says, "think."

In the preceding example, once you have completed the conversions, you can readily reason for the correct amount of tablets to administer. You would give one tablet of phenobarbital.

Step 3. Calculate: Use the ratio-proportion method to calculate the drug dosage.

In Step 3, you will double check your reasonable or estimated answer with the ratio-proportion method. You should always reason (Step 2) for the amount of medicine to administer to the patient before you apply the ratio-proportion method (Step 3).

> **rule**   Ratio for drug you have on hand equals ratio for the desired drug.

Recall that a proportion is a relationship comparing two ratios. When setting up the first ratio to calculate a drug dosage, use the supply dosage or drug concentration information available on the drug label. This is the dosage amount you *have on hand*. Set up the second ratio using the drug order or the *desired dosage* and the amount of volume you will give to the patient (this is the *unknown*, or *X*). Keep the *known* information on the left side of the proportion and the *unknown* on the right. Refer to Chapters 1 and 3 to review information about ratios and proportions, if needed.

remember

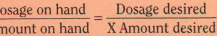

$$\frac{\text{Dosage on hand}}{\text{Amount on hand}} = \frac{\text{Dosage desired}}{X \text{ Amount desired}}$$

In the preceding example, the physician ordered phenobarbital gr $\frac{1}{4}$ (dosage desired) which you converted to 15 mg. You want to know how many tablets to give (*amount desired* or unknown X). The *drug on hand* is labeled 15 mg per each tablet ($\frac{15\ mg}{1\ tab}$). Although the math is obvious, let's apply ratio-proportion to prove your estimate is true. The *dosage desired* is calculated as follows:

$$\frac{15\ mg}{1\ tab} \diagup\!\!\!\!\diagdown \frac{15\ mg}{X\ tab} \qquad \text{(Cross-multiply and solve for X.)}$$

$$15X = 15$$

$$\frac{15\,X}{15} = \frac{15}{15}$$

$$X = 1 \text{ tablet}$$

Remember that proportions compare *like* things. Therefore, you must first convert all units to the same system and to the same size. As pointed out in Chapter 3, notice that the ratio must follow the same sequence. The proportion is set up so that like units are across from each other. The numerators of each ratio represent the *weight* of the drug, and the denominators represent the *amount*. It is important to keep like units in order: mg as the numerators (on top) and tablets or capsules as the denominators (on the bottom). Labeling units when you set up equations helps you to recognize if you have set up the equation in the proper sequence. If you are careful to use the full three-step method and think through or estimate for the logical dosage, you will also minimize the potential for error.

For another example, a medication order is for a *500 milligram dose of Amoxil*. You have *amoxicillin (Amoxil) on hand in 250 milligram capsules;* this means that there are 250 milligrams in each capsule. Use ratio-proportion to determine how many capsules should be administered.

$$\frac{\text{Dosage on hand}}{\text{Amount on hand}} = \frac{\text{Dosage desired}}{\text{X Amount desired}}$$

$$\frac{250\ mg}{1\ cap} \diagup\!\!\!\!\diagdown \frac{500\ mg}{X\ cap} \qquad \text{(Cross-multiply and solve for X.)}$$

$$250X = 500$$

$$\frac{250X}{250} = \frac{500}{250}$$

$$X = 2 \text{ capsules}$$

Steps 1, 2, and 3 can be used to solve all dosage calculation problems encountered. It is important that you develop the ability to reason for the answer logically as well as learn to use the ratio-proportion method.

Errors are often made unknowingly because nurses rely solely on a calculation method rather than asking themselves first what the answer should be. As a nurse you are expected to be able to reason sensibly, problem-solve, and justify your judgments rationally. Use ratio-proportion as a tool to validate the dosage you anticipate should be given. If your reasoning is sound, you will find the dosages you compute make sense and are accurate. For example, if your calculations result in directing you to administer 15 tablets of a medication, you would question this.

EXAMPLE 1:   The drug order is written: *Lopressor 100 mg p.o. b.i.d.* The medicine container is labeled: *Lopressor 50 mg per tablet*

Order: Lopressor 100 mg.
Supply: Lopressor 50 mg tablets

Step 1.   Convert: No conversion is necessary. The units are in the same system and the same size.

Step 2.　Think: You want to administer 100 milligrams, and you have tablets that are 50 milligrams each. You want to give twice the equivalent of each tablet, or you want to administer to the patient 2 tablets per dose.

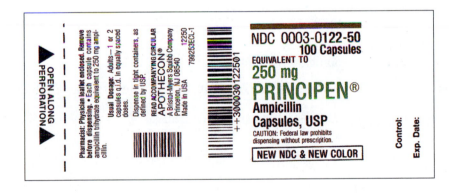

Step 3.　Calculate: $\dfrac{\text{Dosage on hand}}{\text{Amount on hand}} = \dfrac{\text{Dosage desired}}{\text{X Amount desired}}$

$\dfrac{50\text{ mg}}{1\text{ tab}} \diagdown\!\!\!\!\diagup \dfrac{100\text{ mg}}{\text{X tab}}$　　(Cross-multiply and solve for X.)

$50\text{X} = 100$

$\dfrac{50\text{X}}{50} = \dfrac{100}{50}$

X = 2 tablets orally twice daily

Double check to be sure your calculated dosage matches your *reasonable* dosage from Step 2. If for example, you had calculated to give more or less than 2 tablets of Lopressor, you would suspect a calculation error.

EXAMPLE 2:　The physician prescribes *Ampicillin 0.5 g p.o. q.i.d.* The dosage available is *Ampicillin 250 mg per capsule*. How many capsules should the nurse give to the patient per dose?

Step 1.　Convert: Order and supply dosage need to be expressed in the same size units. Cross out 0.5 g and write the equivalent in milligrams above it.

Order: Ampicillin $\overset{500\text{ mg}}{\cancel{0.5\text{ g}}}$　(Equivalent: 1 g = 1000 mg)

$\dfrac{1\text{ g}}{1000\text{ mg}} \diagdown\!\!\!\!\diagup \dfrac{0.5\text{ g}}{\text{X mg}}$　　(Cross-multiply and solve for X.)

$\text{X} = 0.5 \times 1000 = 0.500. = 500\text{ mg}$

Supply: Ampicillin 250 mg capsules

Step 2.　Think: 500 milligrams is twice as much as 250 milligrams. You want to give 2 capsules.

Step 3.   Calculate: $\dfrac{\text{Dosage on hand}}{\text{Amount on hand}} = \dfrac{\text{Dosage desired}}{\text{X Amount desired}}$

$\dfrac{250 \text{ mg}}{1 \text{ cap}} \diagdown\diagup \dfrac{500 \text{ mg}}{\text{X cap}}$ (Cross-multiply and solve for X.)

$250\text{X} = 500$

$\dfrac{250\text{X}}{250} = \dfrac{500}{250}$

X = 2 capsules orally four times daily.

EXAMPLE 3:   The doctor's order reads *Codeine sulfate gr $\frac{3}{4}$ p.o. q.4h p.r.n., pain*. The drug label states *Codeine sulfate 30 mg*.

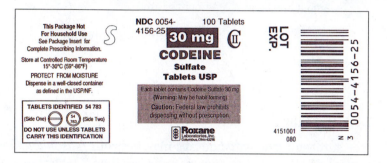

Step 1.   Convert: Order and supply dosage need to be expressed in equivalent units in the same system.

Order: Codeine $\diagdown\begin{smallmatrix}45 \text{ mg}\\ \text{gr } \frac{3}{4}\end{smallmatrix}$ (Equivalent: gr i = 60 mg)

$\dfrac{\text{gr i}}{60 \text{ mg}} \diagdown\diagup \dfrac{\text{gr } \frac{3}{4}}{\text{X mg}}$ (Cross-multiply and solve for X.)

$\text{X} = \dfrac{3}{4} \times 60$

X = 45 mg

Supply: Codeine 30 mg tablets

Step 2.   Think: You want to give more than 1 tablet and less than 2 tablets.

Step 3.   Calculate: $\dfrac{\text{Dosage on hand}}{\text{Amount on hand}} = \dfrac{\text{Dosage desired}}{\text{X Amount desired}}$

$\dfrac{30 \text{ mg}}{1 \text{ tab}} \diagdown\diagup \dfrac{45 \text{ mg}}{\text{X tab}}$ (Cross-multiply and solve for X.)

$30\text{X} = 45$

$\dfrac{30\text{X}}{30} = \dfrac{45}{30}$

$\text{X} = 1\frac{1}{2}$ tablets orally every four hours as needed for pain.

EXAMPLE 4:   *Halcion 0.25 mg tablets available.*

Give *125 mcg Halcion orally h.s.*

Step 1.   Convert: Order and supply dosage need to be expressed in the same size units.
Order: Halcion 125 mcg

Supply: Halcion $\diagdown\begin{smallmatrix}250 \text{ mcg}\\ 0.25 \text{ mg}\end{smallmatrix}$ (Equivalent: 1 mg = 1000 mcg)

$$\frac{1 \text{ mg}}{1000 \text{ mcg}} \bowtie \frac{0.25 \text{ mg}}{\text{X mcg}} \qquad \text{(Cross-multiply and solve for X.)}$$

$$X = 0.25 \times 1000 = 0.250. = 250 \text{ mcg}$$

Step 2.   Think: You want to give less than 1 tablet; in fact you want to give half of 250 mg or $\frac{1}{2}$ tablet.

Step 3.   Calculate: $\dfrac{\text{Dosage on hand}}{\text{Amount on hand}} = \dfrac{\text{Dosage desired}}{\text{X Amount desired}}$

$$\frac{250 \text{ mcg}}{1 \text{ tab}} \bowtie \frac{125 \text{ mcg}}{\text{X tab}} \qquad \text{(Cross-multiply and solve for X.)}$$

$$250X = 125$$

$$\frac{250 \text{ X}}{250} = \frac{125}{250}$$

$$X = \frac{1}{2} \text{ tablet orally at bedtime.}$$

EXAMPLE 5:   Your patient is to receive *Nitrostat gr* $\frac{1}{400}$ *p.r.n.* for angina pain by the sublingual route (under the tongue). The bottle is labeled *1 tablet = 0.3 mg* *(gr* $\frac{1}{200}$ *).*

Step 1.   Convert: The information is available on the label.

Order: Nitrostat $\overset{0.15\,mg}{(\,gr\frac{1}{400}}$ (Equivalent: gr i = 60 mg)

$$\frac{gr\ i}{60\ mg} \diagup\!\!\!\!\diagdown \frac{gr\frac{1}{400}}{X\ mg}$$ (Cross-multiply and solve for X.)

$$X = \frac{1}{400} \times \frac{60}{1}$$

$$X = \frac{60}{400} = \frac{3}{20} = 0.15\ mg$$

Supply: Nitrostat 0.3 mg tablets

Step 2.   Think: 0.3 is equivalent to 0.30 (zero added for comparison). 0.15 is $\frac{1}{2}$ of 0.30. You want to give the equivalent of $\frac{1}{2}$ tablet as needed.

Step 3.   Calculate: $\dfrac{\text{Dosage on hand}}{\text{Amount on hand}} = \dfrac{\text{Dosage desired}}{\text{X Amount desired}}$

$$\frac{0.3\ mg}{1\ tab} \diagup\!\!\!\!\diagdown \frac{0.15\ mg}{X\ tab}$$ (Cross-multiply and solve for X.)

$$0.3X = 0.15$$

$$\frac{0.3\ X}{0.3} = \frac{0.15}{0.30}$$ (Add the zero to compare decimal fractions.)

$$X = \frac{1}{2}\ \text{tablet sublingually as needed.}$$

The following summarizes the three steps to dosage calculation.

quick review

THREE STEPS TO DOSAGE CALCULATION

Step 1.   Convert: to units of the same system and same size.

Step 2.   Think: learn to reason for the logical answer.

Step 3.   Calculate: $\dfrac{\text{Dosage on hand}}{\text{Amount on hand}} = \dfrac{\text{Dosage desired}}{\text{X Amount desired}}$

■ For most problems, convert to:
1.   supply dosage you have on hand (gr → mg)
2.   smaller size unit (g → mg)

review set 21

Calculate the correct number of tablets or capsules to be administered per dose. Tablets are scored.

1. The physician writes an order for Diabinese 0.1 g p.o. q.d. The drug container label reads:
   Diabinese 100 mg tablets
   Give: _____

2. Duricef 500 mg tablets available. Give 0.5 g of Duricef p.o. b.i.d.
   Give: _____

3. Urecholine 10 mg tablets available. 15 mg of Urecholine p.o. t.i.d. is ordered.
   Give: _____

4. Hydrochlorothiazide 12.5 mg p.o. t.i.d. ordered; 25 mg tablets available.
   Give: _____

5. Order: Lanoxin 0.125 mg p.o. q.d.
   Supply: Lanoxin 0.25 mg tablets
   Give: _____

6. Order: Motrin 600 mg p.o. b.i.d.
   Supply: Motrin 300 mg tablets
   Give: _____

7. Order: Slow-K 16 mEq p.o. stat
   Supply: Slow-K 8 mEq tablets
   Give: _____

8. Cytoxan 25 mg tablets available. Give 50 mg of Cytoxan p.o. q.d.
   Give: _____

9. Zaroxolyn 5 mg tablets available. Give 7.5 mg of Zaroxolyn p.o. b.i.d.
   Give: _____

10. Amicar 500 mg tablets available. The doctor orders Amicar 4 g p.o. stat
    Give: _____

11. Drug "X" available in 0.5 g tablets. Dosage is 0.06 g per kg of body weight per day. If a person weighs 145 pounds, what is the total daily dosage? _____ What is the individual q.i.d. dose? _____ How many tablets are needed for each dose? _____

12. Order: Trandate 150 mg p.o. b.i.d.
    Supply: Trandate 300 mg tablets
    Give: _____

13. Order: Duricef 1 g p.o. q.i.d. a.c.
    Supply: Duricef 500 mg capsules
    Give: _____

14. Synthroid 50 mcg tablets available. Give 0.05 mg of Synthroid p.o. q.d.
    Give: _____

15. Tranxene 7.5 mg p.o. q.i.d. is ordered and you have 3.75 mg Tranxene capsules available.
    Give: _____

16. Order: Inderal 15 mg p.o. t.i.d.
    Supply: Inderal 10 mg tablets
    Give: _____

17. The doctor orders Loniten gr $\frac{1}{6}$ p.o. and you have available Loniten 10 mg and 2.5 mg scored tablets. Select _____ mg tablets and give _____ tablet(s).

18. Order: Peritrate gr ss p.o. 1 h a.c. et h.s. You have available Peritrate 10 mg, 20 mg, and 40 mg scored tablets. Select _____ mg tablets and give _____ tablet(s). How many doses of Peritrate will the patient receive in 24 hours?
    _____

19. Order: Phenobarbital gr $\frac{1}{4}$ p.o. q.d.
    Supply: Phenobarbital 15 mg, 30 mg, 60 mg scored tablets.
    Select _____ mg tablets and give _____ tablet(s).

20. Order: Tylenol with codeine gr i p.o. q.4h p.r.n. pain
    Supply: Tylenol with codeine 7.5 mg, 15 mg, 30 mg, and 60 mg tablets.
    Select _____ mg tablets and give _____ tablet(s). How often should the patient receive this medication?

Calculate one dose for each of the medication orders 21 through 30. The labels lettered A through K that follow on pages 111–114 are the drugs you have available. Indicate the letter corresponding to the label you select.

21. Order: Dilatrate-SR 80 mg p.o. b.i.d.
    Select: _____
    Give: _____

22. Order: Carbamazepine 0.2 g p.o. t.i.d.
    Select: _____
    Give: _____

23. Order: Lopressor 50 mg p.o. b.i.d.
    Select: _____
    Give: _____

24. Order: Potassium chloride 16 mEq p.o. q.d.
    Select: _____
    Give: _____

25. Order: Procan SR 1 g p.o. q.6h
    Select: _____
    Give: _____

26. Order: Cephalexin 0.5 g q.i.d.
    Select: _____
    Give: _____

27. Order: Danazol 0.4 g p.o. b.i.d.
    Select: _____
    Give: _____

28. Order: Digoxin 0.5 mg p.o. q.d.
    Select: _____
    Give: _____

29. Order: Meclofenamate sodium 0.1 g p.o. t.i.d.
    Select: _____
    Give: _____

30. Order: Procainamide hydrochloride 50 mg/kg of body weight p.o. q.d. given in equally divided doses q.6h. The patient weighs 176 lb.
    Select: _____
    Give: _____ for *each dose*

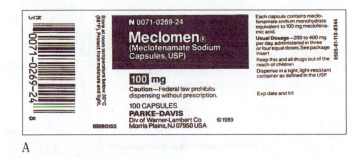

A

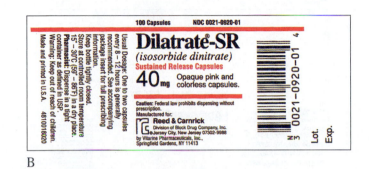

B

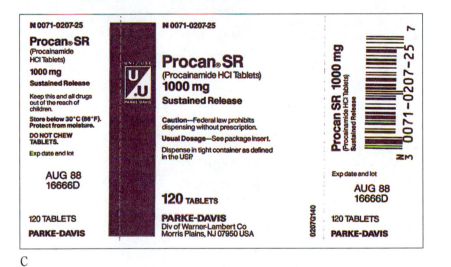

C

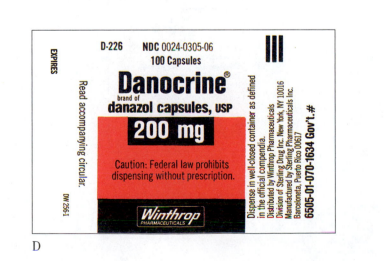

D

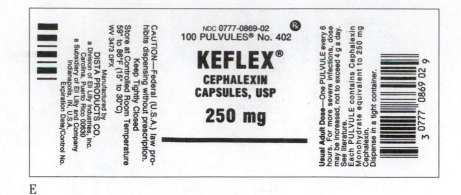

E

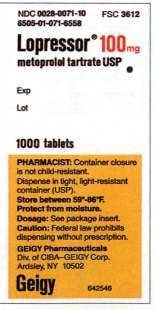

F

NDC 0028-0071-10   FSC 3612
6505-01-071-6558

Lopressor® 100mg
metoprolol tartrate USP •

Exp

Lot

1000 tablets

PHARMACIST: Container closure
is not child-resistant.
Dispense in tight, light-resistant
container (USP).
Store between 59°-86°F.
Protect from moisture.
Dosage: See package insert.
Caution: Federal law prohibits
dispensing without prescription.
GEIGY Pharmaceuticals
Div. of CIBA–GEIGY Corp.
Ardsley, NY 10502
Geigy   642546

G

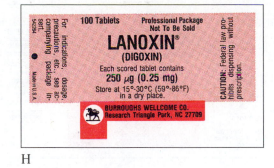

H

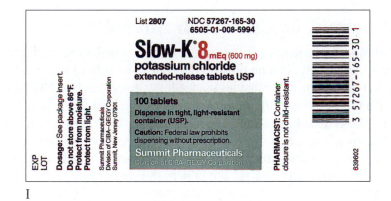

I

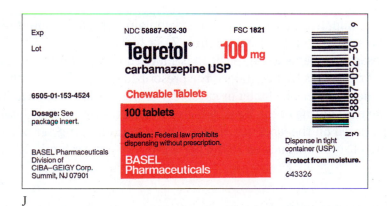

J

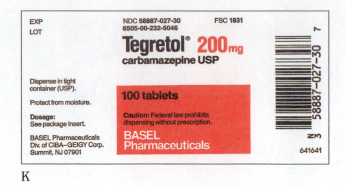

K

After completing these problems, see pages 296 and 297 to check your answers.

Tablets that Cannot Be Crushed or Altered

Children and many elderly patients may need to have a tablet crushed or capsule opened and prepared in a small volume of food or fluid in order to be able to swallow the medication. Also, in order to deliver tablets and capsules via feeding devices such as NG tube, NJ tube, or GT tube, crushing a tablet or opening a capsule is necessary. However, some tablets and capsules should not be crushed or contents opened because such action may interfere with the desired effect of the drug. For example, enteric-coated medications should not be crushed because their special coating prevents destruction by stomach acid, allowing the drug to be dissolved in the duodenum. Sustained-release tablets should not be crushed because the tablet is formulated for gradual release of the drug in the gastrointestinal tract. Crushing these tablets can cause improper release of the drug. Consult a drug reference book or a pharmacist if you are in doubt about the safety of crushing tablets or opening capsules. Figure 7–2 is a list of common tablets and capsules that cannot be crushed or altered.

Oral Liquids

Oral liquids are supplied in solution form and contain a specific amount of drug in a given amount of solution as stated on the label (Figures 7–3a and 7–3b).

In solving dosage problems when the drug is supplied in solid form, you calculated the number of tablets or capsules that contained the prescribed dosage. The supply container gave the amount of medication per one tablet or capsule. For medications supplied in solution form, you must calculate the volume of the liquid which contains the prescribed dosage of the drug. The supply dosage noted on the label may indicate the amount of drug per one milliliter or per multiple milliliters of solution, such as 10 mg per 2 mL, 125 mg per 5 mL, 1.2 g per 30 mL, and so forth.

EXAMPLE 1:   The doctor orders *Betapen-VK 100 mg p.o. q.i.d.* Look at the labels of Betapen-VK available in Figure 7–3(a)(b). You choose *Betapen-VK 125 mg per 5 mL*. Follow the 3 steps to dosage calculations.

Step 1.   Convert: No conversions necessary since the order and supply drug are both in the same units.

Step 2.   Think: You want to give less than 125 mg so you want to give less than 5 mL. Double-check your thinking with the ratio-proportion dosage calculation.

TABLE 1: CHECK OUT THIS LIST BEFORE ALTERING A DRUG.

A. Don't crush or alter these common sustained-release, enteric-coated, and sublingual tablets.

Afrinol Repetabs
Asbron G Inlay-Tabs
Avazyme
Azulfidine EN-tabs

Belladenal-S
Bellergal-S
bisacodyl
Bronkodyl S-R

Chlor-Trimeton
   Repetabs
Choledyl SA
Constant-T

Diamox Sequels
Dimetane Extentabs
Dimetapp Extentabs
Donnatal Extentabs
Donnazyme
Drixoral
Dulcolax

Easprin
Ecotrin
E-Mycin
Eskalith CR

Fero-Grad-500
Fero-Gradumet
Festal II

Hydergine (Sublingual)

Iberet Filmtabs
Iberet-500 Filmtabs

Ilotycin
Indocin SR
Isordil (Sublingual)
Isuprel Glossets

Kaon-Cl
Kaon-Cl-10
K-Dur
Klor-Con
Klotrix
K-Tab

Lithobid

Mestinon Timespan
Micro-K Extencaps
MS Contin

Nico-Span
Nitro-Bid
Nitrostat
Norflex

Pabalate
Pancrease
Peritrate SA
Permitil Chronotab
Phazyme-PB
Phyllocontin
Polaramine Repetab
Preludin Enduret
Procan SR
Pronestyl-SR

Quibron-T/SR
Quinaglute Dura-Tabs
Quinidex Extentabs

Ritalin SR
Roxanol SR

Slow-K

Sorbitrate SA
Sustaire

Tedral SA
Theo-Dur
Theolair-SR
Trilafon Repetabs

B. You can open these sustained-release capsules and carefully mix the contents in a liquid or with a soft food, such as applesauce. Vigorous mixing, however, could alter the rate of release.

Artane Sequels

Combid Spansules
Compazine Spansules

Dexedrine Spansules

Feosol Spansules

Inderal LA
Inderide LA
Isordil Tembids
(capsules)

Nicobid
Nitrostat SR

Ornade Spansules

Pavabid

Slo-bid Gyrocaps
Slo-Phyllin Gyrocaps
Sudafed SA

Temaril Spansules
Theobid
Theo-Dur Sprinkle
Thorazine Spansules
Tuss-Ornade Spansules

Valrelease

C. Because of the makeup of these miscellaneous drugs, you shouldn't crush or alter them.

• *Accutane* (liquid-filled capsule). Liquid can irritate mucous membrane.

• *Chymoral*. Crushing may interfere with enzymatic activity.

• *Depakene* (liquid-filled capsule). Liquid can irritate mucous membrane.

• *Feldene*. Powder from this capsule can irritate mucous membrane.

• *Klorvess* (effervescent tablet). If this tablet isn't dissolved before it's given, gastrointestinal upset will occur, and gastrointestinal damage may occur.

TABLE 2: WATCH FOR THESE NAMES AS A TIP-OFF.

A. These drug manufacturers' names indicate a sustained-release or an enteric-coated form of a drug.

BidCap
Cenule
Chronosule
Chronotab
D-Lay
Dospan

Duracap
Dura-tab
Enduret
Enseal
EN-tab
Extencap
Extentab
Gradumet
Granucap
Gyrocap
Kronocap
Lanacap

Lontab
Repetab
Sequel
Spansule
Tab-in
Tembid
Tempule
Tentab
TimeCap
Timecelle
Timespan

B. When attached to a drug name, these terms indicate a sustained-release form of a drug.

Bid
Dur
Plateau Cap
SA
Span
SR

Fig. 7–2 Tablets That Cannot Be Crushed or Altered *(Courtesy of Springhouse Corporation)*

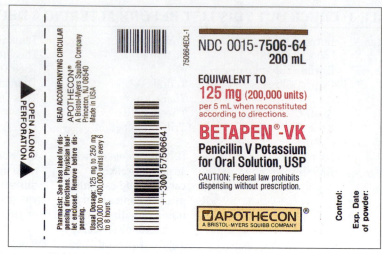

Fig. 7–3(a) Oral Liquid: Betapen-VK 125 mg per 5 mL

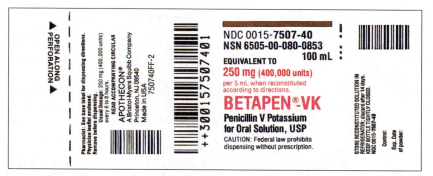

Fig. 7–3(b) Oral Liquid: Betapen-VK 250 mg per 5 mL

Step 3.   Calculate: $\dfrac{\text{Dosage on hand}}{\text{Amount on hand}} = \dfrac{\text{Dosage desired}}{\text{X Amount desired}}$

$\dfrac{125 \text{ mg}}{5 \text{ mL}} \diagdown\diagup \dfrac{100 \text{ mg}}{\text{X mL}}$ (Cross-multiply and solve for X.)

$125X = 500$

$\dfrac{125 \text{ X}}{125} = \dfrac{500}{125}$

$X = 4 \text{ mL}$

You will give 4 mL of the Betapen-VK with the dosage strength of 125 mg per 5 mL. Double check to be sure your calculated dosage matches your *reasonable* dosage from Step 2. If, for instance, you calculate to give more than 5 mL, then you know there must be an error.

remember

- It is important to use your power of reasoning before you apply any formula. In this way, if you make a careless error in math or if you set up the problem incorrectly, your thinking will alert you to try again.

EXAMPLE 2: The doctor orders *potassium chloride 40 mEq p.o.* The label on the package reads *potassium chloride oral solution 20 mEq per 15 mL.* How many mL should you administer?

Step 1. Convert: No conversion necessary.

Step 2. Think: You want to give more than 15 mL. In fact, you want to give exactly twice as much as 15 mL.

Step 3. Calculate: $\dfrac{\text{Dosage on hand}}{\text{Amount on hand}} = \dfrac{\text{Dosage desired}}{\text{X Amount desired}}$

$$\frac{20\ \text{mEq}}{15\ \text{mL}} \underset{\longleftarrow}{\overset{\longrightarrow}{\times}} \frac{40\ \text{mEq}}{\text{X mL}}$$

$$20X = 600$$

$$\frac{20X}{20} = \frac{600}{20}$$

$$X = 30\ \text{mL}$$

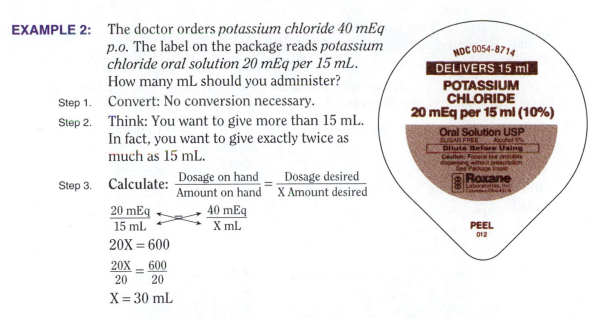

NDC 0054-8714
DELIVERS 15 ml
POTASSIUM
CHLORIDE
20 mEq per 15 ml (10%)
Oral Solution USP
SUGAR FREE   Alcohol 5%
Dilute Before Using
Caution: Federal law prohibits
dispensing without prescription.
See Package Insert
Roxane
Laboratories, Inc
Columbus, Ohio 43216

PEEL
012

quick review

Look again at Steps 1 through 3 as a valuable dosage calculation checklist.

- Step 1. Convert: Be sure that all measures are in the same system, and all units are in the same size.

- Step 2. Think: Carefully consider the reasonable amount of the drug that should be administered.

- Step 3. Calculate: $\dfrac{\text{Dosage on hand}}{\text{Amount on hand}} = \dfrac{\text{Dosage desired}}{\text{X Amount desired}}$

review set 22

Calculate one dose of the drugs ordered.

1. Order: Demerol syrup 75 mg p.o. q.4h p.r.n. pain
   Supply: Demerol syrup 50 mg per 5 mL

   Give: _____ mL

2. Order: Phenergan c̄ codeine gr $\frac{1}{6}$ p.o. q.4–6h p.r.n. cough
   Supply: Phenergan c̄ codeine solution 10 mg per 5 mL

   Give: _____ mL

3. Order: Pen-Vee K 1 g p.o. 1h pre-op dental surgery
   Supply: Pen-Vee K oral suspension 250 mg (400,000 U) per 5 mL

   Give: _____ mL

4. Order: Amoxicillin 100 mg p.o. q.i.d.
   Supply: 80 mL bottle of Amoxil (amoxicillin) oral pediatric suspension 125 mg per 5 mL

   Give: _____ mL

5. Order: Tylenol 0.5 g p.o. q.4h p.r.n. pain
   Supply: Tylenol (acetaminophen) liquid 500 mg in 5 mL

   Give: _____ t

6. Order: Promethazine HCl 25 mg p.o. h.s. pre-op
   Supply: Phenergan Plain (promethazine HCl) 6.25 mg per teaspoon

   Give: _____ mL

7. Order: Pathocil 125 mg p.o. q.6h a.c.
    Supply: Pathocil oral suspension 62.5 mg per 5 mL
    Give: _____ t

Use the labels A, B, and C to calculate one dose of the following orders (8, 9, and 10). Indicate the letter corresponding to the label you select.

8. Order: Erythromycin 125 mg p.o. t.i.d.
    Select: _____
    Give: _____

9. Order: Keflex 50 mg p.o. q.6h
    Select: _____
    Give: _____

10. Order: Vistaril 10 mg p.o. q.i.d.
    Select: _____
    Give: _____

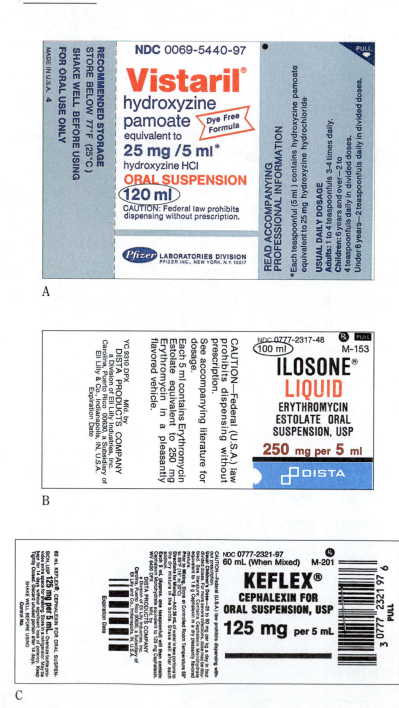

A

B

C

Calculate the information requested based on the drugs ordered. The labels provided are the drugs available.

11.   Order: Lanoxin elixir 0.25 mg p.o. q.d.
Give: _____ mL

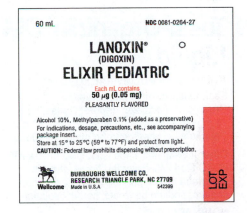

12.   Order: Lactulose 20 g via gastric tube b.i.d. today
Give: _____ mL

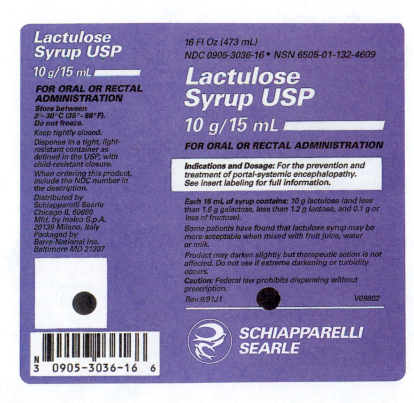

13. Order: Tussi-Organidin DM 10 mL p.o. q. 4h p.r.n. cough
    How many full doses are available in this bottle? _____

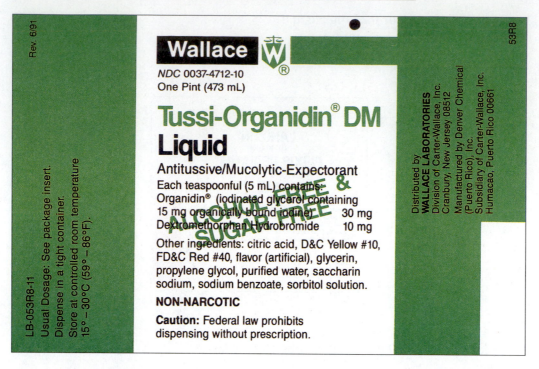

Rev. 6/91

53R8

Wallace Ⓦ

NDC 0037-4712-10
One Pint (473 mL)

Tussi-Organidin® DM
Liquid

Antitussive/Mucolytic-Expectorant

Each teaspoonful (5 mL) contains:
Organidin® (iodinated glycerol containing
15 mg organically bound iodine)   30 mg
Dextromethorphan Hydrobromide   10 mg

Other ingredients: citric acid, D&C Yellow #10,
FD&C Red #40, flavor (artificial), glycerin,
propylene glycol, purified water, saccharin
sodium, sodium benzoate, sorbitol solution.

NON-NARCOTIC

Caution: Federal law prohibits
dispensing without prescription.

LB-053R8-11
Usual Dosage: See package insert.
Dispense in a tight container.
Store at controlled room temperature
15° – 30°C (59° – 86°F).

Distributed by
WALLACE LABORATORIES
Division of Carter-Wallace, Inc.
Cranbury, New Jersey 08512
Manufactured by Denver Chemical
(Puerto Rico), Inc.
Subsidiary of Carter-Wallace, Inc.
Humacao, Puerto Rico 00661

ALCOHOL-FREE &
SUGAR-FREE

14. Order: Lomotil 2.5 mg p.r.n. q. 8h
    Give: _____

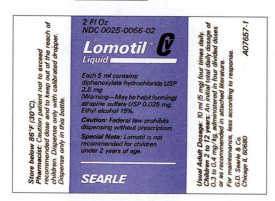

2 Fl Oz
NDC 0025-0066-02

Lomotil® Ⓒ
Liquid

A07657-1

Each 5 ml contains:
diphenoxylate hydrochloride USP
2.5 mg
(Warning—May be habit forming)
atropine sulfate USP 0.025 mg.
Ethyl alcohol 15%.

Caution: Federal law prohibits
dispensing without prescription.

Special Note: Lomotil is not
recommended for children
under 2 years of age.

SEARLE

Store below 86°F (30°C).
Pharmacist: Caution patient not to exceed
recommended dose and to keep out of the reach of
children. Dispense only with calibrated dropper.
Dispense only in this bottle.

Usual Adult Dosage: 10 ml (5 mg) four times daily.
Children 2 to 12 years: An initial total daily dosage of
0.3 to 0.4 mg/kg. administered in four divided doses
or as recommended in attached literature.
For maintenance, less according to response.
G.D. Searle & Co.
Chicago IL 60680

15. Order: Maalox Plus 30 mL 30 min. p.c. and h.s.
    How many containers will be needed for a 24-hour
    period? _____ containers. Meals
    are served at 8 AM, 12 noon, and 6 PM. Using
    24-hour time what are the administration
    times for the p.c. dosages? _____

    HINT: Medication is administered 30 min
    after the meal is completed. Allow 30 min
    for each meal to be eaten.

1 FL OZ (30 mL)

UNIT DOSE NDC 0067-0332-22

**Maalox®
Plus** ALUMINA,
MAGNESIA
AND
SIMETHICONE
ORAL SUSPENSION/ROFER

FOR INSTITUTIONAL USE ONLY
Store at room temperature.
Use as directed by physician.

Lot

SPECIMEN

RORER CONSUMER PHARMACEUTICALS
Fort Washington, PA. U.S.A. 19034

SHAKE WELL
Peel Back

After completing these problems, see page 298 to check
your answers.

You may recall from Chapter 5, "Interpreting Drug Orders," that you were shown how to read a physician's order sheet and how to complete the time schedule for recording on the medication administration record (MAR). For instance, a medication ordered b.i.d. (twice a day) might be timed on the medication administration record as 0800 or 8 AM and 2000 or 8 PM. It is important for you to understand that some oral medications cannot be given at the same time because they may inactivate each other. Also, some medications are to be given on an empty stomach, whereas others should be given with meals. In addition to calculating and administering the correct dosage of medications, the nurse is responsible for knowing the actions (both the desired and adverse effects) of drugs administered. Consulting a drug reference will ensure that you know whether medications have special timing requirements to achieve the desired effect.

critical thinking skills

Inaccuracy in dosage calculation is often attributed to errors in setting up ratio-proportion problems. Often, by first asking the question, "What is the reasonable dose?" many medication errors can be avoided.

■ error 1

Incorrect calculation and not assessing the reasonableness of the calculation before administering the medication.

possible scenario

The physician ordered phenobarbital 60 mg p.o. b.i.d. for a patient with seizures. The pharmacy supplied phenobarbital 30 mg per tablet. The nurse did not use Step 2 to think about the reasonable dosage and calculated the dosage this way:

Calculate: $\dfrac{\text{Dosage on hand}}{\text{Amount on hand}} = \dfrac{\text{Dosage desired}}{\text{X Amount desired}}$

$$\dfrac{30 \text{ mg}}{1 \text{ tab}} \underset{\longrightarrow}{\overset{\longrightarrow}{\times}} \dfrac{60 \text{ mg}}{\text{X tab}}$$

$$30X = 60 \text{ mg}$$

$$\dfrac{30\,X}{30} = \dfrac{60}{30}$$

$$X = 20 \text{ tablets}$$

Suppose the nurse then gave the patient 20 tablets of the 30 mg per tablet phenobarbital. The patient would have received 600 mg of phenobarbital, or 10 times the correct dosage.

potential outcome

The patient would likely develop signs of phenobarbital toxicity such as nystagmus (rapid eye movement), ataxia (lack of coordination), central nervous system depression, respiratory depression, hypothermia, and hypotension. When the error was caught and the physician notified, the patient would likely be given doses of charcoal to hasten elimination of the drug. Depending on the severity of the symptoms, the patient would likely be moved to the intensive care unit for monitoring of respiratory and neurological status.

prevention

This medication error could have been prevented if the nurse used the three-step method and thought about the reasonable dosage of the drug to give. The order is for 60 mg of phenobarbital and the available drug has 30 mg per tablet, so the nurse should give 2 tablets. A dose of 20 tablets should automatically be questioned. Ratio-proportion should be used to verify thinking about the *reasonable* dosage. Learn to trust your thinking. The correct dosage calculation is:

$$\frac{30 \text{ mg}}{1 \text{ tab}} \overset{\longrightarrow}{\underset{\longrightarrow}{\times}} \frac{60 \text{ mg}}{X \text{ tab}}$$

$$30X = 60$$

$$\frac{30 X}{30} = \frac{60}{30}$$

X = 2 tablets, not 20 tablets

It is the nurse's responsibility to know the desired action of medications and to time their administration to achieve the desired effect.

■ error 2

Administration of oral medications that inactivate each other when given at the same time.

possible scenario

Suppose the physician ordered Zantac (anti-ulcer medication) 150 mg p.o. b.i.d. and Maalox (antacid) 30 cc q.i.d. for a patient with a duodenal ulcer. The orders were transferred to the medication administration record like this:

	Time Schedule			
Zantac 150 mg p.o. b.i.d.	8 AM			8 PM
Maalox 30 mL p.o. q.i.d.	8 AM	12 PM	4 PM	8 PM

You will notice that the Zantac was scheduled to be given at 8 AM and 8 PM and that the patient also was to receive Maalox at these same times. However, if you look up Zantac in a drug reference guide you will note that antacids decrease the action of Zantac, and the two should not be given at the same time. The drug reference suggests that the Zantac be given with meals, and the antacid should be given 1 hour before or 1 hour after the Zantac. Suppose at this hospital meals were served at 9 AM, 1 PM, and 5 PM. A better schedule for these medications would have been:

	Time Schedule			
Zantac 150 mg p.o. b.i.d.	9 AM		5 PM	
Maalox 30 mL p.o. q.i.d.		10 AM 2 PM	6 PM	10 PM

potential outcome

When a medication that interferes with the action of another medication is scheduled to be given at the same time, a delay in drug action may delay healing of the patient's ulcer. This may also result in a longer hospital stay.

prevention

This medication error could be prevented by knowing the action of the medications you are giving and timing them appropriately. You cannot assume that just because two medications are ordered, you can always follow the routine administration schedules the hospital has set. When in doubt about the desired effect and interfering actions of medications, consult your drug reference or pharmacist.

Summary

Let's consider where you are in mastering the skill of dosage calculations. You have learned to convert equivalent units within systems of measurements and from one system to another. You have also applied this conversion skill to the calculation of oral dosages—both solid and liquid forms. By now, you know that solving dosage problems requires that all units first be expressed in the same system and same size.

Basically, two methods of calculating dosages have been presented. The first method requires you to think through the dosage ordered and dosage supplied to estimate the amount to be given to the patient. *To minimize medication errors, it is essential that you consider the reasonableness of the amount first, rather than rely solely on calculation methods.*

Second, you have learned the dosage calculation ratio-proportion method: ratio for known equivalent equals ratio for unknown equivalent.

Try the practice problems for Chapter 7. If you are having difficulty, get help from an instructor before proceeding to Chapter 8. Continue to concentrate on accuracy. Keep in mind that one error can be a serious mistake when you are calculating the dosages of medicines.

practice problems—chapter 7

Calculate one dose of the following drug orders. The tablets are scored in half.

1. Order: Orinase 250 mg p.o. b.i.d.
   Supply: Orinase 0.5 g tablets
   Give: _____

2. Order: Codeine gr ss p.o. q.4h p.r.n., pain
   Supply: Codeine 15 mg tablets
   Give: _____

3. Order: Levothyroxine sodium 0.075 mg
   Supply: Synthroid (levothyroxine sodium) 150 mcg tablets
   Give: _____

4. Order: Phenobarbital gr $\frac{1}{6}$ p.o. t.i.d.
   Supply: Phenobarbital elixir 20 mg/5 mL
   Give: _____

5. Order: Keflex 500 mg suspension p.o. q.i.d.
   Supply: Keflex, reconstituted with 62 mL H_2O, 5 mL = 250 mg
   Give: _____

6. Order: Inderal 20 mg p.o. q.i.d.
   Supply: Inderal 10 mg tablets
   Give: _____

7. Order: Amoxil suspension 500 mg p.o. q.6h
   Supply: Amoxil (amoxicillin) 250 mg = 5 mL
   Give: _____

8. Order: Diabenese 150 mg p.o. b.i.d.
   Supply: Diabenese 0.1 g tablets
   Give: _____

9. Order: Phenobarbital gr $\frac{3}{4}$ p.o. q.i.d.
   Supply: Phenobarbital 30 mg tablets
   Give: _____

10. Order: Codeine gr $\frac{1}{4}$ p.o. q.d.
    Supply: Codeine 30 mg tablets
    Give: _____

11. Order: Inderal 30 mg p.o. q.i.d. p.c.
    Supply: Inderal 20 mg tablets
    Give: _____

12. Order: Synthroid 300 mcg p.o. q.d.
    Supply: Synthroid 0.3 mg tablets
    Give: _____

13. Order: Lasix 60 mg p.o. q.d.
    Supply: Lasix 40 mg tablets
    Give: _____

14. Order: Tylenol with codeine gr $\frac{1}{8}$ p.o. q.d.
    Supply: Tylenol with 7.5 mg codeine tablets
    Give: _____

15. Order: Penicillin G 400,000 U p.o. q.i.d.
    Supply: Pentids (Penicillin G) 250 mg = 400,000 U tablets
    Give: _____

16. Order: Vasotec 7.5 mg p.o. q.d.
    Supply: Vasotec 5 mg and 10 mg tablets
    Select: _____ mg tablets
    and give _____ tablet(s)

17. Order: V-Cillin K 300,000 U p.o. q.i.d.
    Supply: V-Cillin K 200,000 U = 5 mL
    Give: _____

18. Order: Neomycin 0.75 g p.o. b.i.d.
    Supply: Neomycin 500 mg tablets
    Give: _____

19. Order: Halcion 0.25 mg p.o. h.s.
     Supply: Halcion 0.125 mg tablets
     Give: _____

20. Order: Dilantin gr i p.o. t.i.d.
     Supply: Dilantin 30 mg capsules
     Give: _____ capsule(s)

21. Order: Decadron 750 mcg p.o. b.i.d.
     Supply: Decadron 0.75 mg and 1.5 mg
         tablets
     Select: _____ mg tablets
     and give _____ tablet(s)

22. Order: Edecrin 12.5 mg p.o. b.i.d.
     Supply: Edecrin 25 mg tablets
     Give: _____

23. Order: Urecholine 50 mg p.o. t.i.d.
     Supply: Urecholine 25 mg tablets
     Give: _____

24. Order: Robaxin 1.5 g p.o. stat
     Supply: Robaxin 750 mg tablets
     Give: _____

25. Order: Robaxin 1 g p.o. q.i.d.
     Supply: Robaxin 500 mg tablets
     Give: _____

See the three medication administration records (MARs) and accompanying labels on the following pages for problems 26 through 40.

Calculate one dose of each of the drugs prescribed. The labels provided are the drugs you have available. Indicate the letter corresponding to the label you select. Record your answers.

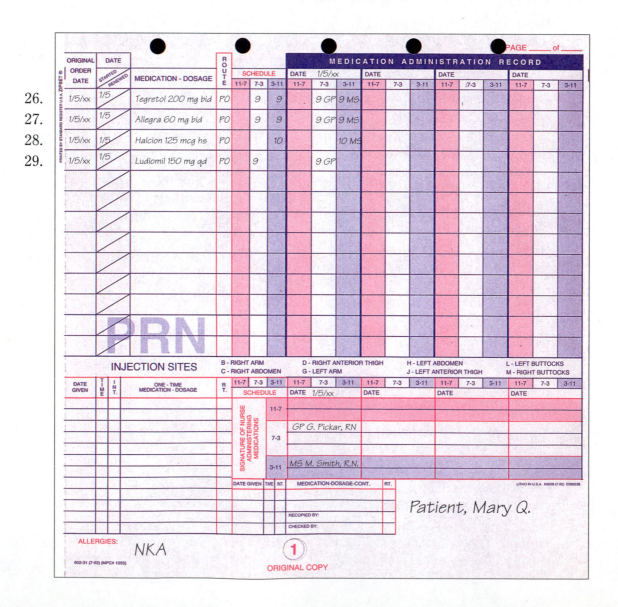

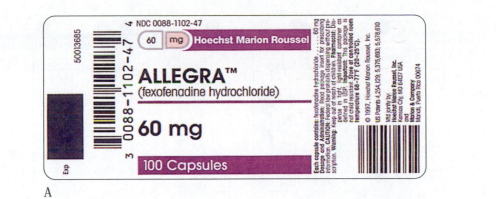

A

26. Select: _____
    Give: _____

27. Select: _____
    Give: _____

28. Select: _____
    Give: _____

29. Select: _____
    Give: _____

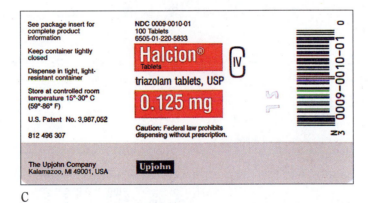

B

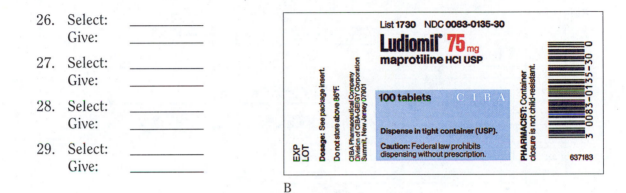

C

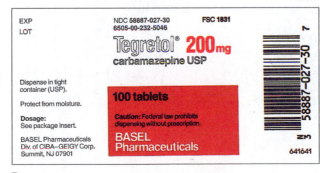

D

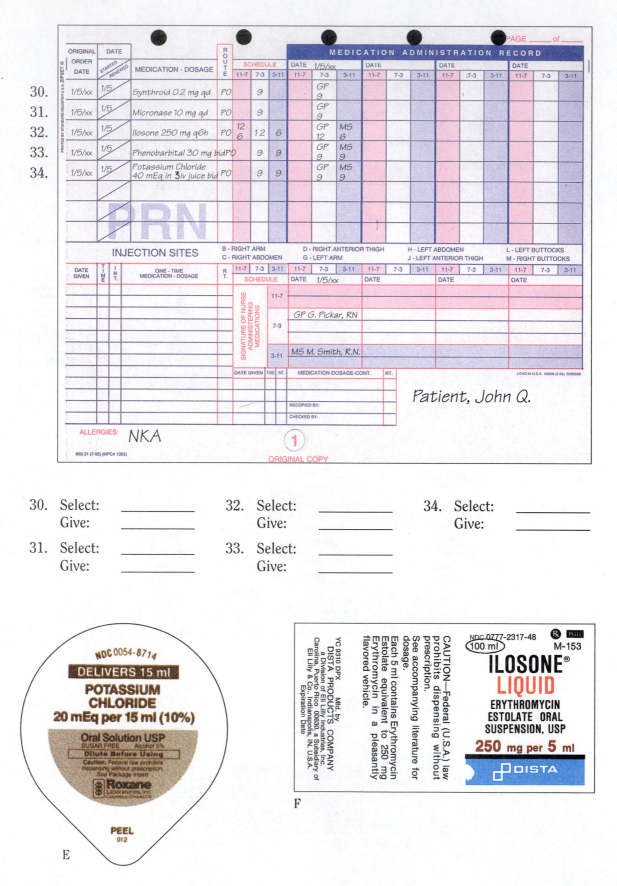

30. Select: _____   32. Select: _____   34. Select: _____
    Give: _____   Give: _____   Give: _____

31. Select: _____   33. Select: _____
    Give: _____   Give: _____

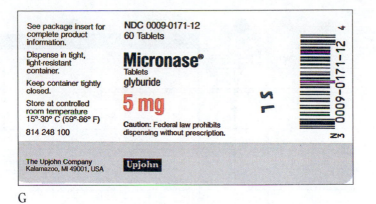

See package insert for
complete product
information.

Dispense in tight,
light-resistant
container.

Keep container tightly
closed.

Store at controlled
room temperature
15°-30° C (59°-86° F)

814 248 100

NDC 0009-0171-12
60 Tablets

Micronase®
Tablets
glyburide

5 mg

Caution: Federal law prohibits
dispensing without prescription.

The Upjohn Company
Kalamazoo, MI 49001, USA

Upjohn

G

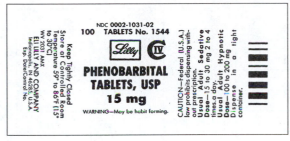

Keep Tightly Closed
Store at Controlled Room
Temperature 59° to 86°F (15°
to 30°C)
WV 2031 AMX
ELI LILLY AND COMPANY
Indianapolis, IN 46285, U.S.A.
Exp. Date/Control No.

NDC 0002-1031-02
100 TABLETS No. 1544

Lilly **C IV**

**PHENOBARBITAL
TABLETS, USP**

15 mg

WARNING—May be habit forming.

CAUTION—Federal (U.S.A.)
law prohibits dispensing with-
out prescription.
Usual Adult Sedative
Dose—15 to 30 mg 2 to 4
times a day.
Usual Adult Hypnotic
Dose—100 to 200 mg
Dispense in a tight
container.

H

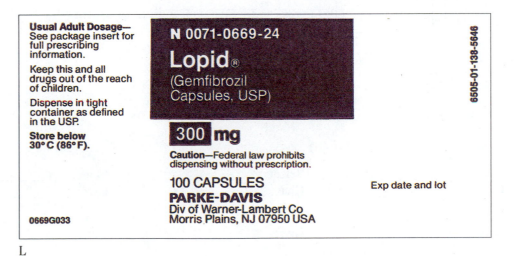

NDC 0048-1070-03
NSN 6505-01-145-8137
Code 3P1073

SYNTHROID®
(Levothyroxine Sodium
Tablets, USP)

100 mcg   (0.1 mg)

100 TABLETS

CAUTION: Federal (USA) law
prohibits dispensing without
prescription.

See full prescribing
information for dosage
and administration.

Dispense in a tight,
light-resistant container
as described in USP.

Store at controlled
room temperature.
15°-30°C (59°-86°F).

Boots
Pharmaceuticals, Inc.
Lincolnshire, IL 60069
USA

7885-01

J

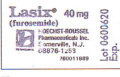

Lasix® 40 mg
(furosemide)
HOECHST-ROUSSEL
Pharmaceuticals Inc.
Somerville, N.J.
08876-1258
760011889

Lot 0600620
Exp.

K

Usual Adult Dosage—
See package insert for
full prescribing
information.

Keep this and all
drugs out of the reach
of children.

Dispense in tight
container as defined
in the USP.

Store below
30° C (86° F).

N 0071-0669-24

Lopid®
(Gemfibrozil
Capsules, USP)

300 mg

Caution—Federal law prohibits
dispensing without prescription.

100 CAPSULES

PARKE-DAVIS
Div of Warner-Lambert Co
Morris Plains, NJ 07950 USA

6505-01-138-5646

Exp date and lot

0669G033

L

ORIGINAL ORDER DATE	DATE STARTED / RENEWED	MEDICATION - DOSAGE	ROUTE	SCHEDULE 11-7 / 7-3 / 3-11			DATE 1/5/xx 11-7 / 7-3 / 3-11			DATE 11-7 / 7-3 / 3-11			DATE 11-7 / 7-3 / 3-11			DATE 11-7 / 7-3 / 3-11		
35. 1/5/xx	1/5	Nitroglycerin 5 mg q8h	PO	6	2	10		2 GP	10 MS									
36. 1/5/xx	1/5	Potassium Chloride gr x tid	PO		8 2	8		8 GP 2 GP	8 MS									
37. 1/5/xx	1/5	Lopid 0.6g bid ac	PO		7³⁰	4³⁰		7⁰⁰ GP	4⁰⁰ MS									
38. 1/5/xx	1/5	Furosemide 40 mg qd	PO		9			9 GP										
39. 1/5/xx	1/5	Lopressor 100 mg bid	PO		9	9		9 GP	9 MS									
PRN **40.** 1/5/xx	1/5	Darvocet-N 100 1 tab q4h prn headache	PO					7³⁰ GP 11³⁰ GP										

INJECTION SITES

B - RIGHT ARM	D - RIGHT ANTERIOR THIGH	H - LEFT ABDOMEN	L - LEFT BUTTOCKS
C - RIGHT ABDOMEN	G - LEFT ARM	J - LEFT ANTERIOR THIGH	M - RIGHT BUTTOCKS

DATE GIVEN	TIME	INT.	ONE - TIME MEDICATION - DOSAGE	R.T.	SCHEDULE 11-7 / 7-3 / 3-11			DATE 1/5/xx 11-7 / 7-3 / 3-11			DATE 11-7 / 7-3 / 3-11			DATE 11-7 / 7-3 / 3-11		

SIGNATURE OF NURSE ADMINISTERING MEDICATIONS

11-7	
7-3	GP G. Pickar RN
3-11	MS M. Smith, R.N

DATE GIVEN	TIME	INT.	MEDICATION-DOSAGE-CONT.	RT.

RECOPIED BY:

CHECKED BY:

Doe, Jane Q.

LITHO IN U.S.A. K6508 (7-92) D395538

ALLERGIES: NKA

602-31 (7-92) (MPC# 1355)

① ORIGINAL COPY

MEDICATION ADMINISTRATION RECORD   PAGE ____ of ____

---

35. Select: _____   37. Select: _____   39. Select: _____
    Give: _____   Give: _____   Give: _____

36. Select: _____   38. Select: _____   40. Select: _____
    Give: _____   Give: _____   Give: _____

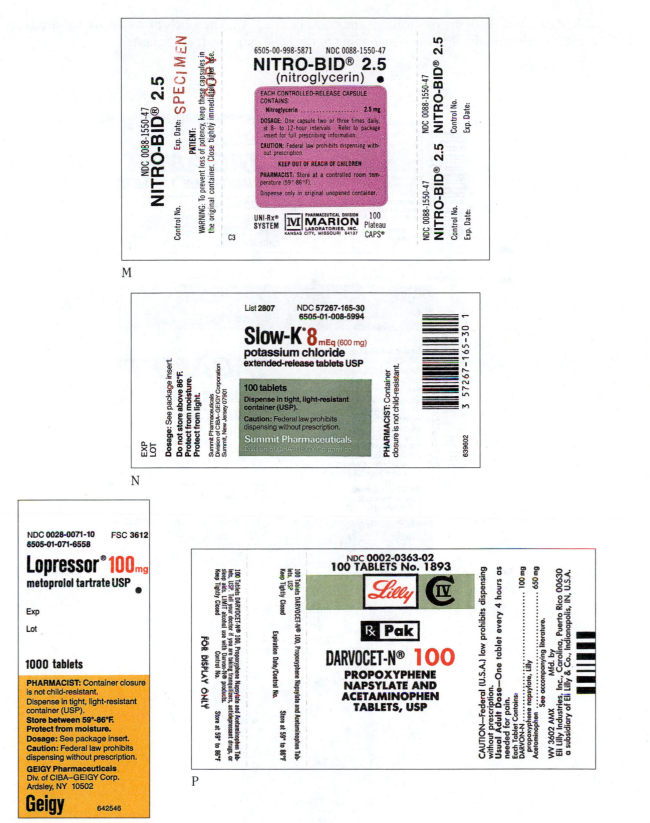

M

NDC 0088-1550-47

NITRO-BID® 2.5

Control No.

Exp. Date: SPECIMEN

PATIENT:

WARNING: To prevent loss of potency, keep these capsules in the original container. Close tightly immediately after use.

C3

6505-00-998-5871   NDC 0088-1550-47

NITRO-BID® 2.5
(nitroglycerin)

EACH CONTROLLED-RELEASE CAPSULE CONTAINS:

Nitroglycerin .... 2.5 mg

DOSAGE: One capsule two or three times daily, at 8- to 12-hour intervals. Refer to package insert for full prescribing information.

CAUTION: Federal law prohibits dispensing without prescription.

KEEP OUT OF REACH OF CHILDREN

PHARMACIST: Store at a controlled room temperature (59°-86°F).

Dispense only in original unopened container.

UNI-Rx® SYSTEM

M MARION PHARMACEUTICAL DIVISION LABORATORIES, INC.
KANSAS CITY, MISSOURI 64137

100 Plateau CAPS®

NDC 0088-1550-47

NITRO-BID® 2.5

Control No.

Exp. Date:

NDC 0088-1550-47

NITRO-BID® 2.5

Control No.

Exp. Date:

N

List 2807   NDC 57267-165-30
6505-01-008-5994

Slow-K® 8 mEq (600 mg)

potassium chloride
extended-release tablets USP

100 tablets

Dispense in tight, light-resistant container (USP).

Caution: Federal law prohibits dispensing without prescription.

Summit Pharmaceuticals
Division of CIBA-GEIGY Corporation

EXP
LOT

Dosage: See package insert.
Do not store above 86°F.
Protect from moisture.
Protect from light.

Summit Pharmaceuticals
Division of CIBA-GEIGY Corporation
Summit, New Jersey 07901

PHARMACIST: Container closure is not child-resistant.

3 57267-165-30 1

639602

O

NDC 0028-0071-10   FSC 3612
6505-01-071-6558

Lopressor® 100 mg

metoprolol tartrate USP

Exp

Lot

1000 tablets

PHARMACIST: Container closure is not child-resistant.
Dispense in tight, light-resistant container (USP).
Store between 59°-86°F.
Protect from moisture.
Dosage: See package insert.
Caution: Federal law prohibits dispensing without prescription.
GEIGY Pharmaceuticals
Div. of CIBA-GEIGY Corp.
Ardsley, NY 10502

Geigy   642546

P

FOR DISPLAY ONLY

100 Tablets DARVOCET-N® 100, Propoxyphene Napsylate and Acetaminophen Tablets, USP. Tell your doctor if you are taking tranquilizers, antidepressant drugs, or sleep aids. LIMIT alcohol use with Darvon-N products.
Keep Tightly Closed

Control No.   Store at 59° to 86°F

100 Tablets DARVOCET-N® 100, Propoxyphene Napsylate and Acetaminophen Tablets USP.
Keep Tightly Closed

Expiration Date/Control No.   Store at 59° to 86°F

NDC 0002-0363-02
100 TABLETS No. 1893

Lilly C IV

Rx Pak

DARVOCET-N® 100
PROPOXYPHENE NAPSYLATE AND ACETAMINOPHEN TABLETS, USP

CAUTION—Federal (U.S.A.) law prohibits dispensing without prescription.
Usual Adult Dose—One tablet every 4 hours as needed for pain.
Each Tablet Contains:
DARVON-N
propoxyphene napsylate, Lilly .... 100 mg
Acetaminophen .... 650 mg
See accompanying literature.

WV 3602 AMX   Mfd. by
Eli Lilly Industries, Inc., Carolina, Puerto Rico 00630
a subsidiary of Eli Lilly & Co., Indianapolis, IN, U.S.A.

Calculate one dose of the medications indicated on the MAR. The labels provided are the drugs available. Indicate the letter corresponding to the label you select, as requested.

41. Select: _____
     Give: _____

42. Give: _____

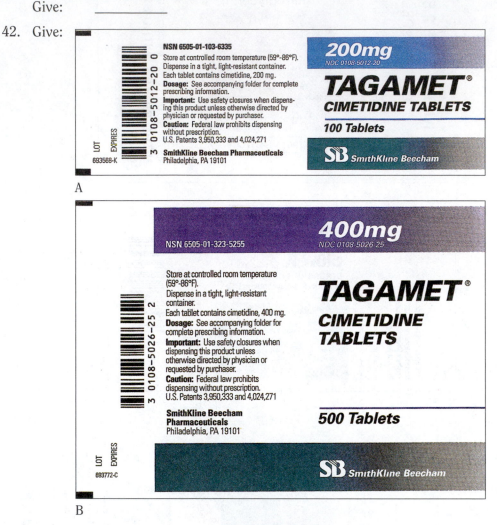

A

B

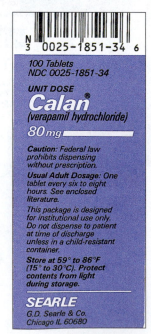

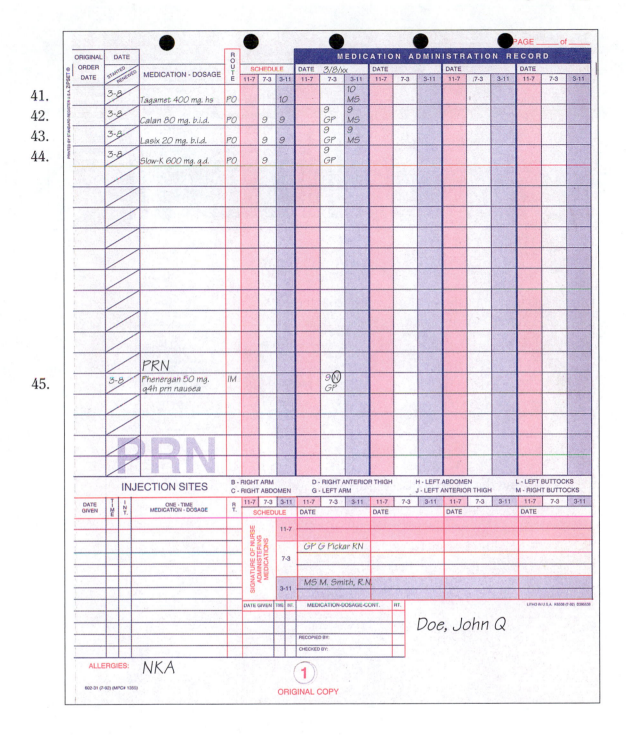

ORIGINAL ORDER DATE	DATE STARTED / RENEWED	MEDICATION - DOSAGE	ROUTE	SCHEDULE 11-7	7-3	3-11	DATE 3/8/xx 11-7	7-3	3-11	DATE 11-7	7-3	3-11	DATE 11-7	7-3	3-11	DATE 11-7	7-3	3-11
41.	3-8	Tagamet 400 mg. hs	PO			10			10 MS									
42.	3-8	Calan 80 mg. b.i.d.	PO		9	9		9 GP	9 MS									
43.	3-8	Lasix 20 mg. b.i.d.	PO		9	9		9 GP	9 MS									
44.	3-8	Slow-K 600 mg. q.d.	PO		9			9 GP										
		PRN																
45.	3-8	Phenergan 50 mg. q4h prn nausea	IM					9 N GP										

PRN

INJECTION SITES		B - RIGHT ARM	D - RIGHT ANTERIOR THIGH	H - LEFT ABDOMEN	L - LEFT BUTTOCKS
		C - RIGHT ABDOMEN	G - LEFT ARM	J - LEFT ANTERIOR THIGH	M - RIGHT BUTTOCKS

DATE GIVEN	TIME	INT.	ONE - TIME MEDICATION - DOSAGE	RT.	SCHEDULE	11-7	7-3	3-11	11-7	7-3	3-11	11-7	7-3	3-11	11-7	7-3	3-11
						DATE			DATE			DATE			DATE		
					11-7												
					7-3	GP G Pickar RN											
					3-11	MS M. Smith, R.N.											

SIGNATURE OF NURSE ADMINISTERING MEDICATIONS

DATE GIVEN	TIME	INT.	MEDICATION-DOSAGE-CONT.	RT.

LITHO IN U.S.A. K6508 (7-92) D395538

RECOPIED BY:

CHECKED BY:

Doe, John Q

ALLERGIES: NKA

602-31 (7-92) (MPC# 1355)

(1)

ORIGINAL COPY

43.   Select: _____
       Give: _____

Lasix® 20 mg (furosemide)
HOECHST-ROUSSEL Pharmaceuticals Inc.
Somerville, N.J. 08876-1258
767010689
Lot 0676080 Exp.

A

Lasix® 40 mg (furosemide)
HOECHST-ROUSSEL Pharmaceuticals Inc.
Somerville, N.J. 08876-1258
760011889
Lot 0600620 Exp.

B

44. Give: _____

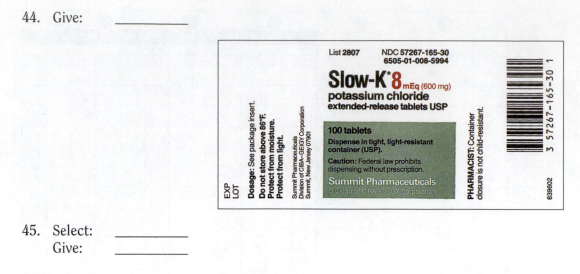

45. Select: _____
    Give: _____

(HINT: This is an introduction to the next chapter.)

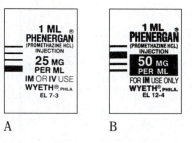

A   B

After completing these problems, see pages 321 and 322 to check your answers.

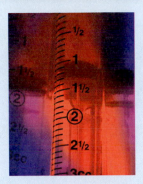

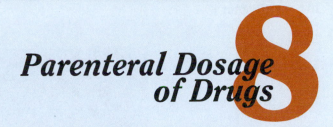

Parenteral Dosage of Drugs

objectives

Upon mastery of Chapter 8, you will be able to calculate the parenteral dosages of drugs. To accomplish this you will also be able to:

- Convert all units of measurement to the same system and size units.
- Analyze the dosage problem after conversion in order to estimate the amount of medication to be administered.
- Apply the ratio-proportion dosage calculation method to check the accuracy of your thinking.
- Reconstitute and label medications supplied in powder or dry form.
- Differentiate between varying directions for reconstitution and select the correct set to prepare the dosage ordered.
- Measure insulin in a matching insulin syringe.

The term *parenteral* is used to designate routes of administration other than gastrointestinal, such as the injection routes of IM, SC, ID, and IV. In this chapter intramuscular (IM) and subcutaneous (SC) injections will be emphasized. Intravenous (IV) drug calculations are discussed in Chapters 11 and 12. Intramuscular indicates an injection given into a muscle, such as Demerol given IM for pain. Subcutaneous means an injection given into the subcutaneous tissue, such as an insulin injection given SC for the management of diabetes. Intradermal (ID) means an injection given under the skin such as an allergy test or tuberculin skin testing.

Injectable Solutions

Most parenteral medications are prepared in liquid or solution form, and packaged in dosage vials, ampules, or prefilled syringes (Figure 8–1). Injectable drugs are measured in syringes.

> **rule** The maximum dosage volume to be administered per intramuscular injection site for:
> 1. An average 150 lb adult = 3 mL
> 2. Children age 6 to 12 years = 2 mL
> 3. Children birth to age 5 years = 1 mL

For example, if you must give an adult patient 4 milliliters of a drug, divide the dose into two injections of 2 milliliters each. The condition of the patient must be considered when applying this rule. Adults or children who have decreased muscle or subcutaneous tissue mass or poor circulation may not be able to tolerate the maximum dosage volumes.

To solve parenteral dosage problems, apply the same steps used for the calculation of oral dosages.

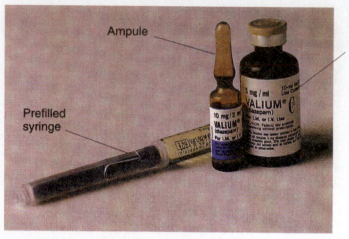

Fig. 8–1 Parenteral Solutions

remember

- Step 1.   **Convert:** all units to the same system, and all units to the same size
- Step 2.   **Think:** estimate the logical amount
- Step 3.   **Calculate:** $\dfrac{\text{Dosage on hand}}{\text{Amount on hand}} = \dfrac{\text{Dosage desired}}{\text{X Amount desired}}$

Use the following rules to help you decide which size syringe to select to administer parenteral dosages.

rule   As you calculate parenteral dosages:

1. Round "X" (amount to be administered) to tenths if the amount is greater than 1 mL and measure it in a 3-cc syringe.
2. Measure amounts of less than 1 mL calculated in hundredths in a tuberculin syringe.
3. Amounts of 0.5–1 mL, calculated in tenths, can be accurately measured in either a tuberculin or 3-cc syringe.
4. Amounts of less than 0.5 mL are preferably measured in a 0.5-mL tuberculin syringe.

Let's look at some examples of appropriate syringe selections for the dosages to be measured.

EXAMPLE 1:   Measure 0.33 mL in a Lo-Dose or 0.5-mL tuberculin syringe.

EXAMPLE 2:   Round 1.33 mL to 1.3 mL and measure in a 3-cc syringe.

EXAMPLE 3:   Measure 0.6 mL in either a 1-mL tuberculin or 3-cc syringe. (Notice that the amount is calculated in tenths.)

EXAMPLE 4:   Measure 0.65 mL in a 1-mL tuberculin syringe. (Notice that the amount is calculated in hundredths and is less than 1 mL.)

An amber color has been added to selected syringe drawings throughout the text *to simulate a specific amount of medication*, as indicated in the example or problem. Since the color used may not correspond to the actual color of the medications named, **it must not be used as a reference for identifying medications.**

Let's look at some examples of parenteral dosage calculations.

EXAMPLE 1:   The doctor's order reads: *Bentyl 20 mg IM q.i.d.* Available is *Bentyl injection 10 mg/mL* in a 10 mL multiple dose vial. How many milliliters should be administered to the patient?

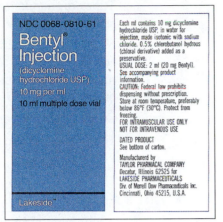

NDC 0068-0810-61

**Bentyl®
Injection**

(dicyclomine
hydrochloride USP)

10 mg per ml

10 ml multiple dose vial

Lakeside

Each ml contains 10 mg dicyclomine hydrochloride USP, in water for injection, made isotonic with sodium chloride. 0.5% chlorobutanol hydrous (chloral derivative) added as a preservative.
USUAL DOSE: 2 ml (20 mg Bentyl). See accompanying product information.
CAUTION: Federal law prohibits dispensing without prescription.
Store at room temperature, preferably below 86°F (30°C). Protect from freezing.
FOR INTRAMUSCULAR USE ONLY NOT FOR INTRAVENOUS USE

DATED PRODUCT
See bottom of carton.

Manufacturerd by
TAYLOR PHARMACAL COMPANY Decatur, Illinois 62525 for LAKESIDE PHARMACEUTICALS Div. of Merrell Dow Pharmaceuticals Inc. Cincinnati, Ohio 45215, U.S.A.

Step 1.   Convert: No conversion is necessary.

Step 2.   Think: You want to give more than 1 mL. In fact, you want to give twice as much, since 20 mg is twice as much as 10 mg.

Step 3.   Calculate: $\dfrac{\text{Dosage on hand}}{\text{Amount on hand}} = \dfrac{\text{Dosage desired}}{\text{X Amount desired}}$

$\dfrac{10 \text{ mg}}{1 \text{ mL}} \rightleftarrows \dfrac{20 \text{ mg}}{\text{X mL}}$ (Cross-multiply and solve for X.)

$10X = 20$

$\dfrac{10X}{10} = \dfrac{20}{10}$

X = 2 mL given intramuscularly four times daily

Select a *3-cc syringe and measure 2 mL* of Bentyl 10 mg per mL.

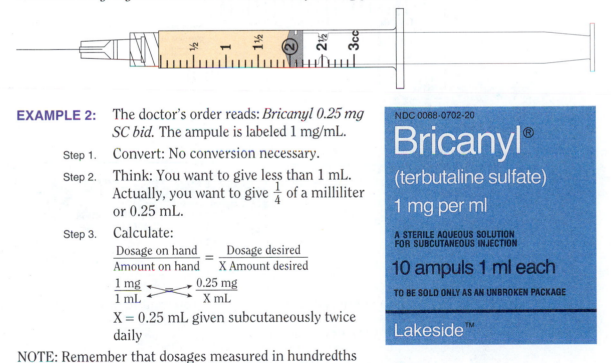

EXAMPLE 2:   The doctor's order reads: *Bricanyl 0.25 mg SC bid.* The ampule is labeled 1 mg/mL.

Step 1.   Convert: No conversion necessary.

Step 2.   Think: You want to give less than 1 mL. Actually, you want to give $\frac{1}{4}$ of a milliliter or 0.25 mL.

Step 3.   Calculate:

$\dfrac{\text{Dosage on hand}}{\text{Amount on hand}} = \dfrac{\text{Dosage desired}}{\text{X Amount desired}}$

$\dfrac{1 \text{ mg}}{1 \text{ mL}} \rightleftarrows \dfrac{0.25 \text{ mg}}{\text{X mL}}$

X = 0.25 mL given subcutaneously twice daily

NDC 0068-0702-20

Bricanyl®

(terbutaline sulfate)

1 mg per ml

A STERILE AQUEOUS SOLUTION
FOR SUBCUTANEOUS INJECTION

10 ampuls 1 ml each

TO BE SOLD ONLY AS AN UNBROKEN PACKAGE

Lakeside™

NOTE: Remember that dosages measured in hundredths (such as 0.25 mL) and all amounts less than 0.5 mL should be prepared in a tuberculin syringe, which is calibrated in hundredths.

Select a *0.5-cc tuberculin syringe and measure 0.25 mL* of Bricanyl 1 mg per mL.

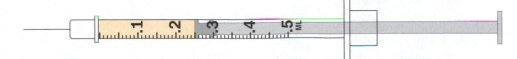

EXAMPLE 3:   Drug order: *Demerol (meperidine hydrochloride) 35 mg IM q.3–4h p.r.n.*, pain

Tubex on hand: *Meperidine HCl 50 mg per mL*

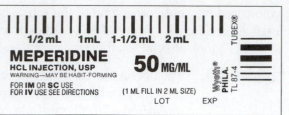

Note: The statement on the label "(1 ML FILL IN 2 ML SIZE)" means that the total capacity of the Tubex syringe is 2 mL, but it is filled with 1 mL of meperidine.

Step 1.   Convert: No conversion necessary.

Step 2.   Think: You want to give less than 1 mL. (Actually, you want to give $\frac{35}{50}$ or 0.7 mL)

Step 3.   Calculate: $\dfrac{\text{Dosage on hand}}{\text{Amount on hand}} = \dfrac{\text{Dosage desired}}{\text{X Amount desired}}$

$$\frac{50 \text{ mg}}{1 \text{ mL}} \quad\times\quad \frac{35 \text{ mg}}{\text{X mL}}$$

$$50X = 35$$

$$\frac{50X}{50} = \frac{35}{50}$$

X = 0.7 mL given intramuscularly every 3–4 hours as needed for pain

Select the *2 mL-Tubex and discard 0.3 mL to leave 0.7 mL* of meperidine (Demerol) 50 mg/mL.

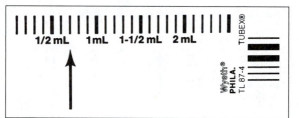

EXAMPLE 4:   Ordered: *Heparin 8,000 U SC b.i.d.*

Available: A vial of *heparin sodium injection 10,000 U per mL*

Step 1.   Convert: No conversion necessary.

Step 2.   Think: You want to give less than 1 mL. Actually, you want to give

$\frac{8,000}{10,000}$ or $\frac{8}{10}$ of the 1 mL or 0.8 mL

Step 3.   Calculate: $\dfrac{\text{Dosage on hand}}{\text{Amount on hand}} = \dfrac{\text{Dosage desired}}{\text{X Amount desired}}$

$$\frac{10,000 \text{ U}}{1 \text{ mL}} \quad\times\quad \frac{8000 \text{ U}}{\text{X mL}}$$

$$10,000X = 8000$$

$$\frac{10,000X}{10,000} = \frac{8000}{10,000}$$

X = 0.8 mL given subcutaneously twice daily

Select a *1-mL* or a *3-cc syringe and measure 0.8 mL* of heparin 10,000 U/mL.

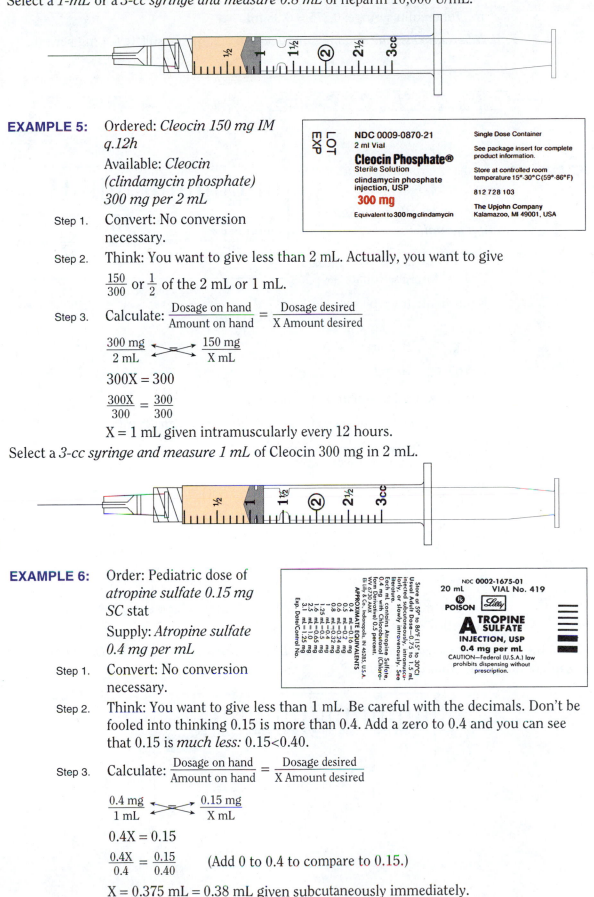

EXAMPLE 5: Ordered: *Cleocin 150 mg IM q.12h*

Available: *Cleocin (clindamycin phosphate) 300 mg per 2 mL*

Step 1. Convert: No conversion necessary.

Step 2. Think: You want to give less than 2 mL. Actually, you want to give $\frac{150}{300}$ or $\frac{1}{2}$ of the 2 mL or 1 mL.

Step 3. Calculate: $\dfrac{\text{Dosage on hand}}{\text{Amount on hand}} = \dfrac{\text{Dosage desired}}{\text{X Amount desired}}$

$$\frac{300 \text{ mg}}{2 \text{ mL}} \diagdown\diagup \frac{150 \text{ mg}}{\text{X mL}}$$

$$300X = 300$$

$$\frac{300X}{300} = \frac{300}{300}$$

X = 1 mL given intramuscularly every 12 hours.

Select a *3-cc syringe and measure 1 mL* of Cleocin 300 mg in 2 mL.

EXAMPLE 6: Order: Pediatric dose of *atropine sulfate 0.15 mg SC stat*

Supply: *Atropine sulfate 0.4 mg per mL*

Step 1. Convert: No conversion necessary.

Step 2. Think: You want to give less than 1 mL. Be careful with the decimals. Don't be fooled into thinking 0.15 is more than 0.4. Add a zero to 0.4 and you can see that 0.15 is *much less*: 0.15<0.40.

Step 3. Calculate: $\dfrac{\text{Dosage on hand}}{\text{Amount on hand}} = \dfrac{\text{Dosage desired}}{\text{X Amount desired}}$

$$\frac{0.4 \text{ mg}}{1 \text{ mL}} \diagdown\diagup \frac{0.15 \text{ mg}}{\text{X mL}}$$

$$0.4X = 0.15$$

$$\frac{0.4X}{0.4} = \frac{0.15}{0.40} \qquad \text{(Add 0 to 0.4 to compare to 0.15.)}$$

X = 0.375 mL = 0.38 mL given subcutaneously immediately.

This is a small pediatric dosage, so round to hundredths and measure in a 0.5 mL tuberculin syringe: 0.375 = 0.38 mL.

Select a *0.5 mL tuberculin syringe and measure 0.38 mL* of atropine sulfate 0.4 mg per mL.

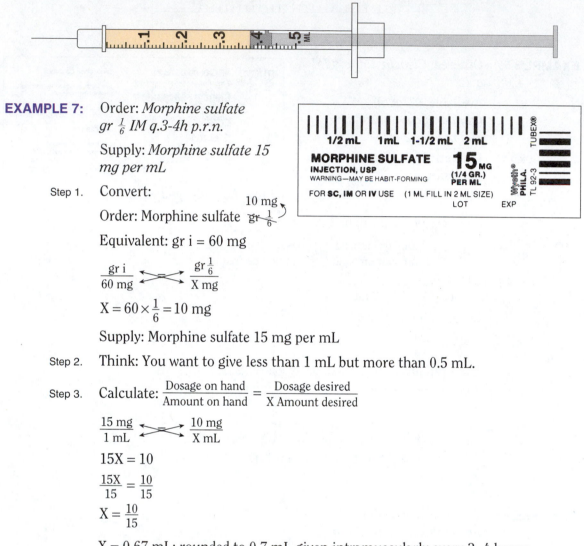

EXAMPLE 7:   Order: *Morphine sulfate gr $\frac{1}{6}$ IM q.3-4h p.r.n.*

Supply: *Morphine sulfate 15 mg per mL*

Step 1.   Convert:

Order: Morphine sulfate gr $\frac{1}{6}$ 10 mg

Equivalent: gr i = 60 mg

$$\frac{\text{gr i}}{60 \text{ mg}} \underset{\longleftarrow}{\overset{\longrightarrow}{\times}} \frac{\text{gr}\frac{1}{6}}{\text{X mg}}$$

$$X = 60 \times \frac{1}{6} = 10 \text{ mg}$$

Supply: Morphine sulfate 15 mg per mL

Step 2.   Think: You want to give less than 1 mL but more than 0.5 mL.

Step 3.   Calculate: $\dfrac{\text{Dosage on hand}}{\text{Amount on hand}} = \dfrac{\text{Dosage desired}}{\text{X Amount desired}}$

$$\frac{15 \text{ mg}}{1 \text{ mL}} \underset{\longleftarrow}{\overset{\longrightarrow}{\times}} \frac{10 \text{ mg}}{\text{X mL}}$$

$$15X = 10$$

$$\frac{15X}{15} = \frac{10}{15}$$

$$X = \frac{10}{15}$$

X = 0.67 mL; rounded to 0.7 mL given intramuscularly every 3–4 hours as needed.

Select the *2 mL Tubex syringe and discard 0.3 mL of the prefilled amount (1 mL)* and give 0.7 mL of morphine sulfate 15 mg/mL.

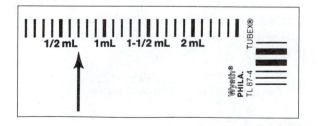

review set 23 _____

Calculate the amount you will prepare for each dose. Draw an arrow to the syringe calibration that corresponds to the amount you will administer. Indicate dosages that need to be divided.

1. Order: Codeine gr $\frac{1}{4}$ SC q.4h p.r.n., pain
    Supply: 20 mL vial codeine labeled 30 mg per mL
    Give: _____

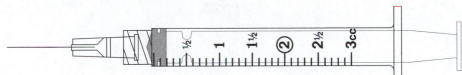

2. Order: Bicillin 2,400,000 U IM stat
    Supply: 10 mL vial of Bicillin containing 600,000 U per mL
    Give: _____

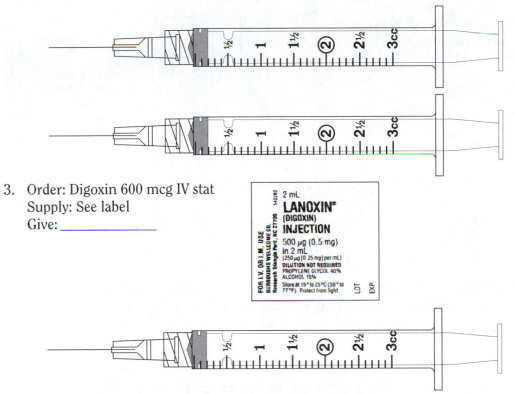

3. Order: Digoxin 600 mcg IV stat
    Supply: See label
    Give: _____

2 mL
LANOXIN®
(DIGOXIN)
INJECTION
500 µg (0.5 mg)
in 2 mL
(250 µg [0.25 mg] per mL)
DILUTION NOT REQUIRED
PROPYLENE GLYCOL 40%
ALCOHOL 10%
Store at 15° to 25°C (59° to
77°F). Protect from light.

FOR I.V. OR I.M. USE
BURROUGHS WELLCOME CO.
Research Triangle Park, NC 27709   542282
LOT   EXP.

4. Order: Procaine penicillin G 2.4 million U IM stat
    Supply: Wycillin (Procaine penicillin G) containing 2,400,000 U/2 mL
    Give: _____

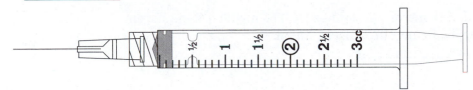

5. Order: Tigan 200 mg IM stat, then 100 mg q.6h p.r.n. nausea
    Supply: 2 mL ampule Tigan containing 100 mg per mL
    Give: _____ stat and _____ q.6h

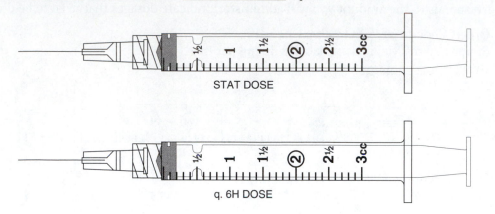

STAT DOSE

q. 6H DOSE

6. Order: Heparin 8000 U SC q.8h
    Supply: See label
    Give: _____

NDC 0002-7217-01
VIAL No. 520
5 ml

Lilly
HEPARIN SODIUM
INJECTION, USP
10,000 USP
Units per ml
Multiple Dose

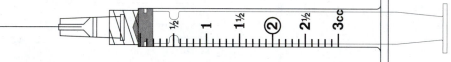

7. Order: Potassium chloride 15 mEq added to each 1000 mL IV fluid container
    Supply: Potassium chloride 30 mL vial containing 2 mEq/mL
    Give: _____

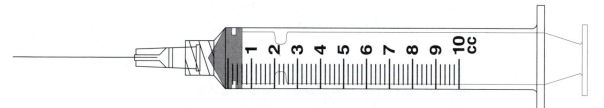

8. Order: Demerol (meperidine HCl) 60 mg IM q.4h p.r.n. pain
    Supply: Demerol 75 mg per 1.5 mL
    Give: _____

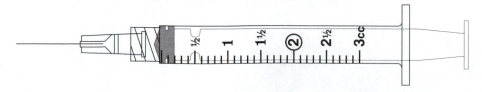

9. Order: Atropine gr $\frac{1}{100}$ IM on call
preoperatively
Supply: See label
Give: _____

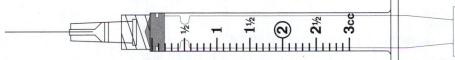

10. Order: Morphine sulfate gr $\frac{1}{6}$ IM q.3–4h p.r.n.
Supply: Morphine sulfate 10 mg per mL
Give: _____

11. Order: Procaine penicillin G 400,000 U IM t.i.d.
Supply: See label
Give: _____

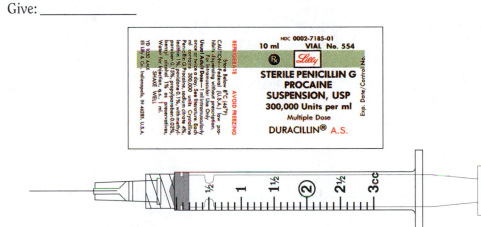

12. Order: Heparin 4500 U SC q.d.
Supply: See label
Give: _____

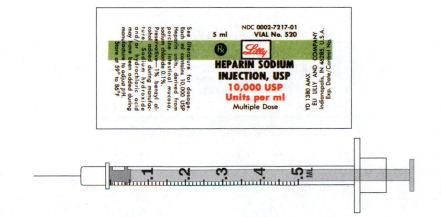

13.   Order: Compazine 7.5 mg IM q.3–4h p.r.n. nausea and vomiting
       Supply: 10 mL vial Compazine containing 5 mg per mL
       Give: _____

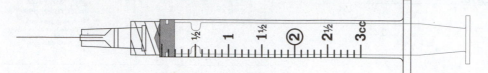

14.   Order: Vistaril 20 mg IM q.4h p.r.n. nausea
       Supply: 10 mL vial of Vistaril 25 mg/mL
       Give: _____

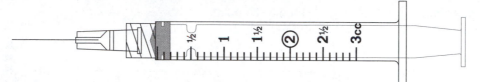

15.   Order: Gentamicin sulfate 60 mg IM b.i.d.
       Supply: 2 cc vial Garamycin (gentamicin sulfate) 40 mg/cc
       Give: _____

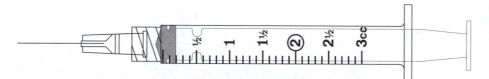

16.   Order: Ativan 3 mg IM on-call pre-operatively
       Supply: 10 mL vial of Ativan 2 mg per mL
       Give: _____

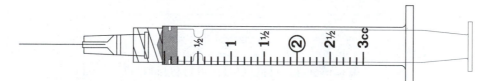

17.   Order: Vit. B$_{12}$ 0.5 mg IM once/week
       Supply: See label
       Give: _____

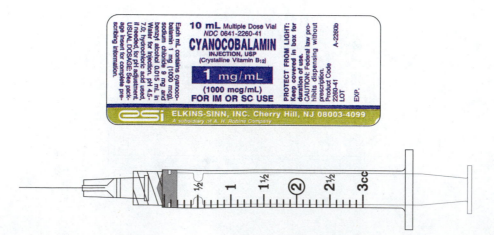

18. Order: Zantac 20 mg IM q.6h
     Supply: See label
     Give: _____

19. Order: Phenergan 12.5 mg IM stat

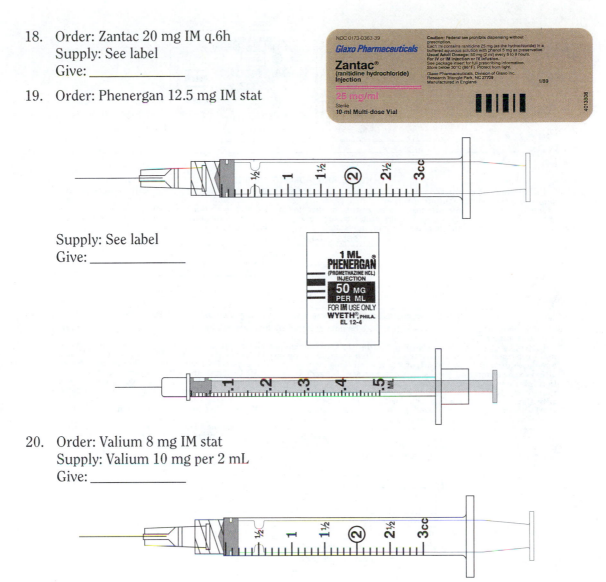

     Supply: See label
     Give: _____

20. Order: Valium 8 mg IM stat
     Supply: Valium 10 mg per 2 mL
     Give: _____

After completing these problems, see pages 298–301 to check your answers.

Injectable Medications in Powder Form

Some medications are unstable when stored in solution form and are therefore packaged in powder form (Figure 8–2). Powders must be dissolved with a sterile diluent before use. Usually sterile water or 0.9% sodium chloride (normal saline) is used as the diluent. The dissolving procedure is referred to as *reconstitution*. In reconstituting the drug, read and follow the directions carefully.

Instructions supplied with the vial state the volume of diluent that should be added. The resulting volume of the reconstituted drug is also given. Often the powdered drug adds volume to the solution in addition to the amount of diluent added.

When you reconstitute or mix a multiple-dose vial of medication in powdered form, it is important that it is clearly *labeled* with the *date* and *time* of preparation and your *initials* as the one responsible for the reconstitution. Since the medication becomes unstable after storage for long periods, the date and time are especially important. Most reconstituted drugs retain their potency for up to one week and should be stored under refrigeration. Check the drug label, package information sheet, or *Hospital Formulary* for how long the drug may be used. (NOTE: The length of potency is different from the expiration date. The expiration date would indicate the *last* date the drug may be reconstituted and used.)

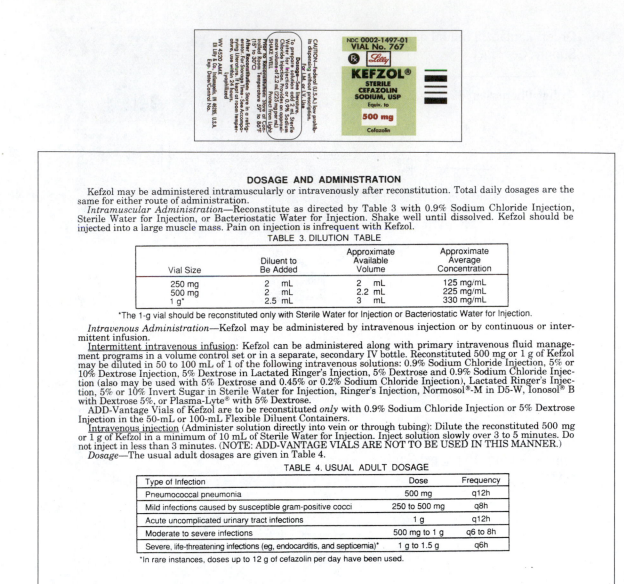

Fig. 8–2 Kefzol Label with Portion of the Package Insert

Note: Figure 8–2 and subsequent reproductions of package inserts represent only the portion of the information relative to the specific problem under study.

EXAMPLE 1:   Order: *Ancef 750 mg IM q.8h*

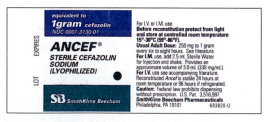

Supply: *1 g vial of powdered Ancef* with directions on the right side of the label as follows: "For IM use, add 2.5 mL sterile water. . . . Provides an approximate volume of 3.0 mL (330 mg/mL)."

This means you have available a vial of 1 gram of *Ancef* to which you will add 2.5 milliliters of diluent (sterile water). The powdered drug displaces 0.5 mL. Then each 3 milliliters contains 1 g of the drug, and there are 330 mg in each 1 mL.

Step 1.   Convert: No conversion necessary.

Order: *Ancef 750 mg*

Supply: 330 mg = 1 mL

Step 2.   Think: You want to give more than 1 mL.

Step 3.   Calculate: $\dfrac{\text{Dosage on hand}}{\text{Amount on hand}} = \dfrac{\text{Dosage desired}}{\text{X Amount desired}}$

$$\dfrac{330 \text{ mg}}{1 \text{ mL}} \xrightarrow{\hspace{1cm}} \dfrac{750 \text{ mg}}{\text{X mL}}$$

$$330X = 750$$

$$\dfrac{330X}{330} = \dfrac{750}{330}$$

X = 2.27 mL; rounded to 2.3 mL

Give 2.3 mL of Ancef intramuscularly every 8 hours.

Label: "1/30/xx, 8 AM, G.D.P." Also notice how long this drug may be kept at room temperature or refrigerated.

Select a *3-cc syringe and measure 2.3 mL* of Ancef reconstituted to 330 mg/mL.

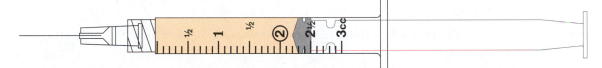

Some medications are supplied with several different directions for reconstitution. Be sure to read all instructions carefully!

EXAMPLE 2:   Order: *Penicillin G potassium 300,000 U IM q.i.d.*

Supply: *Penicillin G potassium 1,000,000 U vial*

This means there is a *total* of 1,000,000 U of penicillin in the vial. The reconstitution instructions are listed on the left side of the label. Choose the solution strength that will result in a reasonable amount to be given to the patient.

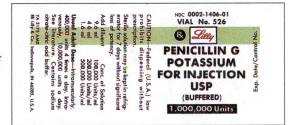

Refer to the directions on the left side of the label which state "Add diluent 4.6 mL (for a) concentration of solution 200,000 units/mL."

This means when you add 4.6 milliliters of sterile diluent to a vial of powdered penicillin, the result is 1,000,000 units of penicillin in 5 milliliters of solution. The diluent is 4.6 milliliters; the powder displaces 0.4 more milliliters for a total of 1,000,000 units in 5 milliliters for a solution strength of 200,000 units per mL.

Step 1.   Convert: No conversion necessary.

Order: Penicillin 300,000 U   Supply: 200,000 U = 1 mL

Step 2.   Think: You want to give more than 1 mL but less than 2 mL.

Step 3.   Calculate: $\dfrac{\text{Dosage on hand}}{\text{Amount on hand}} = \dfrac{\text{Dosage desired}}{\text{X Amount desired}}$

$$\dfrac{200,000 \text{ U}}{1 \text{ mL}} \xrightarrow{\hspace{1cm}} \dfrac{300,000 \text{ U}}{\text{X mL}}$$

$$200,000X = 300,000$$

$$\dfrac{200,000X}{200,000} = \dfrac{300,000}{200,000}$$

X = 1.5 mL given intramuscularly four times daily

Select a *3-cc syringe and measure 1.5 mL* of penicillin reconstituted to 200,000 units/mL.

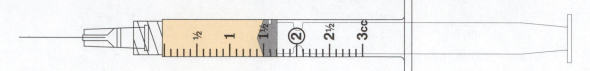

NOTE: You could also reconstitute this drug to a solution strength of 500,000 U/mL by adding 1.6 mL of sterile diluent to the vial and giving 0.6 mL for each dose:

$$\frac{500,000 \text{ U}}{1 \text{ mL}} \xleftrightarrow{\hspace{1cm}} \frac{300,000 \text{ U}}{X \text{ mL}}$$

$$500,000X = 300,000$$

$$\frac{500,000X}{500,000} = \frac{300,000}{500,000}$$

$$X = 0.6 \text{ mL}$$

Select a *3-cc syringe and measure 0.6 mL* of penicillin reconstituted to 500,000 units/mL.

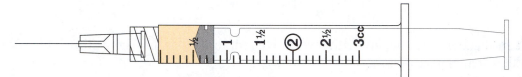

The solution strength of 100,000 U/mL (if 9.6 mL of sterile diluent is added to the vial) would result in a 3-mL dose which is a very large dose per injection site. Although it would be acceptable, it would not be the preferred choice.

Since there are directions for reconstitutions of varying strengths, you must clearly label the vial with the strength you prepared, the date and time of preparation, and your initials. For example: 1 mL = 200,000 U 1/30/xx, 8 AM, G.D.P. Also notice how long this drug retains its potency.

quick review

It is important that you remember the following points when reconstituting drugs:

- If any medicine remains for future use after reconstitution, clearly label:
    1. *strength* or concentration per volume
    2. *date* and *time* of preparation
    3. *initials* of individual performing procedure
- Read all instructions carefully! If no instructions accompany the vial, confer with the pharmacist before proceeding.
- Prepare a maximum of 3 mL per intramuscular injection site for an average size adult, 2 mL per site for children ages 6–12, and 1 mL for an infant to a 5 year old.
- When calculating fractional dosages that will be measured in syringes, give answers in decimal form to the closest amount that can be measured by that syringe, such as 1.5 mL as measured in a 3-cc syringe or 0.25 cc as measured in a tuberculin syringe.
- Round standard injection dosages over 1 mL to tenths and measure in the 3-cc syringe. The 3-cc syringe is calibrated in 0.1 cc increments.
- Round small (less than 1 mL), critical care, or children's dosages to hundredths and measure in the tuberculin syringe. The tuberculin syringes are calibrated in 0.01 mL increments.
- Measure amounts less than 0.5 mL in the tuberculin syringe.

review set 24

Calculate the amount you will prepare for each dose. The labels provided are the drugs available. Draw an arrow to the syringe calibration that corresponds to the amount you will draw up.

1. Order: Ceftazidime 250 mg IM q.i.d.
   Reconstitute with _____ mL diluent
   and give _____ mL.

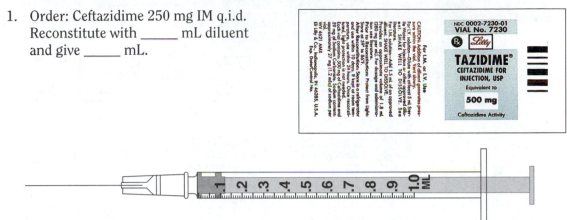

2. Order: Geopen 500 mg IM q.6h
   Reconstitute with _____ mL diluent and give _____ mL.

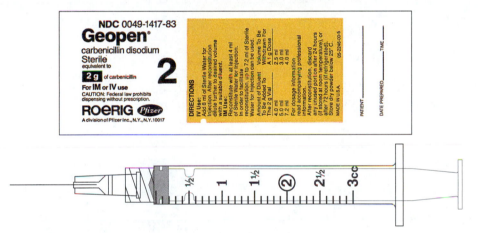

3. Order: Librium 25 mg IM q.6h p.r.n.
   Directions: Add 2 mL special diluent to yield 100 mg per 2 mL.
   Reconstitute with _____ mL diluent and give _____ mL.

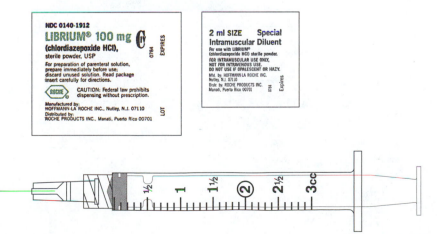

4. Order: Cytoxan 250 mg IV q.d. × 5 days
    Reconstitute with _____ mL diluent and give _____ mL.

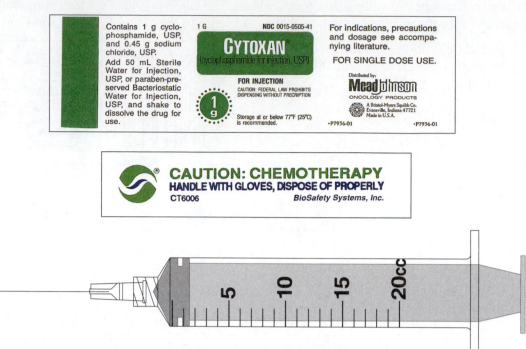

5. Order: Polycillin-N 300 mg IV PB q. 6h in 50 mL D_5W
    Reconstitute with _____ mL diluent and give _____ mL.

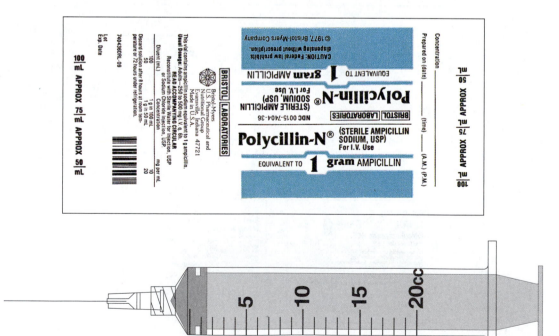

6. Order: Ampicillin 500 mg IM q.6h
    Reconstitute with _____ mL diluent and give _____ mL.

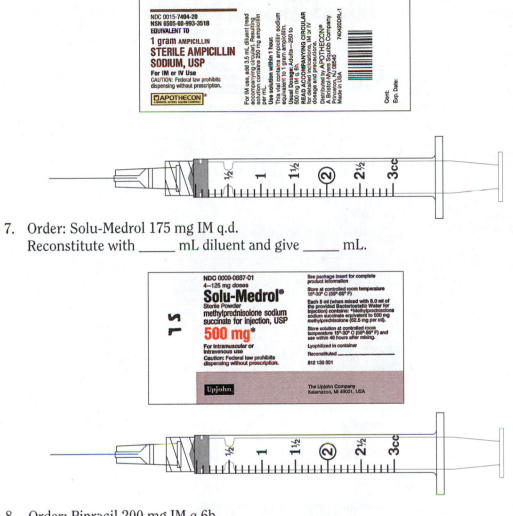

7. Order: Solu-Medrol 175 mg IM q.d.
    Reconstitute with _____ mL diluent and give _____ mL.

8. Order: Pipracil 200 mg IM q.6h
    Directions: Adding 4 cc diluent yields 1 g per 2.5 mL
    Reconstitute with _____ mL diluent and give _____ mL.

9. Order: Penicillin G 500,000 U IM q.6h
    Reconstitute with _____ mL diluent and give _____ mL.

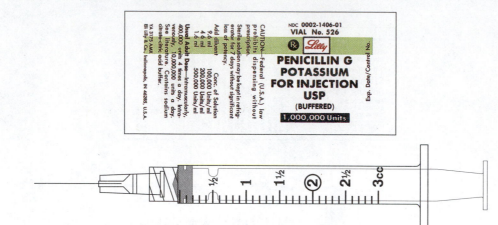

10. Order: Cefadyl 0.5 g IM q.6h
    Reconstitute with _____ mL diluent and give _____ mL.

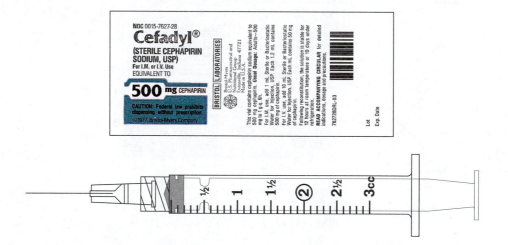

11. Order: Buffered potassium penicillin G 400,000 U IM q.d.
    Reconstitute with _____ mL diluent and give _____ mL.

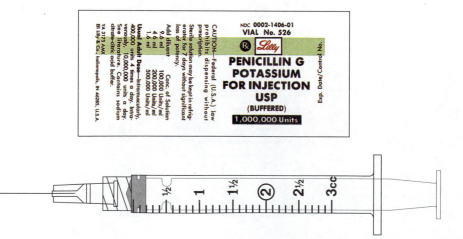

12. Order: Ancef 500 mg IM q.12h
     Reconstitute with _____ mL diluent and give _____ mL.

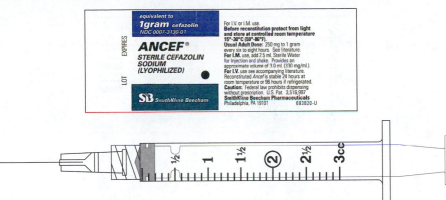

13. Order: Nafcillin sodium 500 mg IM q.i.d.
     Reconstitute with _____ mL diluent and give _____ mL.

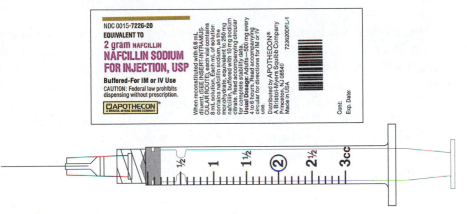

14. Order: Wydase 75 U SC stat
     Directions in package insert: Add 10 mL of diluent to provide a solution containing
          150 U/mL
     Reconstitute with _____ mL diluent and give _____ mL.

15. Order: Kefzol 250 mg IM q.6h
     Reconstitute with _____ mL diluent and give _____ mL.

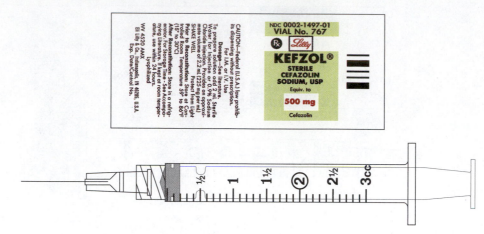

After completing these problems, see pages 302–304 to check your answers.

Insulin

Insulin, a hormone made in the pancreas, is necessary for the metabolism of glucose, proteins, and fats. Patients who are deficient in insulin (insulin-dependent diabetics) are required to take insulin by injection daily. In the United States there are two major manufacturers of insulin: Eli Lilly & Company and Novo Nordisk. Insulins are classified by *type,* such as rapid-, intermediate-, or long-acting; and by origin or *species,* such as human or animal (pork, beef, pork-beef mixture). The patient is instructed to stay with the same manufacturer, type, and species of insulin unless otherwise instructed by the physician. The rationale for this is that different manufacturers of the same type of insulin may vary in the onset, peak, and duration of action. Also, different species of insulins may cause allergy-like symptoms in some patients.

Manufacturers of Insulin in the United States

Examine the following insulin labels (Figure 8–3 and Figure 8–4) to identify the manufacturers.

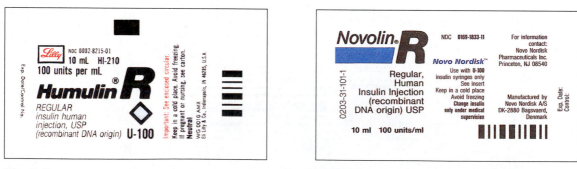

Fig. 8–3   Fig. 8–4

Types of Insulin

Rapid-, intermediate-, and long-acting insulins vary in their action times. The *onset* (when the insulin begins to work), the *peak* (when the insulin is working hardest), and the *duration* (how long the insulin works) are provided in the table in Figure 8-5. You will note

	ONSET	PEAK	DURATION THERAPEUTIC*	PHARMACEUTIC**
Rapid-Acting (Regular, Semilente)	$\frac{1}{2}$–1 h	2–4 h	6–8 h	5–12 h
Intermediate- Acting (NPH, Lente)	1–4 h	8±2 h	10–16 h	16–24 h
Long-Acting	4–6 h	18 h	24–36 h	36+ h

*Therapeutic (or effective duration of action)—the amount of active insulin needed to keep blood glucose levels in normal limits.

**Pharmaceutic (or pharmacokinetic)—the action of insulin on "entrance" into and "exit" from the body.

Source: Adapted from Campbell R.K., *Diabetic management: Insulin, oral agents, and intensified insulin therapy (module 9, table 3)*. Chicago: American Association of Diabetes Educators Continuing Education Self-Study Program. Diabetes Treatment Center. 1988. *Care and control of your diabetes*. Wichita, KS: St. Joseph Medical Center.

Fig. 8–5 Onset, Peak, and Duration of Different Insulins

that there are examples of the different types of insulins. Regular and Semilente are examples of rapid-acting insulins. NPH and Lente are examples of intermediate-acting insulins. Ultralente is an example of a long-acting insulin. The two types of insulin used most often are the rapid-acting Regular insulin and the intermediate-acting NPH insulin. Figure 8–5 describes the action times of various insulins.

Species of Insulin

Insulin comes from various sources:

- beef insulin—from the pancreas of cattle
- pork insulin—from the pancreas of pigs
- beef-pork mixture—a combination of beef and pork insulin
- human insulin
    a. bio-synthetic—bacteria are genetically altered to create human insulin.
    b. semi-synthetic—pork insulin is chemically altered to produce human insulin.

When receiving an insulin order it is necessary to know the manufacturer of the insulin, the species, and the action. Let's look again at the label in Figure 8–3. Eli Lilly Humulin R means the manufacturer is Eli Lilly & Co., and the species is human (Humulin). The designation *R* means Regular, which is a rapid-acting insulin. All of this information is provided on the label, and the label must be read very carefully. This is a critical nursing skill.

70–30 Insulin

A new insulin now available is called 70–30 U-100 insulin (Figure 8–6). The 70–30 insulin concentration means there is 70% NPH insulin and 30% Regular insulin in each unit. Therefore, if the physician orders 10 units of 70–30 insulin, the patient would receive 7 units of NPH insulin (70% or 0.7 × 10 U = 7 U) and 3 units of Regular insulin (30% or 0.3 × 10 U = 3 U) in the 70–30 concentration. If the physician orders 20 units of 70–30 insulin, the patient would receive 14 units (0.7 × 20 = 14) of NPH and 6 units (0.3 × 20 = 6) of Regular insulin, and so on.

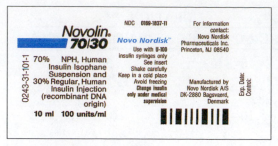

Fig. 8–6 70/30 U-100 Insulin

Measuring Insulin in an Insulin Syringe

The insulin syringe and measurement of insulin were introduced in Chapter 4. This critical skill warrants your attention again. Once you understand how insulin is packaged and how to use the insulin syringe, you will find insulin dosage simple. You need to know:

- Insulin should be measured in insulin syringes.

- Equivalents of insulin units to milliliters: 100 U of U-100 insulin = 1 milliliter (See Figures 8–3, 8–4, and 8–6)

- All insulin dosages should be double-checked by two nurses before administering

Measuring insulin with the insulin syringe is very simple. The insulin syringe makes it possible to obtain a correct dosage without mathematical calculation. Let's look at three different insulin syringes.

EXAMPLE 1:   The standard U-100 syringe in Figure 8–7 has a dual scale; even numbers on one side, and odd numbers on the other side. Each scale is marked for every 2 units up to 100 units. To measure 60 units, withdraw U-100 insulin to the 60-unit mark on the even-numbered scale, Figure 8–7(a). To measure 73 units, withdraw U-100 insulin to the 73-unit mark on the odd-numbered scale, Figure 8–7(b).

NOTE: Look carefully at the calibrations on each scale. Count each calibration (on one side only) as two units. You are probably comfortable counting by twos for even numbers. Pay close attention when counting by twos with odd numbers.

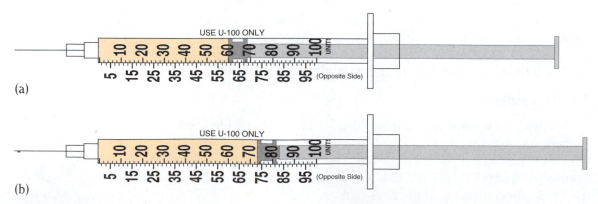

Fig. 8–7 Standard 100-Unit Dual-Scale U-100 Insulin Syringe: Even- and Odd-Numbered Scales

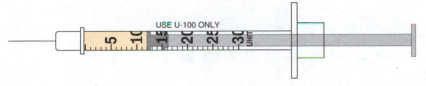

Fig. 8–8 50-U Lo-Dose U-100 Insulin Syringe

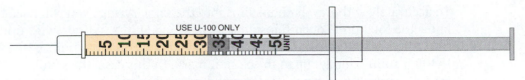

Fig. 8–9 30-U Lo-Dose U-100 Insulin Syringe

EXAMPLE 2: The enlarged scale of the 50-unit Lo-Dose U-100 insulin syringe makes it easier to read and measure low dosages of insulin. It is marked in units up to 50. To measure 32 units, withdraw U-100 insulin to the 32 unit mark on the Lo-Dose syringe (Figure 8–8).

EXAMPLE 3: The 30-unit Lo-Dose U-100 insulin syringe most accurately measures very small amounts of insulin, such as for children. It is marked in units up to 30. To measure 12 units, withdraw U-100 insulin to the 12 unit mark on the 30-unit Lo-Dose syringe. See Figure 8–9.

To be sure you are accurately measuring the correct insulin dosage, always use the smallest capacity insulin syringe possible. Dosages of U-100 insulin under 50 units should be measured in a Lo-Dose U-100 insulin syringe.

NOTE: Although the Lo-Dose U-100 insulin syringes only measure a maximum of 30 or 50 units, they are still intended for the measurement of *U-100 insulin* only.

Combination Insulin Dosage

The patient may have two types of insulin prescribed to be administered at the same time. To avoid injecting the patient twice, it is common practice to draw up both insulins in the same syringe.

▶ *rule* Draw up *clear insulin first,* then draw up cloudy insulin. Regular insulin is clear. NPH insulin is cloudy.

EXAMPLE 1: Order: Novolin R Regular U-100 insulin 12 U c̄ Novolin N NPH U-100 insulin 40 U SC ā breakfast.

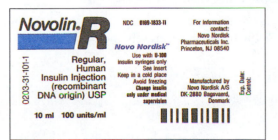

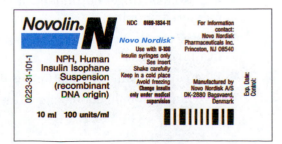

To accurately withdraw both insulins into the same syringe you will need to know the total units of both insulins: 12 + 40 = 52 units. Withdraw 12 units of the Regular U-100 insulin (clear) and then withdraw 40 more units of the NPH U-100 insulin (cloudy) up to the 52 unit mark. In this case, the smallest capacity syringe you can use is the standard U-100 syringe (see Figure 8–10).

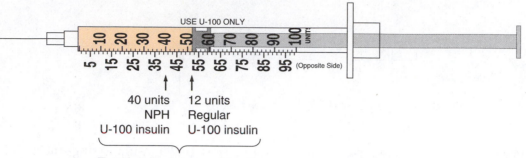

Fig. 8–10 Combination Insulin Dosage

The second example gives step-by-step directions for this procedure.

EXAMPLE 2:   The physician tells you to give 30 units of Novolin N NPH U-100 insulin and 10 units of Novolin R Regular U-100 insulin.

1. Draw back 30 units of air into the insulin syringe.
2. Inject 30 units of air into the NPH insulin vial (cloudy liquid). Remove needle.
3. Draw back and inject 10 units of air into the Regular insulin vial (clear liquid) and leave the needle in the vial.
4. Turn the vial of Regular insulin upside down and draw out the insulin to the 10-unit mark on the syringe. Make sure all air bubbles are removed.
5. Roll the vial of the NPH insulin in your hands to mix; do not shake it.
6. Insert the needle into the NPH insulin vial and draw back to the 40-unit mark: 10 units of Regular + 30 units of NPH = 40 units of insulin total.

quick review

- Always measure insulin in an insulin syringe.
- An insulin syringe is to be used to measure insulin only.
- An insulin syringe must not be used to measure other medications that are measured in units.
- Use the smallest capacity insulin syringe possible to most accurately measure insulin dosages.
- When drawing up combination insulin doses, think: *clear first*; *then cloudy*.
- Two nurses should double-check the insulin dosage.

review set 25

1. Describe the preferred method of measuring U-100 insulin. _____

   _____

2. What would be your preferred syringe choice to measure 24 units of U-100 insulin?

   _____

3. 20 units of U-100 insulin equals _____ mL.

4. 60 units of U-100 insulin equals _____ mL.

5. 25 units of U-100 insulin equals _____ mL.

6. Insulin should be measured in a(an) _____ syringe.

7. True or False. The 50 unit Lo-Dose U-100 insulin syringe is intended to measure U-50 insulin only. _____

Identify the U-100 insulin dosage indicated by the colored area of the syringe.

8.

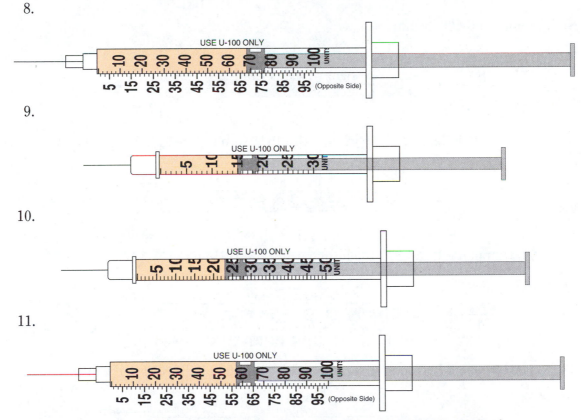

9.

10.

11.

Draw an arrow on the syringe to identify the given dosages. Identify each insulin for combination doses.

12. 80 units U-100 insulin.

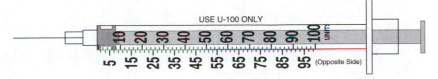

13. 15 units U-100 insulin.

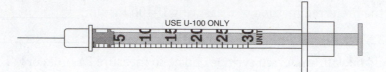

14. 66 units U-100 insulin.

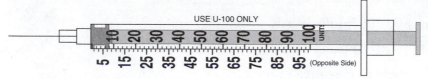

15. 16 units U-100 insulin.

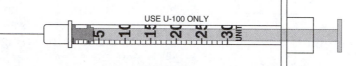

16. 32 units of U-100 insulin

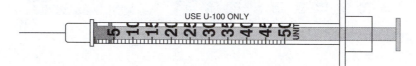

17. 21 U Novolin R Regular U-100 insulin with 15 U Novolin N NPH U-100 insulin SC

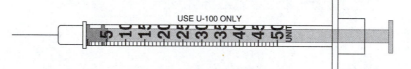

18. 16 U Humulin R Regular U-100 insulin with 42 NPH Humulin N U-100 insulin

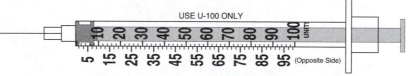

19. 32 U Humulin R Regular U-100 insulin with 40 U Humulin N NPH U-100 insulin

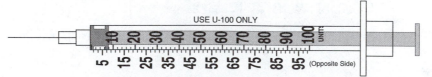

20. 8 U Humulin R Regular U-100 insulin with 12 U Humulin N NPH U-100 insulin

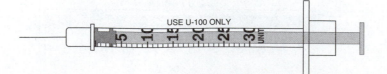

21. 34 U of Novolin N NPH U-100 insulin SC

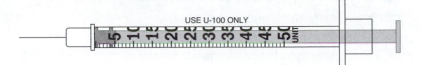

22. 75 U of Novolin R Regular U-100 insulin SC

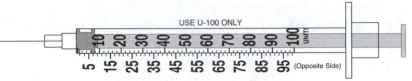

23. 22 U of Humulin N NPH U-100 insulin SC

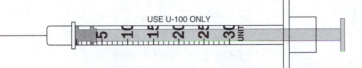

24. 13 U of Novolin N NPH U-100 insulin SC

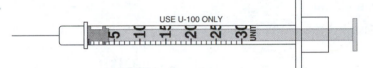

25. 17 U of Humulin R Regular U-100 insulin with 42 U of Humulin N NPH U-100 insulin SC

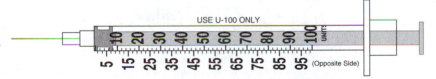

After completing these problems, see pages 304–306 to check your answers.

Calculating Dosage Expressed as a Ratio or Percent

Occasionally, solutions will be ordered and/or supplied in a dosage strength expressed as a ratio or percent.

Percentage (%) solutions express the number of grams of the drug per 100 mL of solution.

EXAMPLES: Calcium gluconate 10% = 10 g of pure drug per 100 mL of solution
Lidocaine 2% = 2 g of pure drug per 100 mL of solution.

Ratio solutions express the number of grams of the drug per total milliliters of solution.

EXAMPLES: Adrenalin 1:1000 = 1 g pure drug per 1000 mL solution.
Prostigmin 1:4000 = 1 g pure drug per 4000 mL solution.

Solving dosage problems expressed in ratio and percent is not difficult. Follow the same steps used to calculate all dosages.

Step 1.   Convert: to units of the same system and same size.

Convert: ratio or percent to g or mg per mL.

Step 2.   Think: estimate the amount to give.

Step 3.   Calculate: $\dfrac{\text{Dosage on hand}}{\text{Amount on hand}} = \dfrac{\text{Dosage desired}}{\text{X Amount desired}}$

EXAMPLE 1:   Order: *Epinephrine 0.4 mg SC q.3h p.r.n.* for asthma.

Supply: *1 mL ampules of epinephrine 1:1000*

Step 1.   Convert: Epinephrine 1:1000 = 1 g of epinephrine per 1000 mL = 1000 mg per 1000 mL = 1 mg per 1 mL

The problem now looks like this:

Order: Epinephrine 0.4 mg

Supply: Epinephrine 1:1000 per 1 mL ampules = 1 mg per 1 mL

Step 2.   Think: You have 1 mg per 1 mL and you want to give 0.4 mg; therefore, you want to give 0.4 mL.

Step 3.   Calculate: $\dfrac{\text{Dosage on hand}}{\text{Amount on hand}} = \dfrac{\text{Dosage desired}}{\text{X Amount desired}}$

$$\dfrac{1\ \text{mg}}{1\ \text{mL}} \;\rightleftharpoons\; \dfrac{0.4\ \text{mg}}{\text{X mL}}$$

X = 0.4 mL

Give 0.4 mL of the 1 mL ampule measured in a 0.5 mL tuberculin syringe.

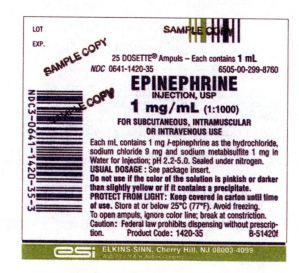

EXAMPLE 2:   Order: *Calcium gluconate 1 g IV stat*

Supply: *10 mL ampule of 10% calcium gluconate*

Step 1.   Convert: 10% calcium gluconate = 10 g in 100 mL.

Order: Calcium gluconate 1 g

Supply: 10 mL ampule of calcium gluconate 10% = 10 g in 100 mL

NOTE: "10 mL ampule" simply refers to the volume size of the ampule. The 10% = 10 g per 100 mL.

Step 2.   Think: If there are 10 g in 100 mL and you want to give 1 g or one-tenth of the supply, then you want to give one-tenth of 100 mL or 10 mL.

Step 3. Calculate: $\dfrac{\text{Dosage on hand}}{\text{Amount on hand}} = \dfrac{\text{Dosage desired}}{\text{X Amount desired}}$

$$\dfrac{10\text{ g}}{100\text{ mL}} \underset{\times}{\overset{\times}{\rightleftarrows}} \dfrac{1\text{ g}}{\text{X mL}}$$

$$10\text{X} = 100$$

$$\dfrac{10\text{X}}{10} = \dfrac{100}{10}$$

$$\text{X} = 10\text{ mL}$$

Give 10 mL or all of the 10 mL ampule measured in a 10-cc syringe.

review set 26 _____

Calculate the amount you will prepare for one dose.

1. Order: Magnesium sulfate 4 g IV
   Supply: 10 mL vials of 20% magnesium
      sulfate solution
   Give: _____

2. Order: Adrenalin 0.5 mg SC q.3h p.r.n.
   Supply: 30 mL vial of epinephrine
      (Adrenalin) 1:2000
   Give: _____

3. Order: Epinephrine 0.3 mg IM
   Supply: Epinephrine solution 1: 1000
   Give: _____

4. Order: Prostigmin 0.25 mg IM
   Supply: Prostigmin 1:2000 solution
   Give: _____

5. Order: Calcium gluconate gr viiss IV
   Supply: Calcium gluconate 25%
      solution
   Give: _____

   Watch this one, it's a little tricky.

   HINT: Convert gr to g first.

After completing these problems, see page 306 to check your answers.

critical thinking skills

Insulin errors are all too common in nursing practice. Let's look at an example in which the nurse was careless in preparing two types of insulin in the same syringe.

■ error 1

Drawing up the wrong amount of insulin.

possible scenario

Suppose the physician ordered Humulin R insulin 20 units mixed with Humulin N insulin 40 units to be administered before breakfast. The nurse selected the vials of Humulin R and Humulin N from the medication drawer and injected 20 units of air in the Humulin N vial and 40 units of air in the Humulin R vial, drew up 40 units of Humulin R and then drew up 20 units of Humulin N. The nurse gave the AM dose of insulin without having the dose double checked by another nurse (as required by hospital policy).

potential outcome

The patient received the incorrect dose of insulin because the nurse drew up 40 units of Humulin R and 20 units of Humulin N instead of the dosage that was ordered: 20 units of Humulin R and 40 units of Humulin N. Because the patient received too much short-acting insulin (twice the amount ordered), the patient would likely show signs of hypoglycemia such as shakiness, confusion, and diaphoresis.

prevention

This error could have been avoided had the nurse been more careful checking the label of the insulin vial and comparing the label to the order. Had the nurse checked the label three times as taught in nursing school, this error would not have occurred. In addition, had the nurse asked another nurse to double-check her as she was drawing up the insulin, this error could have been avoided. Such hospital policies and procedures are written to protect the patient and the nurse.

critical thinking skills

Many insulin errors occur when the nurse fails to clarify an incomplete order. Let's look at an example of an insulin error when the order did not include the type of insulin to be given.

■ error 2

Failing to clarify an insulin order when the type of insulin is not specified.

possible scenario

Suppose the physician wrote an insulin order this way:

Humulin insulin 50 U ā breakfast

Since the physician did not specify the type of insulin, the nurse assumed it was Regular insulin and noted that on the medication administration record. Suppose the patient was given the Regular insulin for three days. On the morning of the third day, the patient developed signs of hypoglycemia (low blood glucose), including shakiness, tremors, confusion, and sweating.

potential outcome

A stat blood glucose would likely reveal a dangerously low glucose level. The patient would be given a glucose infusion to increase the blood sugar. The nurse may not have realized the error until she and the doctor checked the original order and found that the incomplete order had been filled in by the nurse. When the doctor did not specify the type of insulin, the nurse assumed the physician meant Regular, which is short-acting, when in fact intermediate-acting NPH insulin was desired.

prevention

This error could have been avoided by remembering all the essential components of an insulin order: species, type of insulin (such as Regular or NPH), the amount to give in units, and the frequency. When you fill in an incomplete order, you are essentially practicing medicine without a license. This would be a clear malpractice incident. It does not make sense to put you and your patient in such jeopardy. A simple phone call would clarify the situation for everyone involved.

critical thinking skills

Insulin errors are very likely to occur if the correct syringe is not used. Let's look at an example in which the nurse selects the incorrect syringe to give insulin.

■ error 3

Selecting the wrong syringe to give insulin.

possible scenario

Suppose the physician ordered 10 units of Novolin R insulin for a patient with a blood glucose of 300. The nurse selected the Novolin R from the patient's medication drawer and selected a tuberculin syringe to administer the dose, even though insulin syringes were available. The nurse looked at the syringe for the 10-unit mark and was confused as to how much should have been drawn up. The nurse finally decided to draw up 1 mL of insulin into the tuberculin syringe, administered the dose, and then began to question whether the correct dosage was administered. The nurse called the supervisor for advice.

potential outcome

The patient would have received 10 times the correct dosage of insulin. Because this was a short-acting insulin, the patient would likely show signs of severe hypoglycemia, such as loss of consciousness and seizures. The likelihood of a successful outcome is questionable.

prevention

This insulin error should never occur. It is obvious that the nurse did not use Step 2 of the three-step method. The nurse did not stop to think of the reasonable dosage. If so, the nurse would have realized that 1 mL = 100 U, not 10 U; 10 U is $\frac{1}{10}$, or 0.1 mL.

If you are unsure of what you are doing, you need to ask before you act. Insulin is best given in an insulin syringe only. The likelihood of the nurse needing to give insulin in a TB syringe because an insulin syringe was unavailable is almost nonexistent today. In our scenario, insulin syringes were available, but the nurse chose the incorrect syringe. Whenever you are in doubt you should ask for help. If the nurse had asked another nurse to double check the dosage, the error could have been found before the patient received the wrong dosage of insulin. After giving the insulin, it may be too late to rectify the error.

Many injection medication errors occur by not reading the directions on the label for the correct dilution. Let's look at an example in which the nurse did not select the correct dilution for the amount of medication to be given.

■ error 4

Choosing the incorrect dilution for injection.

possible scenario

Suppose a physician ordered 1,000,000 U of Penicillin G IM stat for a patient with a severe staph infection. Look at the label of the medication available on hand.

The nurse in a hurry to give the stat medication selected the first concentration given on the label: 100,000 Units/mL concentration. Next the nurse calculated the dosage using ratio-proportion.

$$\frac{100,000 \text{ U}}{1 \text{ mL}} = \frac{1,000,000 \text{ U}}{X \text{ mL}}$$

$$100,000X = 1,000,000$$

$$\frac{100,000X}{100,000} = \frac{1,000,000}{100,000}$$

$$X = 10 \text{ mL}$$

The nurse added 9.6 mL to the vial and drew up 10 mL of medication. It was not until the nurse drew up the 10 mL that the error was recognized. The nurse realized that 10 mL IM should not be administered in one or even in two injection sites. The nurse called the pharmacy for another vial of Penicillin G and prepared the dose again, using 1.6 mL of diluent for a concentration of 500,000 Units/mL. To give 1,000,000 U the nurse easily calculated to give 2 mL, which was a safe volume of medication for IM injection in adults.

potential outcome

Had the nurse given the 10-mL intramuscular injection, the patient would likely have developed an abscess at the site due to the excessive volume of medication being given into the muscle. The patient's hospital stay would likely have been lengthened. Further, the nurse and the hospital may have faced a malpractice suit. The alternative would have been to divide the dose into four injections. Although the patient would have received the correct dosage, to give four injections would have been poor nursing judgment.

prevention

This type of error could have been prevented had the nurse read the label carefully for the correct amount of diluent for the dosage of medication to be prepared. Had the nurse read the label carefully the first time he or she prepared the medication, he or she would have prevented having to waste both the medication and valuable time in preparing a stat dose for injection. Additionally, if the nurse had used Step 2 of the three-step method, he or she would have realized sooner (before preparing it) that 10 mL would be an unreasonable volume for an IM injection.

Summary

You are now prepared to solve most of the dosage calculations you will encounter in your health care career. Oral and parenteral drug orders, written in the forms presented thus far, account for the largest percentage of prescriptions. You have learned to think through the process from order to supply to amount administered and to use the ratio-proportion dosage calculation method.

Work the practice problems for Chapter 8. After completing the practice problems, you should feel comfortable and confident working dosage calculations. If not, seek additional instruction. Concentrate on accuracy. Remember, one error in dosage calculation can be a serious mistake for your patient.

practice problems—chapter 8

Calculate the amount you will prepare for one dose. Indicate the syringe you will select to measure the medication.

1. Order: Demerol 20 mg IM q.3–4h p.r.n.
    Supply: Demerol 50 mg/cc
    Give: _____   Select _____ syringe

2. Order: Morphine sulfate 15 mg IM stat
    Supply: Morphine sulfate gr $\frac{1}{4}$ per mL
    Give: _____   Select _____ syringe

3. Order: Lanoxin 0.6 mg IV
    Supply: Lanoxin 500 mcg/2 mL
    Give: _____   Select _____ syringe

4. Order: Vistaril 15 mg IM stat
    Supply: Vistaril 25 mg/mL
    Give: _____   Select _____ syringe

5. Order: Penicillin G 500,000 U
    Supply: Penicillin G 1,000,000 U in 10 mL vial
    Directions: Add 3.6 mL diluent and each mL = 250,000 U
    Give: _____   Select _____ syringe

6. Order: Cleocin 300 mg IM q.i.d.
    Supply: Cleocin 0.6 g = 4 mL
    Give: _____   Select _____ syringe

7. Order: Isuprel 3 mg IV drip in 500 mL dextrose and water
   Supply: Isuprel 1 mg = 5 mL
   Add: _____ to IV   Select_____ syringe

8. Order: Ampicillin 500 mg IM q.4h
   Supply: Polycillin N (ampicillin) 500 mg
   Directions: Reconstitute with 1.8 mL diluent for volume of 2 mL with concentration of 250 mg/mL.
   Give: _____   Select_____ syringe

9. Order: Potassium chloride 30 mEq added to each 1000 mL IV fluids
   Supply: 30 mL multiple dose vial potassium chloride 2 mEq/mL
   Give: _____   Select_____ syringe

10. Order: Atarax 40 mg IM p.r.n.
    Supply: Atarax 50 mg/cc
    Give: _____   Select_____ syringe

11. Order: Valium 5 mg IM q.4–6h p.r.n., restlessness
    Supply: Valium 10 mg/2 cc
    Give: _____   Select_____ syringe

12. Order: Tigan 100 mg IM q.6h p.r.n., nausea and vomiting
    Supply: Tigan 200 mg = 2 mL
    Give: _____   Select_____ syringe

13. Order: Dilantin 25 mg IV q.8h
    Supply: Dilantin 100 mg/2 mL ampule
    Give: _____   Select_____ syringe

14. Order: Atropine gr $\frac{1}{100}$ IM on call to O.R.
    Supply: Atropine 0.4 mg/mL
    Give: _____   Select_____ syringe

15. Order: Valium 3 mg IV stat
    Supply: Valium 10 mg/2 mL
    Give: _____   Select_____ syringe

16. Order: Heparin 6000 U SC q.12h
    Supply: Heparin 10,000 U/mL vial
    Give: _____   Select_____ syringe

17. Order: Tobramycin sulfate 75 mg IM q.8h
    Supply: Nebcin (tobramycin sulfate) 80 mg/2 mL
    Give: _____   Select_____ syringe

18. Order: Morphine sulfate gr $\frac{1}{10}$ IM q.3h p.r.n., pain
    Supply: Morphine sulfate 10 mg/cc ampule
    Give: _____   Select_____ syringe

19. Order: Atropine gr $\frac{1}{150}$ IM on call to O.R.
    Supply: Atropine 0.4 mg/cc
    Give: _____   Select_____ syringe

20. Order: Terramycin 120 mg IM q.d.
    Supply: Terramycin 100 mg/mL
    Give: _____   Select_____ syringe

21. Order: Ancef 500 mg IV q.6h
    Supply: Ancef 1g
    Directions: Reconstitute with 2.5 mL diluent to yield 3.0 mL = 330 mg/mL.
    Give: _____   Select _____ syringe

22. Order: Garamycin 40 mg IM q.8h
    Supply: Garamycin 80 mg = 2 mL
    Give: _____   Select _____ syringe

23. Order: Demerol 60 mg IM q.3h p.r.n., pain
    Supply: Demerol 75 mg = 1.5 cc
    Give: _____   Select _____ syringe

24. Order: Demerol 35 mg IM q.4h p.r.n., pain
    Supply: Demerol 50 mg = 1 cc
    Give: _____   Select _____ syringe

25. Order: Vitamin B_{12} 0.75 mg IM q.d.
    Supply: Vitamin B_{12} 1000 mcg/mL
    Give: _____   Select _____ syringe

26. Order: Aquamephyton 15 mg IM stat
    Supply: Aquamephyton 10 mg per mL
    Give: _____   Select _____ syringe

27. Order: Phenergan 35 mg IM q.4h p.r.n., nausea
    Supply: Phenergan 50 mg = 1 cc
    Give: _____   Select _____ syringe

28. Order: Heparin 8000 U SC stat
    Supply: Heparin 10,000 U = 1 cc
    Give: _____   Select _____ syringe

29. Order: Morphine sulfate gr $\frac{1}{10}$ SC q.4h p.r.n.
    Supply: Morphine sulfate 6 mg = 1 cc
    Give: _____   Select _____ syringe

30. Order: Cefadyl 750 mg IV PB in 50 mL D_5W q.6h
    Supply: Cefadyl 2 g
    Directions: Reconstitute with 10 mL diluent and 1 g = 5 mL.
    Give: _____   Select _____ syringe

31. Order: Omnipen N 100 mg IM q.8h
    Supply: Omnipen N 125 mg
    Directions: Reconstitute with 1 mL of sterile water
    Give: _____   Select _____ syringe

32. Order: Lanoxin 0.4 mg IV stat
    Supply: Lanoxin 500 mcg/2 cc
    Give: _____   Select _____ syringe

33. Order: Lasix 60 mg IV stat
    Supply: Lasix 20 mg per 2 mL ampule
    Give: _____   Select _____ syringe

34. Order: Heparin 4000 U SC q.6h
    Supply: Heparin 5000 U = 1 mL
    Give: _____   Select _____ syringe

35. Order: Apresoline 30 mg IV
    Supply: Hydralazine (Apresoline) 20 mg per mL
    Give: _____   Select _____ syringe

36. Order: Calcium gluconate 0.5 g IV stat
    Supply: Calcium gluconate 10%
    Give: _____   Select _____ syringe

37. Order: Potassium penicillin G 400,000 U IM qd × 10 days
    Supply: 10 cc reconstituted vial potassium penicillin G, 300,000 U = 1 mL
    Give: _____   Select _____ syringe

38. Order: Calan 2.5 mg IV push, stat
    Supply: Calan 10 mg = 4 mL
    Give: _____   Select _____ syringe

39. Order: Heparin 3500 U SC q.12h
    Supply: Heparin 5000 U = 1 mL
    Give: _____   Select _____ syringe

40. Order: Neostigmine 0.5 mg IM t.i.d.
    Supply: Neostigmine 1:2000
    Give: _____   Select _____ syringe

41. Order: KCl 60 mEq added to 1000 mL IV fluid
    Supply: KCl 2 mEq = 1 mL
    Give: _____   Select _____ syringe

42. Order: 16 U of U-100 Novolin R Regular insulin SC ac
    Supply: U-100 insulin and standard 100 U and Lo-Dose 50 U and 30 U insulin syringes
    Give: _____   Select _____ syringe

43. Order: 70 U of U-100 Humulin R Regular insulin SC stat
    Supply: U-100 insulin and standard 100 U and Lo-Dose 50 U and 30 U insulin syringes
    Give: _____   Select _____ syringe

44. Order: 25 U of U-100 Novolin N NPH insulin SC a.c. breakfast
    Supply: U-100 insulin and standard 100 U and Lo-Dose 50 U and 30 U insulin syringes
    Give: _____   Select _____ syringe

Calculate one dose of each of the drug orders numbered 45–62. Draw an arrow indicating the calibration line on the syringe that corresponds to the dose to be administered. Identify each insulin for combination insulin dosages. The labels provided on pages 171–174 are the medications you have available. Indicate dosages that need to be divided.

45. Vistaril 35 mg IM stat
    Give: _____

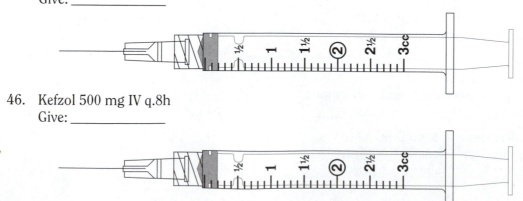

46. Kefzol 500 mg IV q.8h
    Give: _____

47. Nebcin 65 mg IM q.8h
    Give: _____

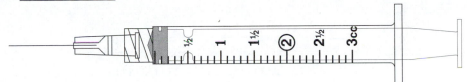

48. Carbenicillin disodium 2 g IM q.6h
    Give: _____

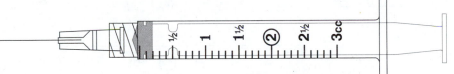

49. Vitamin B$_{12}$ 0.5 mg IM stat
    Give: _____

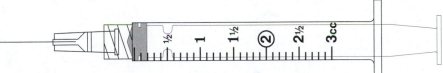

50. Procaine penicillin G 400,000 U IM q.d.
    Give: _____

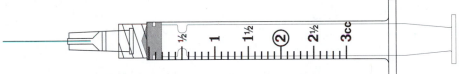

51. Humulin R Regular U-100 insulin 22 units SC stat
    Give: _____

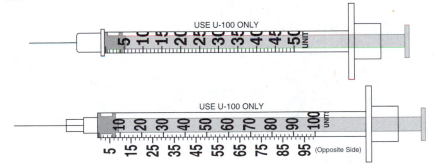

52. Bentyl 15 mg IM q.i.d.
    Give: _____

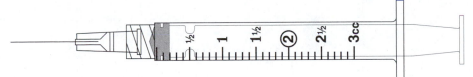

53. Heparin 8000 U SC q.12h
    Give: _____

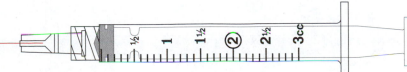

54. Tazidime 300 mg IM q.12h
    Give: _____

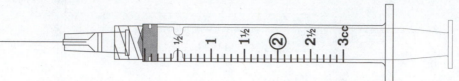

55. Moxam 0.5 g IM q.8h
    Give: _____

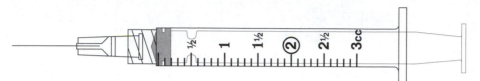

56. Methylprednisolone 200 mg IM stat
    Give: _____

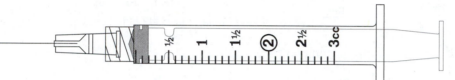

57. Nafcillin 500 mg IM q.6h
    Give: _____

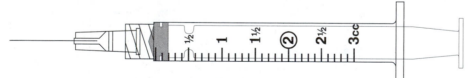

58. Atropine gr $\frac{1}{300}$ SC stat
    Give: _____

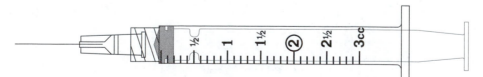

59. Terramycin 60 mg IM q.12h
    Give: _____

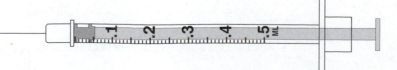

60. Bricanyl 0.25 mg SC q.30 min × 2 doses
    Give: _____

61. Novolin R Regular U-100 insulin 32 units with U-100 Novolin N NPH insulin 54 units SC before breakfast

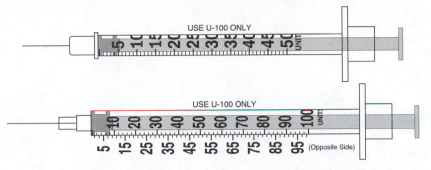

62. Novolin 70/30 U-100 70% NPH + 30% regular insulin 46 units SC before dinner

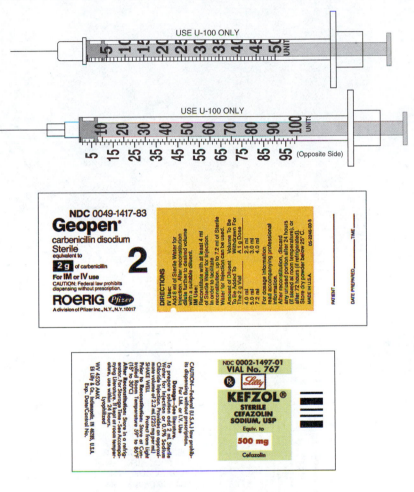

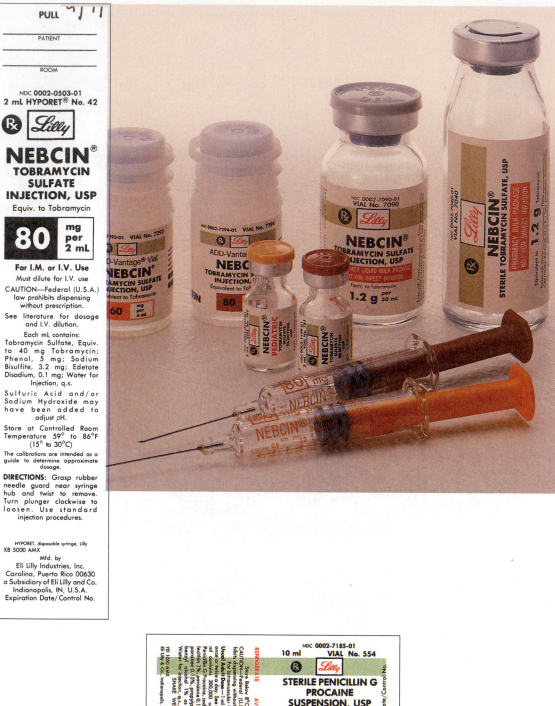

PULL _____

PATIENT _____

ROOM _____

NDC 0002-0503-01
2 mL HYPORET® No. 42

℞ Lilly

NEBCIN®
TOBRAMYCIN
SULFATE
INJECTION, USP
Equiv. to Tobramycin

80 mg per 2 mL

For I.M. or I.V. Use

Must dilute for I.V. use

CAUTION—Federal (U.S.A.) law prohibits dispensing without prescription.

See literature for dosage and I.V. dilution.

Each mL contains: Tobramycin Sulfate, Equiv. to 40 mg Tobramycin; Phenol, 5 mg; Sodium Bisulfite, 3.2 mg; Edetate Disodium, 0.1 mg; Water for Injection, q.s.

Sulfuric Acid and/or Sodium Hydroxide may have been added to adjust pH.

Store at Controlled Room Temperature 59° to 86°F (15° to 30°C)

The calibrations are intended as a guide to determine approximate dosage.

DIRECTIONS: Grasp rubber needle guard near syringe hub and twist to remove. Turn plunger clockwise to loosen. Use standard injection procedures.

HYPORET, disposable syringe, Lilly
XB 5000 AMX

Mfd. by
Eli Lilly Industries, Inc.
Carolina, Puerto Rico 00630
a Subsidiary of Eli Lilly and Co.
Indianapolis, IN, U.S.A.
Expiration Date/Control No.

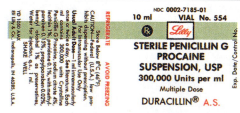

NDC 0002-7185-01
10 ml   VIAL No. 554

℞ Lilly

STERILE PENICILLIN G PROCAINE SUSPENSION, USP
300,000 Units per ml
Multiple Dose
DURACILLIN® A.S.

REFRIGERATE   AVOID FREEZING

Exp. Date/Control No.

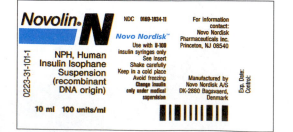

Novolin® N

Novo Nordisk™

NDC 0169-1834-11

NPH, Human Insulin Isophane Suspension (recombinant DNA origin)

10 ml   100 units/ml

0223-31-101-1

Use with U-100 insulin syringes only
See insert
Shake carefully
Keep in a cold place
Avoid freezing
Change insulin only under medical supervision

For information contact:
Novo Nordisk Pharmaceuticals Inc.
Princeton, NJ 08540

Manufactured by
Novo Nordisk A/S
DK-2880 Bagsvaerd,
Denmark

Exp. Date:
Control:

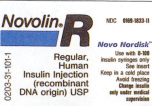
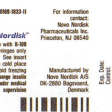

Novolin® R

Novo Nordisk™

NDC 0169-1833-11

Regular, Human Insulin Injection (recombinant DNA origin) USP

10 ml   100 units/ml

0203-31-101-1

Use with U-100 insulin syringes only
See insert
Keep in a cold place
Avoid freezing
Change insulin only under medical supervision

For information contact:
Novo Nordisk Pharmaceuticals Inc.
Princeton, NJ 08540

Manufactured by
Novo Nordisk A/S
DK-2880 Bagsvaerd,
Denmark

Exp. Date:
Control:

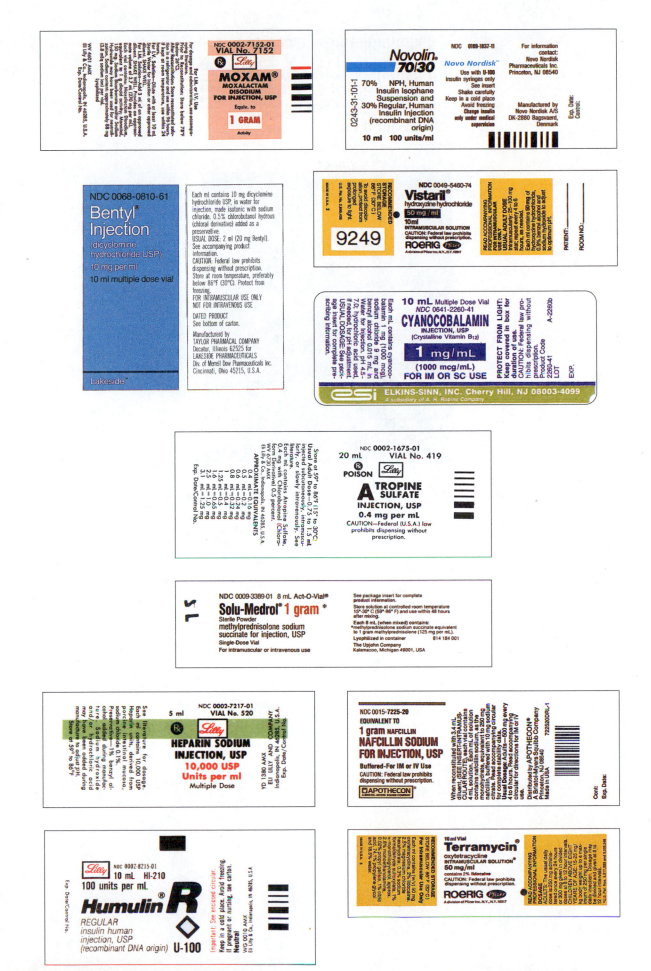

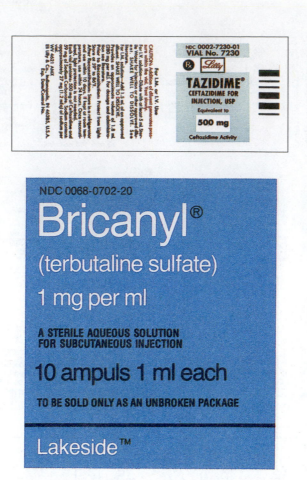

After completing these problems, see pages 323–326 to check your answers.

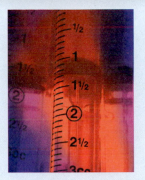

Using the Formula Method to Calculate Dosages

9

objectives

Upon mastery of Chapter 9, you will be able to calculate the dosages of drugs using the formula method. To accomplish this, you will also be able to:

■ Use the conversion factor method to convert all units of measurement to the same system and same size units.
■ Consider the reasonable amount of the drug to be administered.
■ Use the formula $\frac{D}{H} \times Q = X$ to calculate drug dosages.

You may prefer to calculate drug dosages by the formula method: $\frac{D}{H} \times Q = X$. It is presented here as an alternative to using the dosage calculation ratio-proportion method that you learned in Chapters 7 and 8.

If you preferred to perform conversions by the conversion factor method found in Chapter 3, then you will likely want to use the formula method to solve dosage problems. Try both methods: ratio-proportion and $\frac{D}{H} \times Q = X$. *Choose the one that is easiest and most logical to you.*

▶ **rule**   The formula method for dosage calculations is: $\frac{D}{H} \times Q = X$

$$\frac{Desired \text{ dosage}}{\text{Dosage you } have \text{ on hand}} \times Quantity \text{ you have on hand} = \text{Amount to give}$$

In this formula the *dosage desired* (D) is the same as the drug dosage ordered. The *dosage you have on hand* (H) and the *quantity you have on hand* (Q) represent the supply dosage or the concentration of the drug available to fill the order. Recall from Chapter 6 that the supply dosage or dosage strength may be per one, more than one, or less than one; such as 100 mg per one tablet or 125 mg per 5 mL.

The formula method is based on the same ratio and proportion you have already learned. Let's examine this.

Recall that the ratio for the drug you have on hand equals the ratio for the desired drug or $\frac{H}{Q} = \frac{D}{X}$ where H is the dosage you *have* on hand, Q is the *quantity* you have on hand, D is the dosage *desired*, and X is the *amount* you desire to give.

$$\frac{H}{Q} \diagdown \diagup \frac{D}{X}$$

$H \times X = D \times Q$ (Cross-multiply.)

$\frac{H \times X}{H} = \frac{D \times Q}{H}$ (Simplify.)

$X = \frac{D}{H} \times Q$

Therefore, the formula method is really just a shortcut to eliminate the steps of cross-multiplying and simplifying the two ratios.

For example, the physician *orders* 500 milligrams of Amoxil (amoxicillin) and you *have on hand* a drug labeled amoxicillin 250 mg per capsule. The formula method is:

$$\frac{D}{H} \times Q = X \qquad \text{(Amount to give)}$$

$$\frac{500 \text{ mg}}{250 \text{ mg}} \times 1 \text{ capsule} = X$$

$$X = \frac{500}{250} \text{ capsules}$$

$$X = 2 \text{ capsules}$$

Use the same three steps to calculate dosages learned in Chapters 7 and 8. Substitute the formula $\frac{D}{H} \times Q = X$ for the ratio-proportion dosage calculation in Step 3.

remember

1. **Convert**
2. **Think**
3. **Calculate:** $\frac{D}{H} \times Q = X$

EXAMPLE 1: Order: *Thorazine 15 mg IM stat*

Supply: *Thorazine (chlorpromazine) 25 mg per mL*

Step 1. Convert: No conversion necessary.

Step 2. Think: You want to give less than 1 mL; in fact, you want to give $\frac{15}{25}$ of a mL or $\frac{3}{5}$ mL or 0.6 mL.

Step 3. Calculate: $\frac{D}{H} \times Q = X$

$$\frac{15 \text{ mg}}{25 \text{ mg}} \times 1 \text{ mL} = X$$

$$\frac{15}{25} \text{ mL} = X$$

$$X = \frac{3}{5} = 0.6 \text{ mL}$$

EXAMPLE 2: Order: *Ritalin 15 mg p.o. q.d.*

Supply: *Ritalin 10 mg tablets*

Step 1. Convert: No conversion necessary.

Step 2. Think: You want to give more than one tablet. In fact, you want to give $1\frac{1}{2}$ times more or $1\frac{1}{2}$ tablets.

Step 3. Calculate: $\frac{D}{H} \times Q = X$

$$\frac{15 \text{ mg}}{10 \text{ mg}} \times 1 \text{ tab} = X$$

$$\frac{15}{10} \text{ tab} = X$$

$$X = 1\frac{1}{2} \text{ tablets}$$

EXAMPLE 3:   Order: *Motrin 0.6 g p.o. b.i.d.*

                    Available: *Motrin 300 mg tablets*

Step 1.   Convert: Equivalent 1 g = 1000 mg

              g → mg = larger → smaller: multiply

$$0.6 \times 1000 = 0.\underset{\curvearrowright}{600}. = 600 \text{ mg}$$

$$0.6 \text{ g} = 600 \text{ mg}$$

Step 2.   Think: You want to give twice the available dosage or 2 tablets.

Step 3.   Calculate: $\frac{D}{H} \times Q = X$

$$\frac{600 \text{ mg}}{300 \text{ mg}} \times 1 \text{ tablet} = X$$

$$X = 2 \text{ tablets}$$

EXAMPLE 4:   Order: *Phenobarbital suppository gr $\frac{1}{4}$ p.r.*

                    Supply: *Phenobarbital 15 mg per suppository*

Step 1.   Convert: Equivalent gr i = 60 mg

              gr → mg = larger → smaller: multiply

$$\frac{1}{4} \times 60 = 15 \text{ mg}$$

$$\text{gr} \frac{1}{4} = 15 \text{ mg}$$

Step 2.   Think: It is obvious. You want to administer one suppository.

Step 3.   Calculate: $\frac{D}{H} \times Q = X$

$$\frac{15 \text{ mg}}{15 \text{ mg}} \times 1 \text{ suppository} = X$$

$$X = 1 \text{ suppository}$$

EXAMPLE 5:   Order: *Lasix 15 mg IM stat*

                    Supply: *Lasix 20 mg/2 mL*

Step 1.   Convert: No conversions necessary.

Step 2.   Think: You want to give more than 1 mL and less than 2 mL.

Step 3.   Calculate: $\frac{D}{H} \times Q = X$

$$\frac{15 \text{ mg}}{20 \text{ mg}} \times 2 \text{ mL} = X$$

$$\frac{30}{20} \text{ mL} = X$$

$$X = 1.5 \text{ mL}$$

quick review

- You cannot calculate drug dosages unless all units of measure are in the same system and the same size. Regardless of which method you use (formula or ratio-proportion), the first step is to always CONVERT, the second step is to always THINK or reason for the logical answer and the third step is to CALCULATE the amount to give.

review set 27 _____

Use the formula method to calculate the amount you will prepare for each dose.

1. Order: Premarin 1.25 mg p.o. q.d.
   Supply: Premarin 0.625 mg tablets
   Give: _____ tablet(s)

2. Order: Tagamet 150 mg p.o.
   Supply: Tagamet liquid 300 mg per 5 mL
   Give: _____ mL

3. Order: Thiamine 80 mg IM stat
   Supply: Thiamine 100 mg per 1 mL
   Give: _____ mL

4. Order: Demerol 35 mg IM q.4h p.r.n.
   Supply: Demerol 50 mg per 1 mL
   Give: _____ mL

5. Order: Lithium 12 mEq p.o. t.i.d.
   Supply: Lithium 8 mEq per 5 mL
   Give: _____ mL

6. Order: Ativan 2.4 mg IM h.s. p.r.n.
   Supply: Ativan 4 mg per 1 mL
   Give: _____ mL

7. Order: Prednisone 7.5 mg p.o. q.d.
   Supply: Prednisone 5 mg (scored) tablets
   Give: _____ tablet(s)

8. Order: Hydrochlorothiazide 30 mg p.o. b.i.d.
   Supply: Hydrochlorothiazide 50 mg/5 mL
   Give: _____ mL

9. Order: Theophylline oral solution 160 mg p.o. q.6h
   Supply: Theophylline oral solution 80 mg per 15 mL
   Give: _____ mL

10. Order: Tofranil 20 mg IM h.s.
    Supply: Tofranil 25 mg per 2 mL
    Give: _____ mL

11. Order: Indocin 15 mg p.o. t.i.d.
    Supply: Indocin Suspension 25 mg/5 mL
    Give: _____ mL

12. Order: Ativan 2 mg IM 2 hrs pre-op
    Supply: Ativan 4 mg per mL
    Give: _____ mL

13. Order: Luminal gr ss p.o. t.i.d. (30 mg)
    Supply: Phenobarbital (Luminal) 15 mg tablets
    Give: _____ tablet(s)

14. Order: Diabinese 125 mg p.o.
    Supply: Diabinese 100 mg or 250 mg (scored) tablets
    Give: _____ of _____ tablet(s)

15. Order: Thorazine 60 mg IM stat
    Supply: Thorazine 25 mg per mL
    Give: _____ mL

16. Order: Synthroid 0.15 mg p.o. q.d.
    Supply: Synthroid 75 mcg tablets
    Give: _____ tablet(s)

17. Order: Choledyl Elixir 160 mg p.o. q.6h
    Supply: 100 mg per 5 mL
    Give: _____ mL

18. Order: Solu-Medrol 100 mg IV q.6h
    Supply: Methylprednisolone (Solu-Medrol) 80 mg per mL
    Give: _____ mL

19. Order: Prolixin Elixir 8 mg p.o. q.8h
    Supply: Prolixin Elixir 2.5 mg per 5 mL
    Give: _____ mL

20. Order: Trimox 350 mg p.o. q.8h
    Supply: Amoxicillin (Trimox) 250 mg per 5 mL
    Give: _____ mL

After completing these problems, see pages 306 and 307 to check your answers.

For more practice, recalculate the amount you will prepare for each dose in Review Sets 20–23, using the formula method.

critical thinking skills

Medication errors are often attributed to carelessness in the calculation of the dosage. Let's look at an example to identify the nurse's error.

■ *error*

Using the formula method of calculation incorrectly.

possible scenario

Suppose the physician ordered Keflex 80 mg p.o. q.i.d. for a patient with an upper respiratory infection and the Keflex is supplied in an oral suspension with 250 mg per 5 mL. The nurse decided to calculate the dosage using the $\frac{D}{H} \times Q = X$ formula method and set up the problem this way:

$$\frac{250 \text{ mg}}{80 \text{ mg}} \times 5 \text{ mL} = X$$

$$\frac{1250}{80} \text{ mL} = X$$

$$X = 15.6 \text{ mL}$$

The nurse gave the patient 15.6 mL of Keflex for two doses. The next day as the nurse prepared the medication in the medication room, another nurse observed the nurse pour 15.6 mL in a medicine cup and asked what he was giving. Not until the nurse was questioned about the dosage did he realize the error.

potential outcome

The patient would likely have developed complications from overdosage of Keflex such as renal impairment and liver damage. When the physician was notified of the errors, he would likely have ordered the medication be discontinued, and the patient's blood urea nitrogen (BUN) and liver enzymes be monitored. An incident report would be filed and the patient notified of the error.

prevention

This type of calculation error occurred because the nurse applied the formula method incorrectly. It is important to remember the correct interpretation of the components of the formula: D = dosage *desired*, H = dosage *on hand*, Q = *quantity* of the dosage *on hand*, and X = *amount to give*.

$$\frac{D}{H} \times Q = X$$

$$\frac{80 \text{ mg}}{250 \text{ mg}} \times 5 \text{ mL} = X$$

$$X = \frac{400}{250} \text{ mL}$$

$$X = 1.6 \text{ mL}$$

In addition, had the nurse used Step 2 in the calculation process, the nurse would have realized the correct dosage would be less than 5 mL, not more. Consider this: you should estimate the dosage is $\frac{80}{250}$ or less than half of 5 mL. In this scenario the patient would have received more than nine times the amount of medication ordered by the physician each time the nurse committed the error.

Obviously the nurse did not think through for the logical amount, and either miscalculated the dose three times or did not bother to calculate the dose again, preventing identification of the error. The formula method should be used to double-check your thinking, rather than the other way around. Remember to *think first*, then use the formula method to calculate the dosage.

practice problems—chapter 9

Use the formula method to calculate the amount you would prepare for each dose.

1. Order: Lactulose 30 g in 100 mL fluid rectally t.i.d.
   Supply: Lactulose 3.33 g per 5 mL
   Give: _____ mL in 100 mL

2. Order: Penicillin G potassium 500,000 U IM q.i.d.
   Supply: Penicillin G potassium 5,000,000 U per 20 mL
   Give: _____ mL

3. Order: Keflex 80 mg p.o. q.i.d.
   Supply: Keflex oral suspension 250 mg per 5 ml
   Give: _____ mL

4. Order: Amoxicillin 125 mg p.o. q.i.d.
   Supply: Amoxicillin 250 mg/5 mL
   NOTE: You are giving home care instructions.
   Give: _____ t

5. Order: Benadryl 25 mg IM stat
    Supply: Diphenhydramine (Benadryl) 10 mg per 1 mL
    Give: _____ mL

6. Order: Benadryl 40 mg p.o. stat
    Supply: Diphenhydramine (Benadryl) 12.5 mg per 5 mL
    Give: _____ mL

7. Order: Penicillin G potassium 350,000 U IM b.i.d.
    Supply: Penicillin G potassium 500,000 U per 2 mL
    Give: _____ mL

8. Order: Valium 3.5 mg IM q.6h p.r.n.
    Supply: Valium 10 mg per 2 mL
    Give: _____ mL

9. Order: Tobramycin sulfate 90 mg IM q.8h.
    Supply: Nebcin (tobramycin sulfate) 80 mg per 2 mL
    Give: _____ mL

10. Order: Heparin 2,500 U SC b.i.d.
    Supply: Heparin 20,000 U per mL
    Give: _____ mL

11. Order: Compazine 8 mg IM q.6h p.r.n., nausea
    Supply: Compazine 10 mg per 2 mL
    Give: _____ mL

12. Order: Gentamycin 60 mg IM q.6h
    Supply: Garamycin (gentamycin) 80 mg per 2 mL
    Give: _____ mL

13. Order: Pipracil 500 mg IM b.i.d.
    Supply: Pipracil 1 g per 2.5 mL
    Give: _____ mL

14. Order: Nilstat Oral Suspension 250,000 U p.o. q.i.d.
    Supply: Nilstat Oral Suspension 100,000 U per mL
    Give: _____ mL

15. Order: Ilosone 80 mg p.o. q.4h
    Supply: Ilosone 250 mg per 5 mL
    Give: _____ mL

16. Order: Potassium 10 mEq p.o. stat
    Supply: Potassium 20 mEq per 15 mL
    Give: _____ mL

17. Order: Unipen 400 mg IM q.6h
    Supply: Nafcillin (Unipen) 1 g per 4 mL
    Give: _____ mL

18. Order: Synthroid 150 mcg p.o. daily
    Supply: Synthroid 0.075 mg tablets
    Give: _____ tablet(s)

19. Order: Amoxicillin 400 mg p.o. q.8h
    Supply: Amoxicillin 250 mg/5 mL
    Give: _____ mL

20. Order: Dilantin 225 mg IV stat
     Supply: Dilantin 50 mg per mL
     Give: _____ mL

21. Order: Elixophyllin 160 mg p.o. q.6h
     Supply: Elixophyllin 80 mg per 15 mL
     Give: _____ mL

22. Order: Thorazine 35 mg IM stat
     Supply: Chlorpromazine (Thorazine) 25 mg/mL
     Give: _____ mL

23. Order: Add potassium chloride 30 mEq to 1000 mL D_5 W IV
     Supply: KCl (potassium chloride) 40 mEq per 20 mL
     Add: _____ mL KCl to 1000 mL D_5 W

24. Order: Phenergan 25 mg via nasogastric tube h.s.
     Supply: Phenergan 6.25 mg per 5 mL
     Give: _____ mL

25. Order: Ceclor 300 mg p.o. t.i.d.
     Supply: Ceclor 125 mg per 5 mL
     Give: _____ mL

After completing these problems, see pages 326 and 327 to check your answers.

For more practice, recalculate the amount you will prepare for each dose in the Practice Problems for Chapters 7 and 8 using the formula method.

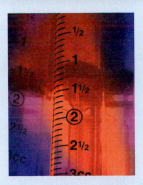

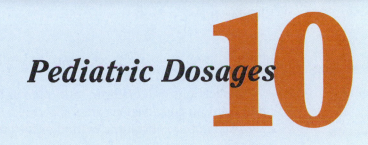

Pediatric Dosages

10

objectives

Upon mastery of Chapter 10, you will be able to calculate the dosages of drugs for children and to double-check pediatric drug orders. To accomplish this you will also be able to:

- Convert pounds to kilograms.
- Determine the recommended safe pediatric dosage per pound or kilogram of body weight from a reputable drug resource (such as standing or routine doctor's order, or drug reference book).
- Compute the amount of drug to be administered per pound or per kilogram of body weight.
- Compute the safe amount of drug to be administered according to the child's body surface area (BSA).

Only a doctor, dentist, or nurse practitioner (in some states) may prescribe the dosage of medications. However, before administering a drug, the nurse should know if the ordered dosage is safe. Those who administer drugs to patients are legally responsible for recognizing incorrect dosage and alerting the physician. The one who administers an incorrect dosage is just as responsible for the patient's safety as the one who prescribes it. For the protection of the patient and yourself, you must familiarize yourself with the usual adult dosage of drugs, or consult a reputable drug reference, such as the *Hospital Formulary* or the *Physicians' Desk Reference*. A drug book especially written for use in pediatrics is: Bindler, Ruth McGillis, and Howry, Linda Berner (1996) *Pediatric Drugs and Nursing Implications,* 2nd edition, Norwalk, CT: Appleton & Lange. There are also a variety of small pocket-size drug handbooks, especially suitable for use in pediatrics, such as Rowe, Peter C. (ed.) (1996) *Johns Hopkins Hospital: The Harriet Lane Handbook*, 14th edition, St. Louis: Mosby.

Dosages for infants and children are a fraction of the amount given adults, and are reduced in proportion to the weight, height, body surface area, age, and condition of the child. Since children are smaller than adults by weight, body size, and body surface area, they may require less medication than adults. Factors related to growth and development significantly affect the child's ability to metabolize and excrete drugs. Immaturity in the processes related to absorption, distribution, metabolism, or excretion can significantly alter the effects of a drug. Newborns and premature infants with immature enzyme systems in the liver, where most drugs are metabolized or broken down, have lower plasma concentrations of protein. Protein is important for binding with drugs. Without this binding action, more drug is in the infant's system. Also, newborns and premature infants can have immature kidney function. The kidneys are where most drugs are eliminated; therefore, these infants are especially susceptible to the harmful effects of medications.

Beyond the newborn period, many drugs are metabolized more quickly by the liver, which may necessitate even larger doses or more frequent administration compared with adults. As a result of increased metabolism in children, the effects of drugs may be achieved more quickly.

Administration of an incorrect dosage to adult patients is dangerous, but with a child the risk is even greater.

Medications ordered by mouth (p.o.) or by feeding tube (NG, GT) are often prepared in a liquid solution and given via an oral syringe. Oral tablets and capsules may need to be crushed and mixed in a small volume of fluid or food to assist the child in taking the medication. Remember to consult a drug reference regarding tablets and capsules that cannot be crushed.

Injections in children require the nurse to take into account the child's growth and development. Injections in infants, for example, are given in the *vastus lateralis* (lateral thigh) because this muscle is more developed than other sites generally used in adults. In addition, the maximum volume an infant can receive in one injection site is limited to 1 mL due to the child's smaller muscle mass. Consult a pediatric reference guide regarding site selection and maximum volume for injection before giving injections to children.

In this chapter, calculating safe dosages of p.o., IM, or IV medications for children is emphasized. Chapter 11 shows some of the equipment used for administering IV medications to children, and Chapter 12 emphasizes additional critical care IV calculations for both the child and the adult.

Body Weight Method

The most common, current method of administering the exact amount of medication that a child needs is to calculate the amount of drug according to the child's body weight. When the physician writes the drug order in this manner, it becomes the nurse's responsibility to weigh the child and then determine how much drug the child should receive. Usually the medication will be ordered according to the **amount of drug per kilogram (or pound) of body weight**. If you have the child's weight in pounds, it may be necessary to convert the pounds to kilograms. (Remember, 1 kg = 2.2 lb.)

> **rule** Ratio for recommended equivalent dosage per body weight equals ratio for desired dosage per body weight.

Usually the order will be given as a **total dosage per day** (24 hours) to be administered or divided over a specified number of doses. Refer to the label in Figure 10–1. Notice the "usual dose" instructions on the left side.

EXAMPLE 1: The recommended dose of Ceclor (Figure 10–1) is 20 mg per kg a day or 20 mg/kg/day in three divided doses. Based on this information, what dosage would a 20-pound child receive?

First, convert pounds to kilograms (1 kg = 2.2 lb).

$$\frac{1 \text{ kg}}{2.2 \text{ lb}} \quad \frac{X \text{ kg}}{20 \text{ lb}}$$

$$2.2X = 20$$

$$\frac{2.2X}{2.2} = \frac{20}{2.2}$$

$$X = 9 \text{ kg}$$

Then calculate the equivalent desired daily dosage based on the recommended dosage of 20 mg/kg.

$$\frac{20 \text{ mg}}{1 \text{ kg}} \quad \frac{X \text{ mg}}{9 \text{ kg}}$$

$$X = 9 \times 20 = 180 \text{ mg}$$

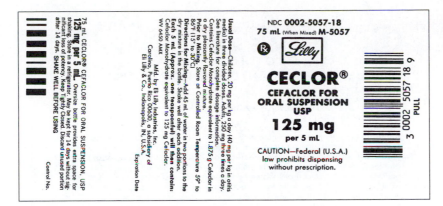

Fig. 10–1 Ceclor Label

The physician would order this daily dosage divided into three doses of $\frac{180}{3} = 60$ mg per dose.

The Ceclor available is 125 mg per 5 mL. Calculate one dose.

Apply the three steps to dosage calculation.

Order: *Ceclor 60 mg p.o. t.i.d.*

Supply: *Ceclor 125 mg/5 mL*

Step 1.　Convert: No conversion necessary.

Step 2.　Think: You want to give less than 5 mL. Estimate that you want to give approximately $\frac{1}{2}$ of 5 mL, since 60 is approximately $\frac{1}{2}$ of 125.

Step 3.　Calculate: $\dfrac{125\text{ mg}}{5\text{ mL}} \diagdown\!\!\!\diagup \dfrac{60\text{ mg}}{X\text{ mL}}$

$125X = 300$

$\dfrac{125X}{125} = \dfrac{300}{125}$

$X = \dfrac{300}{125} = 2.4$ mL

Or, apply the formula method to dosage calculations.

$\dfrac{D}{H} \times Q = \dfrac{60\text{ mg}}{125\text{ mg}} \times 5\text{ mL} = \dfrac{300}{125} = \dfrac{12}{5} = 2\frac{2}{5} = 2.4$ mL

EXAMPLE 2:　The physician orders *Demerol 0.5 mg/lb IM* as a preoperative medication (see Figure 10–2). The child weighs 30 lb. How many milligrams should the child receive? You have *Demerol 50 mg/mL* available. How many milliliters would you give?

No conversions for lb to kg are necessary, since the order is per pound of body weight and the child's weight is given in pounds.

Calculate the equivalent desired dosage based on the recommended dosage of 0.5 mg/lb.

$\dfrac{0.5\text{ mg}}{1\text{ lb}} \diagdown\!\!\!\diagup \dfrac{X\text{ mg}}{30\text{ lb}}$

$X = 30 \times 0.5$

$X = 15$ mg

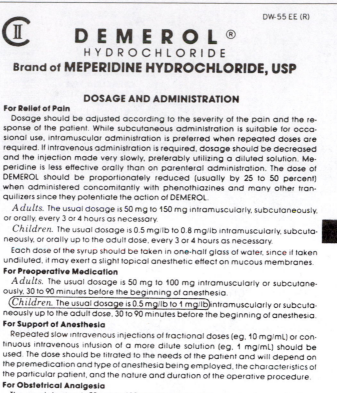

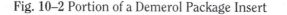

Fig. 10–2 Portion of a Demerol Package Insert

Apply the 3 steps to dosage calculation.

Order: *Demerol 15 mg IM pre op on call*

Supply: *Demerol 50 mg/mL*

Step 1.   Convert: No conversion necessary.

Step 2.   Think: You want to give less than 1 mL.

Step 3.   Calculate: $\dfrac{50\ mg}{1\ mL} \overset{\times}{\longleftrightarrow} \dfrac{15\ mg}{X\ mL}$

$50X = 15$

$\dfrac{50X}{50} = \dfrac{15}{50}$

$X = \dfrac{\overset{3}{\cancel{15}}}{\underset{10}{\cancel{50}}} = 0.3\ mL$

Or, apply the formula method to dosage calculations.

$\dfrac{D}{H} \times Q = \dfrac{15\ mg}{50\ mg} \times 1\ mL = \dfrac{3}{10} = 0.3\ mL$

This is a child's dose and a small dose; measure it in a 0.5 mL tuberculin syringe.

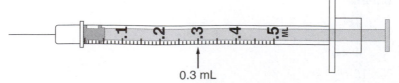

0.3 mL

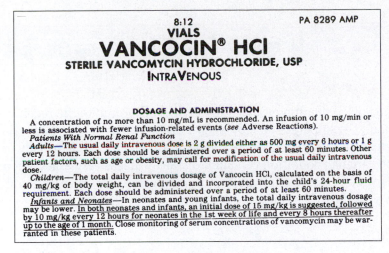

Fig. 10–3 Portion of a Vancocin Package Insert

EXAMPLE 3: The doctor orders *Vancocin (vancomycin) 10 mg/kg q.12h IV* for a newborn (neonate) as recommended in the package insert (Figure 10–3). If the infant weighs 4000 g, how many milligrams should be given per dose?

First, convert grams to kilograms (1 kg = 1000 g)

$$\frac{1 \text{ kg}}{1000 \text{ g}} \diagup\!\!\!\!\diagdown \frac{\text{X kg}}{4000 \text{ g}}$$

$$1000\text{X} = 4000$$

$$\frac{1000\text{X}}{1000} = \frac{4000}{1000}$$

$$\text{X} = 4 \text{ kg}$$

The child weighs 4 kilograms. Calculate the equivalent desired dosage based on the recommended dosage of 10 mg/kg.

$$\frac{10 \text{ mg}}{1 \text{ kg}} \diagup\!\!\!\!\diagdown \frac{\text{X mg}}{4 \text{ kg}}$$

$$\text{X} = 40 \text{ mg}$$

If the medication is supplied in a vial of 500 mg per 10 mL, how much should the infant receive per dose?

Order: *Vancocin 40 mg IM q. 12h*

Supply: *Vancocin 500 mg/10 mL*

Step 1. Convert: No conversion necessary.

Step 2. Think: You want to give less than 10 mL (MUCH LESS).

Step 3. Calculate: $\dfrac{500 \text{ mg}}{10 \text{ mL}} \diagup\!\!\!\!\diagdown \dfrac{40 \text{ mg}}{\text{X mL}}$

$$500\text{X} = 400$$

$$\frac{500\text{X}}{500} = \frac{400}{500}$$

$$\text{X} = \frac{400}{500} = \frac{4}{5} = 0.8 \text{ mL}$$

or, $\dfrac{\text{D}}{\text{H}} \times \text{Q} = \dfrac{40 \text{ mg}}{500 \text{ mg}} \times 10 \text{ mL} = \dfrac{400}{500} = \dfrac{4}{5} = 0.8 \text{ mL}$ measured in a tuberculin syringe

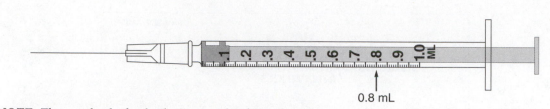

0.8 mL

NOTE: The method of calculating or checking dosages according to the recommended amount of the drug per pound or kilogram of body weight is most often used in pediatrics. However, there may be other situations when you will apply it for adults. This is usually in critical care settings when the patient's condition can only tolerate or needs very exact amounts of medication. Ordinarily, in such cases, the medication is administered by the parenteral routes (IM or IV) by which it is possible to measure most precisely.

Safe Dosages

As noted at the beginning of this chapter, it is the nurse's responsibility, as well as the physician's, to be sure the dosage prescribed and administered is reasonable and safe. When a pediatric medicine is ordered by a specific dosage, verify the amount against the recommended dosage.

EXAMPLE 1:   Order: *Ampicillin 125 mg IM q.6h*

Is this dosage safe? The child weighs 40 pounds.

Look at the label. Notice that the recommended dosage for children is "25 to 50 mg/kg/day in equally divided doses at 6-hour intervals."

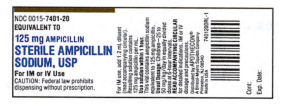

First, calculate the child's weight in kilograms.

$$\frac{1 \text{ kg}}{2.2 \text{ lb}} \quad \frac{X \text{ kg}}{40 \text{ lb}}$$

$$2.2X = 40$$

$$\frac{2.2X}{2.2} = \frac{40}{2.2}$$

$$X = 18 \text{ kg}$$

The child weighs 18 kilograms. Calculate the equivalent desired *daily* dosage based on the recommended minimum dosage of 25 mg/kg/day.

$$\frac{25 \text{ mg}}{1 \text{ kg}} \quad \frac{X \text{ mg}}{18 \text{ kg}}$$

$$X = 25 \times 18$$

$X = 450$ mg divided into 4 q.6h doses: $\frac{450}{4} = 112.5$ mg/dose for the minimum dose.

The maximum dosage is 50 mg/kg/day.

$$\frac{50 \text{ mg}}{1 \text{ kg}} \quad \frac{X \text{ mg}}{18 \text{ kg}}$$

$$X = 50 \times 18$$

$X = 900$ mg; divided into 4 q.6h doses: $\frac{900}{4} = 225$ mg/dose for the maximum dose.

Therefore, the dosage range is 112.5–225 mg/dose. The order of 125 mg is within the recommended range and is safe.

Look at the label again. How would you reconstitute this ampicillin and how much would you prepare to administer to the child? You would add 1.2 mL diluent for a reconstituted solution strength of 125 mg/mL. To give 125 mg, you obviously want to prepare 1 mL. No calculations are necessary.

EXAMPLE 2: Order: *Demerol 25 mg IM q.3h p.r.n. pain*

The child weighs 25 pounds. Is this dosage safe?

Refer back to the Demerol package insert information in Figure 10–2. Notice the recommended dosage for pain relief in children is 0.5 mg/lb to 0.8 mg/lb.

Minimum dosage:

$$\frac{0.5\ mg}{1\ lb} \quad \frac{X\ mg}{25\ lb}$$

$X = 0.5 \times 25 = 12.5\ mg$

Maximum dosage:

$$\frac{0.8\ mg}{1\ lb} \quad \frac{X\ mg}{25\ lb}$$

$X = 0.8 \times 25 = 20\ mg$

Therefore, 25 mg is too high and is not safe. Contact the physician to review the order.

Likewise, what if the order for this same child was for Demerol 8 mg q.3h p.r.n. pain. Would this dosage be reasonable? The answer is still no. Underdosage, as well as overdosage, can be a hazard. If the medication is necessary for the treatment or comfort of the patient, then giving too little can be just as wrong as giving too much.

Combination Drugs

Some medications contain two drugs combined into one solution or suspension. In order to calculate the safe dose of these medications, the nurse should consult a pediatric drug reference. Often, but not always, the nurse will need to calculate the *safe* dosage for each of the medications combined in the solution or suspension.

EXAMPLE 1: The physician orders *Pediazole 6.25 mL p.o. q.6h* for a child weighing 20 kg. The pediatric drug reference states that Pediazole is a combination drug containing 200 mg of erythromycin ethylsuccinate with 600 mg of sulfisoxazole acetyl in every 5 mL oral suspension. The safe dose for Pediazole is 50 mg erythromycin and 150 mg sulfisoxazole/kg/day in equally divided doses administered every 6 hours. Is the dosage safe?

Erythromycin dosage:

$$\frac{50\ mg}{1\ kg} \quad \frac{X\ mg}{20\ kg}$$

$X = 20 \times 50 = 1000\ mg$ divided into 4 q.6h doses $= \dfrac{1000}{4} = 250\ mg/dose$

Now calculate the safe amount of erythromycin:

$$\frac{200\ mg}{5\ mL} \quad \frac{250\ mg}{X\ mL}$$

$200X = 1250$

$\dfrac{200\ X}{200} = \dfrac{1250}{200}$

$X = 6.25\ mL$

Sulfisoxazole dosage:

$$\frac{150 \text{ mg}}{1 \text{ kg}} \times \frac{X \text{ mg}}{20 \text{ kg}}$$

$X = 20 \times 150 = 3000$ mg divided into 4 q.6h doses $= \frac{3000}{4} = 750$ mg/dose

And, calculate the safe amount of sulfisoxazole:

$$\frac{600 \text{ mg}}{5 \text{ mL}} \times \frac{750 \text{ mg}}{X \text{ mL}}$$

$600 \text{ X} = 3,750$

$$\frac{600X}{600} = \frac{3,750}{600}$$

$X = 6.25$ mL

Note: Because this is a combination product, 6.25 mL would contain the safe dosage of both medications delivered in a suspension. Therefore, the combination dosage is safe.

EXAMPLE 2: The physician orders *Septra suspension 7.5 cc p.o. q.12h* for a child weighing 10 kg. The pediatric drug reference states that Septra is a combination drug containing trimethoprim (TMP) 40 mg and sulfamethoxazole (SMZ) 200 mg in 5 mL oral suspension. The pediatric reference guide states the safe dosage of Septra is based on the TMP component and the safe dose is 6–12 mg/kg/day of TMP given q.12h. Is the dosage safe?

Minimum dosage: 6 mg/kg/day

$$\frac{6 \text{ mg}}{1 \text{ kg}} \times \frac{X \text{ mg}}{10 \text{ kg}}$$

$X = 6 \times 10 = 60$ mg/day

60 mg/day is to be administered q.12h; therefore give $\frac{60}{2}$ or 30 mg for each minimum dosage.

Now calculate the safe minimum quantity to administer per dose.

$$\frac{40 \text{ mg}}{5 \text{ mL}} \times \frac{30 \text{ mg}}{X \text{ mL}}$$

$40X = 150$

$$\frac{40X}{40} = \frac{150}{40}$$

$X = 3.75$ mL

Maximum dosage: 12 mg/kg/day

$$\frac{12 \text{ mg}}{1 \text{ kg}} \times \frac{X \text{ mg}}{10 \text{ kg}}$$

$X = 120$ mg/day

120 mg/day is to be administered q.12h; therefore give $\frac{120}{2}$ or 60 mg for each maximum dosage.

And, calculate the safe maximum quantity to administer per dose.

$$\frac{40 \text{ mg}}{5 \text{ mL}} \times \frac{60 \text{ mg}}{X \text{ mL}}$$

$40X = 300$

$$\frac{40X}{40} = \frac{300}{40}$$

$X = 7.5$ mL

The dosage is safe because the order of 7.5 cc is within the recommended allowable range of 3.75–7.5 mL.

review set 28

Calculate the following pediatric dosages.

1. The recommended dosage of Pathocil (dicloxacillin sodium) for children weighing less than 88 lb is 25 mg/kg/day in equally divided doses q.6h for severe infections. Calculate the amount for one dose for a 55 lb child. _____

2. The dicloxacillin sodium is available as an oral suspension of 62.5 mg per 5 mL. Calculate one dose for the child in No. 1. _____

3. A premature infant weighs 2000 g. The order is for Chloromycetin (chloramphenical) IV 25 mg/kg/day administered in 2 equally divided doses. Calculate one dose. _____

4. The chloramphenical is available as a solution for injection of 100 mg/mL. Calculate one dose for the infant in No. 3. _____

5. Order: Geopen (carbenicillin sodium) 100 mg/kg/day IM in equally divided doses q.i.d. The child weighs 33 lbs. Calculate one dose. _____

6. The carbenicillin sodium is available in a solution strength of 1 g per 4 mL. Calculate one dose. _____

7. Order: Panadol 10 mg per kg IM q.4h p.r.n.
    Supply: Panadol 160 mg per 1 mL
    Child's weight: 32 kg
    Give: _____ mL

8. The suggested dosage of tobramycin is 4 mg/kg/day to be administered every 12 hours. A neonate weighing 4000 g should receive _____ mg per dose.

9. Nebcin (tobramycin) is available in a solution strength of 40 mg/mL. How much should you administer to the neonate in No. 8 for each dose? _____ mL

10. How much Keflex should be given to a 44-lb child for one dose, if the recommended dosage is 25 mg/kg/day in four divided doses? _____ Keflex is available in an oral suspension of 250 mg per 5 mL. Give _____ mL.

Order: Polymox suspension 75 mg p.o. q.8h × 10 days for a 15 lb child. The following label represents the medication available.

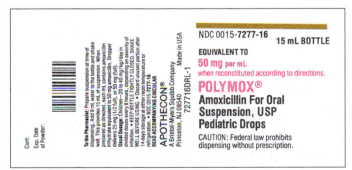

11. What is the recommended dosage range? _____

12. How many doses are recommended per day? _____

13. Is this order safe? _____ Explain. _____

14. How much should you give the child to administer one dose? _____ mL

15. Can you administer the full 10-day order from this bottle? _____
    Explain. _____

Order: Kantrex 30 mg IM b.i.d. for a 9-pound child.

Available:

Kantrex Pediatric Injection

KANAMYCIN SULFATE INJECTION, USP

75 mg per 2 mL

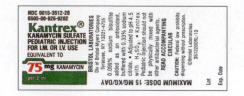

Intramuscular Route: The recommended maximum dosage for adults or children is 15 mg/kg/day in two equally divided doses administered at equally divided intervals.

16. What is the recommended daily dosage? _____

17. Is the order safe? _____

18. How much should you administer per dose? _____ mL

19. The physician orders Claforan 400 mg IV q.6h for a child who weighs 8 kg. The reference guide states the safe dose of Claforan is 100–200 mg/kg/day q.6–8h. What is the low range of safe dosage for this child to be administered over 24 h? _____

20. What is the high range of safe dosage for the child in #19 to be administered over 24 h? _____

21. How much (mg) can the child in #19 receive in each dose if the drug is ordered q.6h? _____

22. Is the dosage ordered in #19 safe for this child? _____

23. The physician orders Septra IV for a child weighing 15 kg. The pediatric reference states that Septra IV solution is a combination medication containing 16 mg/mL of trimethoprim (TMP) and 80 mg/mL of sulfamethoxazole (SMZ). The safe dosage of Septra is based on the TMP component and is recommended at a dose of 6–12 mg/kg of TMP a day. What dosage range of the TMP component of Septra should this child receive daily? _____

24. If the physician ordered 5.6 mL of Septra IV q.12h for the child in #23, is the dosage safe? _____

After completing these problems, see pages 307 and 308 to check your answers.

Body Surface Area (BSA) Method

Another method of calculating a child's dosage or checking for accuracy and safety of the pediatric drug order is to compare it to the usual dosage an adult receives, based on the child's body surface area (BSA). The BSA formula is the more accurate method since BSA is estimated by both height and weight.

The Body Surface Area (BSA) method is used to calculate dosages for infants and children up to 12 years of age. It is also used for calculating chemotherapy drugs for adults and fluid volume for adults after open-heart surgery, burns, or renal disease. This method requires the use of a chart or nomogram that estimates the BSA of the infant or child according to his height and weight (Figure 10–4). The BSA is expressed in square meters (m^2). Follow the directions given in Figure 10–4 to determine the BSA of a child who is 35 inches tall and weighs 30 pounds: $0.6 m^2$.

▶ ***rule***   To calculate child's drug dose using BSA, multiply recommended dose per m^2 times BSA.

$$mg/m^2 \times m^2 = \text{child's dose}$$

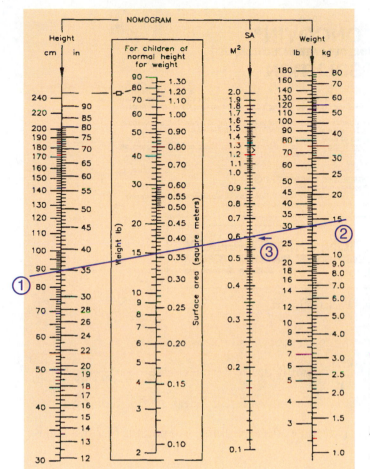

West's Nomogram for Estimation of Body Surface Area

Fig. 10–4 Body surface area (BSA) is determined by drawing a straight line from the patient's height ① in the far left column to his or her weight ② in the far right column. Intersection of the line with the body surface area (BSA) column ③ is the estimated BSA (m²). For infants and children of normal height for weight, BSA may be estimated from weight alone by referring to the enclosed area. *(Reprinted with permission from Behrman, R. E. and Vaughan, V. C., Nelson Textbook of Pediatrics, 15th ed., 1996, W. B. Saunders Company, Philadelphia, PA 19105.)*

EXAMPLE: Use BSA to calculate the correct dosage.

Order: *Oncovin (vincristine) IV* for a child who weighs 28 kilograms and is 100 centimeters tall

Supply: *Oncovin 2 mg/2 mL*

The recommended dosage as noted on the package instructions (Figure 10–5) is 2 mg/m².

The child's BSA is 0.9 m², as determined by the West Nomogram.

mg/m² × m² = child's dose

2 mg/m² × 0.9 m² = 1.8 mg/dose

$$\frac{\overset{1}{\cancel{2}}\,mg}{\underset{1}{\cancel{2}}\,mL} = \frac{1.8\,mg}{X\,mL}$$

$$\frac{1\,mg}{1\,mL} \bowtie \frac{1.8\,mg}{X\,mL}$$

X = 1.8 mL

or, $\dfrac{D}{H} \times Q = \dfrac{1.8\,mg}{2\,mg} \times 2\,mL = 1.8\,mL$

The BSA can also be used to determine a child's dose if the recommended average adult dose is known.

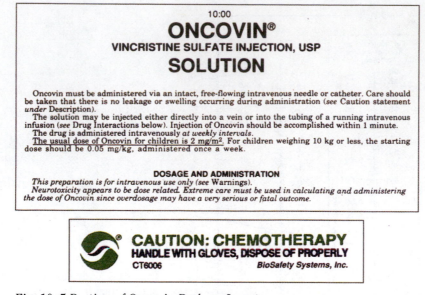

10:00
ONCOVIN®
VINCRISTINE SULFATE INJECTION, USP
SOLUTION

Oncovin must be administered via an intact, free-flowing intravenous needle or catheter. Care should be taken that there is no leakage or swelling occurring during administration (*see* Caution statement *under* Description).
    The solution may be injected either directly into a vein or into the tubing of a running intravenous infusion (*see* Drug Interactions below). Injection of Oncovin should be accomplished within 1 minute.
    The drug is administered intravenously *at weekly intervals.*
    <u>The usual dose of Oncovin for children is 2 mg/m².</u> For children weighing 10 kg or less, the starting dose should be 0.05 mg/kg, administered once a week.

DOSAGE AND ADMINISTRATION
This preparation is for intravenous use only (see Warnings).
Neurotoxicity appears to be dose related. Extreme care must be used in calculating and administering the dose of Oncovin since overdosage may have a very serious or fatal outcome.

CAUTION: CHEMOTHERAPY
HANDLE WITH GLOVES, DISPOSE OF PROPERLY
CT6006   *BioSafety Systems, Inc.*

Fig. 10–5 Portion of Oncovin Package Insert

> ### *rule*
> $$\frac{\text{BSA of child (m}^2)}{1.7 \ (\text{m}^2)} \times \text{Adult dose} = \text{Child's dose}$$

The formula is based on the BSA of an average adult weighing 140 pounds (1.7 m²) and the usual adult dosage.

HINT: Think! Don't panic. Although the formula is different, notice that the format is just like the simple equations you solved in Chapter 1 and the formula method   from Chapter 9.

EXAMPLE: Use BSA to calculate the correct dosage.

Order: *Garamycin IM t.i.d.* for a 3-year-old child who is 35 inches tall and weighs 30 pounds

Supply: *Garamycin 40 mg per mL*

Adult dose: 40 mg

BSA Method: $\dfrac{\text{BSA of child (m}^2)}{1.7 \ (\text{m}^2)} \times \text{Adult dose} = \text{Child's dose}$

Using the BSA nomogram, a child who is 35 inches tall and weighs 30 pounds has a BSA of 0.6 m² (Figure 10–4).

$$\frac{0.6 \ \cancel{m^2}}{1.7 \ \cancel{m^2}} \times 40 \text{ mg} = \frac{24 \text{ mg}}{1.7} = 14.1 \text{ mg} = 14 \text{ mg}$$

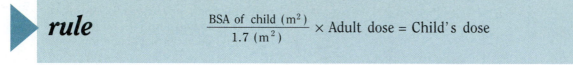

$$\frac{40 \text{ mg}}{1 \text{ mL}} \underset{=}{\overset{}{\rightleftarrows}} \frac{14 \text{ mg}}{X \text{ mL}}$$

$$40X = 14$$

$$\frac{40X}{40} = \frac{14}{40} = 0.35 \text{ mL}$$

$$X = 0.35 \text{ mL}$$

or, $\dfrac{D}{H} \times Q = \dfrac{14 \text{ mg}}{40 \text{ mg}} \times 1 \text{ mL} = 0.35 \text{ mL}$ to be measured in a tuberculin syringe.

Alternate BSA Method

For a child of fairly normal height and weight, the BSA can be determined using the weight alone. Notice in Figure 10–4 that the enclosed column to the left demonstrates that the BSA (m^2) for a 30-pound child of normal height would be 0.6 m^2. This is the same BSA determined for the 30-lb, 35-inch tall child described in the preceding example, using the height and weight columns.

If you are unsure of normal growth and development standards, do not guess. Use both the height and weight columns to determine BSA (m^2).

review set 29

Refer to West's Nomogram in Figure 10–4 to answer these items.

1. Calculate the BSA of a child who is 15 kg and 65 cm. _____ m^2

2. What is the pediatric dosage (in mg) for the child described in No. 1 if the usual adult dosage is 1 g? _____ mg

3. What is the pediatric dosage of an infant of normal proportions who weighs 10 lbs when the usual adult dosage is 250 mg. _____ mg

4. What is the BSA of a child who is 55 inches tall and weighs 60 pounds? _____ m^2

5. What is the dosage of acyclovir required for the child in No. 4, if the recommended dose is 250 mg/m^2? _____ mg

6. Order: Child is 30 inches tall and weighs 25 pounds.
   Give Zovirax (acyclovir) 250 mg/m^2 IV q.8h
   Supply: Acyclovir 50 mg/mL
   NOTE: The required dose must be diluted in a proper solution prior to IV administration.
   Give: _____ mL

7. Order: Child is 45 inches tall and weighs 55 pounds.
   Methotrexate 3.3 mg/m^2 IV q.d.
   Supply: Methotrexate 5 mg/2 mL
   Give: _____ mL

8. What is the dosage of Unipen appropriate for a 45-lb child who is 45 inches tall, if the usual adult dosage is 500 mg? _____ mg

After completing these problems, see page 308 to check your answers.

quick review

To calculate and check pediatric dosages:

■ Calculate the amount of drug per pound or kilogram of body weight as ordered by the doctor and recommended by a reputable drug reference:

$$mg/kg \times kg \ \text{ or } \ mg/lb \times lb$$

■ Or, calculate the amount of drug by the BSA methods:

$$mg/m^2 \times m^2$$

$$\text{or,} \ \frac{\text{BSA of child (m}^2)}{1.7 \ (\text{m}^2)} \times \text{Adult dose} = \text{Child's dose}$$

- The BSA (m²) can be determined for children of normal height and weight by the "normal height and weight" column on the West Nomogram.
- The "normal height and weight" column on the West Nomogram for estimating BSA (m²) should *only* be used when the child's height and weight is within normal limits.
- If you are unsure of normal growth and development standards, do not guess. Use both the height and weight columns to determine BSA (m²).
- Double-check against a reputable drug reference to be sure dosages are safe and reasonable. If not, notify the physician.

critical thinking skills

Medication errors in pediatrics are often caused by failure to calculate the safe dosage of medication for a child.

■ *error 1*

Failing to calculate the safe dosage of medication for a child.

possible scenario

Suppose the family practice resident ordered Tobramycin 110 mg IV q.8h for a child with cystic fibrosis who weighs 10 kilograms. The pediatric reference guide states that the safe dosage of Tobramycin for a child with severe infections is 7.5 mg/kg/day. The nurse received five admissions the evening of this order and thought, "I'm too busy to calculate the safe dosage this time." The pharmacist prepared and labeled the medication in a syringe and the nurse administered the first dose of the medication. Two hours later the resident arrived on the pediatric unit and inquired if the nurse had given the first dose. When the nurse replied "yes," the resident became pale and stated, "I ordered an adult dose of Tobramycin. But if you had double checked my order against the safe pediatric dosage, my error would have been corrected."

potential outcome

The resident's next step would likely have been to discontinue the Tobramycin and order a stat Tobramycin level. The level would most likely be elevated and the child would have required close monitoring for renal damage and hearing loss.

prevention

The child should have received 75 mg a day, and no more than 25 mg per dose. The child received more than four times the safe dosage of Tobramycin. Had the nurse calculated the safe dosage, the error would have been caught sooner, and the dosage could have been adjusted before the child ever received the first dose. The pharmacist also should have caught the error but did not. In this scenario the resident, pharmacist, and nurse all committed medication errors. If the resident had not noticed the error as soon as he did, one can only wonder how many doses the child would have received. The nurse is the last safety net for the child when it comes to a dosage error.

In addition, the nurse has to reconcile the fact she actually gave the overdose. The nurse is responsible for whatever dosage she administers. We are all accountable for our actions. Taking shortcuts in administering medications to children can be disastrous. The time the nurse saved by not calculating the safe dosage was more than lost in the extra monitoring, not to mention cost of follow-up to the medication error, *and most importantly*, the risk to the child.

critical thinking skills

Medication errors in pediatrics often occur when the nurse fails to properly identify the child before administering the dose.

■ *error 2*

Failing to identify the child before administering a medication.

possible scenario

Suppose the physician ordered Ampicillin 500 mg IV q.6h for a child with pneumonia. The nurse calculated the dosage to be safe, checked to be sure the child had no allergies, and prepared the medication. The child had been assigned to a semi-private room. The nurse entered the room and noted only one child in the room and administered the IV Ampicillin to that child, without checking the identification of the child. Within an hour of the administered Ampicillin the child began to break out in hives and had signs of respiratory distress. The nurse asked the child's mother, "Does Johnny have any known allergies?" The mother replied, "This is James, not Johnny, and yes, James is allergic to penicillin. His roommate, Johnny, is in the playroom." At this point the nurse realized he gave the Ampicillin to the wrong child, who was allergic to penicillin.

potential outcome

James' physician would have been notified and orders received for epinephrine SC stat (given for anaphylactic reactions), followed by close monitoring of the child. Anaphylactic reactions can range from mild to severe. Ampicillin is a derivative of penicillin and would not have been prescribed for a child such as James.

prevention

This error could have easily been avoided had the nurse remembered the cardinal rule of identifying the child before administering any and all medications. Children are very mobile, and you cannot assume the identity of a child simply because he is in a particular room. The correct method of identifying the child is to check the wrist or ankle band and compare it to the medication administration record with the child's name, room number, physician, and account number. Finally, remember that the first of the Five Rights of medication administration is the *right patient*.

*practice problems—chapter 10*_____

Calculate the following dosages. Refer to the West Nomogram on page 199 as needed.

1. Order: (20-lb child) Gentamicin 2 mg/kg of body weight IVPB q.8h
   Supply: Gentamicin 20 mg/2 mL
   Give: _____ mL

2. The doctor orders Somophyllin 105 mg orally every six hours for a 66-lb child. The drug insert recommends 3 mg/kg per dose. Somophyllin is supplied in a dosage strength of 105 mg per 5 mL. Is the order safe and reasonable according to the recommended dosage? _____ What would you do next? _____

   _____

3. Order: (Child of normal proportions who weighs 25 pounds) phenobarbital IM stat
      computed per BSA
   Usual adult dosage: 100 mg
   Supply: 50 mg/mL
   Give: _____ mL

4. Order: (1-year-old child, 25 inches tall, weighs 20 pounds) Sulfadiazine IM t.i.d.
      computed per BSA
   Usual adult dosage: 500 mg
   The child should receive _____ milligrams.

5. Sulfadiazine is available in a solution strength of 250 mg per mL. Calculate one dose for the child in No. 4. _____ mL

6. Use the BSA method to calculate the dosage of IM ampicillin for a child who is 36 inches tall and weighs 30 pounds. Adult dose: 0.5 g. Give: _____ mg

7. Ampicillin is supplied in ampules of 250 mg per mL. Calculate one dose for the child in No. 6. _____ mL

8. Use the BSA method to determine the dosage of IM Prostaphlin (oxacillin) for a child who is normal height and weighs 44 pounds. The adult dosage is 500 mg. _____ mg

9. Oxacillin is reconstituted to 250 mg per 1 mL. Calculate one dose for the child in No. 8. _____ mL

10. Order: 55-lb child. Sandoglobulin 0.2 g/kg IV
    Supply: Sandoglobulin 6 g/100 mL
    Give: _____ mL

11. Order: 26-lb child. Ampicillin 50 mg/kg/day p.o. in equally divided doses q.6h
    Supply: Ampicillin 125 mg/5 mL
    Give: _____ mL for one dose

12. Order: Child is 55 inches tall and weighs 90 lbs.
    Adriamycin 20 mg/m^2 IV stat
    Supply: Adriamycin 2 mg/mL
    Give: _____ mL

13. Order: Child is 45 inches tall and weighs 55 pounds.
    Vincristine (oncovin) 2 mg/m^2 IV weekly
    Supply: Oncovin 1 mg/mL
    Give: _____ mL

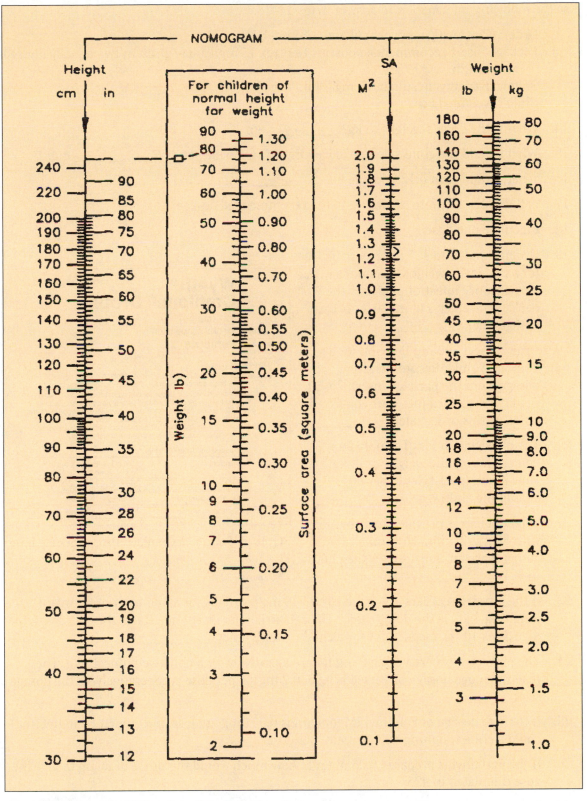

West's Nomogram for Estimation of Body Surface Area
(Reprinted with permission from Behrman, R. E. and Vaughan, V. C., Nelson Textbook of Pediatrics, *15th ed., 1996, W. B. Saunders Company, Philadelphia, PA 19105.)*

Use the following information to answer items 14–18.

> Order: Kantrex (kanamycin sulfate) 37.5 mg b.i.d.
> Package insert recommended dosage: Kantrex 15 mg/kg/day given in two equally divided doses q.12h
> Supply: Kanamycin sulfate 75 mg/2 mL
> Child's weight: 11 lb

14. What is the child's weight in kg? _____ kg

15. What should the child's dosage of kanamycin sulfate be per day? _____ mg

16. What should each q.12h dosage be? _____ mg

17. Is the order accurate according to the recommended dosage? _____

18. Calculate one dose: _____ mL

19. Order: Ampicillin 125 mg p.o. q. 6h for a child who weighs 22 pounds with a respiratory infection. Refer to the package insert in Figure 10–6. Is this dosage safe? _____

20. Order: Ancef 300 mg IM q. 6h for a 44-pound child. Recommended dosage from the package insert: 25–50 mg/kg/day divided into four equal doses. Is this order safe? _____

21. The physician orders Tylenol 10 mg/kg/dose for a child weighing 12 kg. How much (mg) Tylenol per dose should the child receive? _____

22. Tylenol elixir is provided in a solution with 80 mg/2.5 mL. How much would you prepare for one dose for the child in #21? _____

Wyeth®
Omnipen® Drops
(ampicillin)
for oral suspension
Pediatric

A.H.F.S. Category 8:12.16

Description
Omnipen (ampicillin) is a semisynthetic penicillin derived from the basic penicillin nucleus, 6-amino-penicillanic acid.
Omnipen Pediatric Drops for oral administration is a powder which when reconstituted as directed yields a suspension of 100 mg ampicillin per mL. The inactive ingredients present are artificial and natural flavors, colloidal silicon dioxide, D&C Yellow 10, methylparaben, propylparaben, simethicone, sodium benzoate, sodium citrate, sucrose, and water.

Dosage and Administration

Infection	Total Daily Dose* (Give in equal doses q. 6h.)
Respiratory Tract	50 mg/kg/24 hours
Gastrointestinal Tract	100 mg/kg/24 hours
Genitourinary Tract	100 mg/kg/24 hours

Fig. 10–6 Portion of Omnipen Drops Package Insert

23. If the physician orders digoxin elixir 0.048 mg p.o. daily for a one-month-old infant weighing 4 kg, is the dosage safe? The pediatric reference guide states the safe dosage of digoxin is 10–12 mcg/kg/day for a child under 2 years. _____

24. The physician orders Versed 2 mg IM preoperatively for a child weighing 14 kg. The recommended dosage of Versed is 0.08–0.2 mg/kg per dose preoperatively. Is the dosage safe? _____

25. If the safe dosage of Fentanyl IM for pain is 0.001 mg/kg/dose, how much Fentanyl (mg) could a child weighing 40 kg receive per dose? _____

26. If the Fentanyl is prepared 0.05 mg/mL, how much would the nurse draw up to give the dose calculated in #25? _____

27. The safe dosage of Tobramycin is 7.5 mg/kg/day given q.8h. Calculate the safe daily dosage for a child weighing 15 kg. _____

28. How much (mg) Tobramycin should the child receive per dose in #27? _____

29. Calculate the safe dosage of SoluMedrol for a child weighing 22 kg. The safe dosage range is 1–2 mg/kg/day up to 1–2 mg/kg/dose. _____

30. What is the BSA for a child weighing 6 kg and measuring 60 cm? _____

31. Calculate the safe dosage of Retrovir for the child in #30 if the recommended safe dosage of Retrovir is 180 mg/m²/dose given q.6h.

32. The physician orders Septra IV for a child weighing 25 kg. The pediatric reference guide states that Septra IV solution is a combination medication containing 16 mg/mL of trimethroprim (TMP) and 80 mg/mL of sulfamethoxazole (SMZ). The dose of Septra is based on the TMP component and is recommended at a dosage range of 6–12 mg/kg/day of TMP given q.12h. What dosage range of the TMP component should a child who weighs 25 kg receive daily? _____

33. What dosage range (mg) of TMP should the child in #32 receive for each dose?

    _____

34. If the physician ordered 9.3 mL of Septra IV q.12h for the child in #32, is the dosage safe? _____

After completing these problems, see pages 327–329 to check your answers.

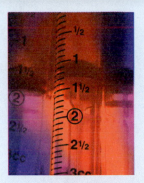

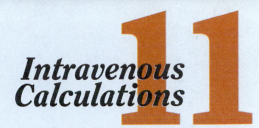
objectives

Upon mastery of Chapter 11, you will be able to calculate intravenous solution flow rate for electronic or manual infusion systems. To accomplish this you will also be able to:

- Identify common IV solutions.
- Calculate the amount of specific components in common IV fluids.
- Define the following terms: IV, peripheral line, central line, primary IV, secondary IV, and saline/heparin locks.
- Calculate milliliters per hour: mL/h.
- Recognize the calibration or drop factor in gtt/mL as stated on the IV tubing package.
- Calculate IV flow rate in gtt/min.:

$$\frac{V \text{ (volume)}}{T \text{ (time in min)}} \times C \text{ (drop factor calibration)} = R \text{ (rate of flow)}$$

- Use the short cut method to calculate IV flow rate in gtt/min.:

$$\frac{mL / h}{\text{drop factor constant}} = \text{gtt/min}$$

- Recalculate the flow rate when the IV is off schedule.
- Calculate small volume piggyback IVs (IV PB).

    Intravenous means the administration of fluids or medication through a vein. Intravenous (IV) fluids are ordered for a variety of reasons. They may be ordered for replacement of lost fluids, to maintain electrolyte balance, or to keep the vein open (KVO). *Replacement fluids* are often ordered due to losses that may occur from hemorrhage, vomiting, or diarrhea. *Maintenance fluids* sustain normal fluid and electrolyte balance. They may be used for the patient who is not yet depleted but is beginning to show symptoms of depletion. They may also be ordered for the patient who has the potential to become depleted, such as the patient who is allowed nothing by mouth (NPO) for surgery. *KVO fluids* are often ordered at a very low rate to keep an IV line accessible should the patient require emergency fluids or IV medications.

IV Solutions

    IV solutions are ordered by the physician; however, they are administered and monitored by the nurse. It is the responsibility of the nurse to ensure that the correct IV fluid is administered to the correct patient. IV fluids may be prepared in plastic solution bags or glass bottles with the volume of the IV fluids varying from 50 mL to 1000 mL. The IV solution bag or bottle will be labeled with the exact components of the IV solution. The physician and nursing staff often use abbreviations to indicate the IV solution.

In IV abbreviations *letters* indicate the solution components, and *numbers* indicate the percentage (%) or concentration strength. Remember the following common IV solution abbreviations.

remember

ABBREVIATION	IV COMPONENT
D	Dextrose
W	Water
S	Saline
NS	Normal Saline
RL	Ringer's Lactate
LR	Lactated Ringer's

EXAMPLE 1:   Dextrose 5% in Water is abbreviated as D_5W.

EXAMPLE 2:   Dextrose 5% in Lactated Ringer's is abbreviated as either D_5LR or D_5RL.

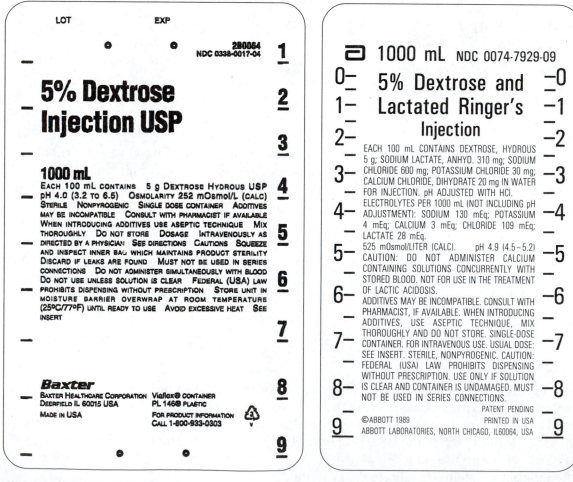

(Courtesy of Baxter Health Care Corporation)   (Courtesy of Abbott Laboratories)

Different Concentrations of IV Fluids

A common IV solution is normal saline (NS). NS has a concentration of 0.9% sodium chloride (NaCl). Other common saline IV fluids include 0.45% NS (usually written as $\frac{1}{2}$ NS) and 0.225% NS (usually written as $\frac{1}{4}$ NS). Notice that 0.45% is $\frac{1}{2}$ of 0.9% NaCl, and 0.225% is $\frac{1}{4}$ of 0.9% NaCl.

EXAMPLE: Dextrose 5% with 0.225% normal saline is abbreviated as:

$$D_5 \tfrac{1}{4} NS$$

IV fluids may be *isotonic*, meaning the solution has the same osmolarity as the serum and other body fluids; *hypotonic*, meaning the solution has a lower osmolarity than serum and other body fluids; or *hypertonic*, meaning the solution has a higher osmolarity than serum and other body fluids. Isotonic solutions exert no pull on the cells and simply expand the intravascular compartment. Examples of isotonic fluids are Lactated Ringer's and normal saline (0.9% NaCl).

Hypotonic solutions cause fluid from the intravascular compartment to move into the cell, thereby depleting the intravascular compartment but hydrating the cell. This type of solution would be used in a patient who needs cellular hydration, such as a patient with a high blood glucose level. An example of a hypotonic solution is 0.45% normal saline ($\frac{1}{2}$NS). Hypertonic solutions cause fluid to move from interstitial and cellular space into the intravascular space. These fluids are often ordered for patients with edema or to maintain adequate urinary output and blood pressure. Examples of hypertonic solutions are $D_5 \tfrac{1}{2} NS$ and $D_5 NS$.

IV Fluid Additives

Electrolytes also may be added to the basic IV fluid. Potassium chloride (KCl) is commonly added to the basic fluid and is measured in milliequivalents (mEq). The order is usually written to indicate the amount of milliequivalents per liter to be added to the IV fluid.

EXAMPLE: Dextrose 5% normal saline with 20 mEq per liter of potassium chloride is abbreviated as: $D_5 NS \ \bar{c} \ 20$ mEq KCl/L.

review set 30

For each of the following IV solutions:

  a. List the components and concentration strengths of the solutions.

  b. Match the correct fluid from the illustrations labeled A–H.

		Components and Strength	Matching Illustration
1.	NS	_____	_____
2.	$D_5 W$	_____	_____
3.	$D_5 NS$	_____	_____
4.	$D_5 \tfrac{1}{2} NS$	_____	_____
5.	$D_5 \tfrac{1}{4} NS$	_____	_____
6.	$D_5 RL$	_____	_____
7.	$D_5 \tfrac{1}{2} NS \ \bar{c} \ 20$ mEq KCl/L	_____	_____
8.	$D_5 NS \ \bar{c} \ 20$ mEq KCl/L	_____	_____

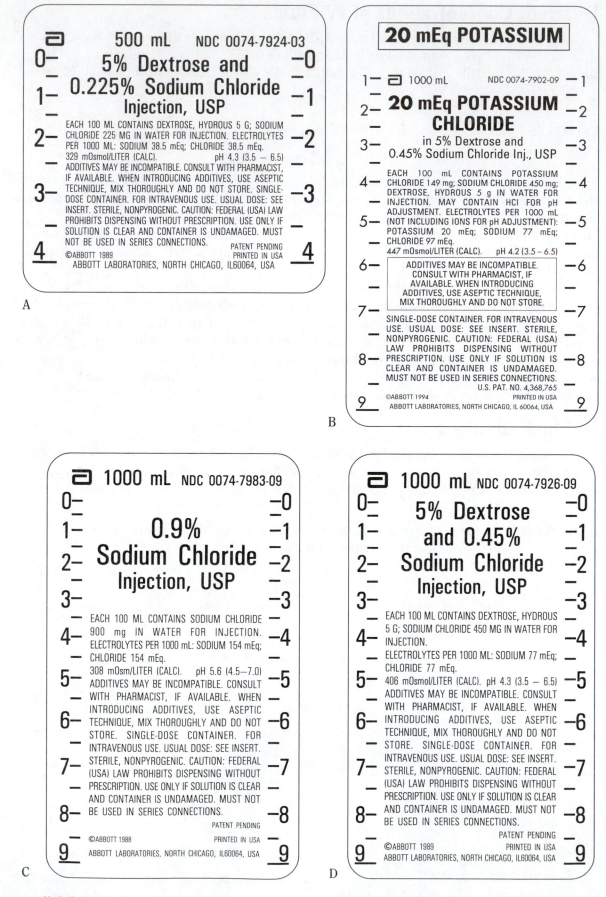

A

500 mL   NDC 0074-7924-03

5% Dextrose and 0.225% Sodium Chloride
Injection, USP

EACH 100 ML CONTAINS DEXTROSE, HYDROUS 5 G; SODIUM CHLORIDE 225 MG IN WATER FOR INJECTION. ELECTROLYTES PER 1000 ML: SODIUM 38.5 mEq; CHLORIDE 38.5 mEq. 329 mOsmol/LITER (CALC).   pH 4.3 (3.5 – 6.5)
ADDITIVES MAY BE INCOMPATIBLE. CONSULT WITH PHARMACIST, IF AVAILABLE. WHEN INTRODUCING ADDITIVES, USE ASEPTIC TECHNIQUE, MIX THOROUGHLY AND DO NOT STORE. SINGLE-DOSE CONTAINER. FOR INTRAVENOUS USE. USUAL DOSE: SEE INSERT. STERILE, NONPYROGENIC. CAUTION: FEDERAL (USA) LAW PROHIBITS DISPENSING WITHOUT PRESCRIPTION. USE ONLY IF SOLUTION IS CLEAR AND CONTAINER IS UNDAMAGED. MUST NOT BE USED IN SERIES CONNECTIONS.
PATENT PENDING
©ABBOTT 1989   PRINTED IN USA
ABBOTT LABORATORIES, NORTH CHICAGO, IL60064, USA

B

20 mEq POTASSIUM

1000 mL   NDC 0074-7902-09

20 mEq POTASSIUM CHLORIDE
in 5% Dextrose and 0.45% Sodium Chloride Inj., USP

EACH 100 mL CONTAINS POTASSIUM CHLORIDE 149 mg; SODIUM CHLORIDE 450 mg; DEXTROSE, HYDROUS 5 g IN WATER FOR INJECTION. MAY CONTAIN HCl FOR pH ADJUSTMENT. ELECTROLYTES PER 1000 mL (NOT INCLUDING IONS FOR pH ADJUSTMENT): POTASSIUM 20 mEq; SODIUM 77 mEq; CHLORIDE 97 mEq.
447 mOsmol/LITER (CALC).   pH 4.2 (3.5 – 6.5)

ADDITIVES MAY BE INCOMPATIBLE. CONSULT WITH PHARMACIST, IF AVAILABLE. WHEN INTRODUCING ADDITIVES, USE ASEPTIC TECHNIQUE, MIX THOROUGHLY AND DO NOT STORE.

SINGLE-DOSE CONTAINER. FOR INTRAVENOUS USE. USUAL DOSE: SEE INSERT. STERILE, NONPYROGENIC. CAUTION: FEDERAL (USA) LAW PROHIBITS DISPENSING WITHOUT PRESCRIPTION. USE ONLY IF SOLUTION IS CLEAR AND CONTAINER IS UNDAMAGED. MUST NOT BE USED IN SERIES CONNECTIONS.
U.S. PAT. NO. 4,368,765
©ABBOTT 1994   PRINTED IN USA
ABBOTT LABORATORIES, NORTH CHICAGO, IL 60064, USA

C

1000 mL   NDC 0074-7983-09

0.9% Sodium Chloride
Injection, USP

EACH 100 ML CONTAINS SODIUM CHLORIDE 900 mg IN WATER FOR INJECTION. ELECTROLYTES PER 1000 mL: SODIUM 154 mEq; CHLORIDE 154 mEq.
308 mOsm/LITER (CALC).   pH 5.6 (4.5–7.0)
ADDITIVES MAY BE INCOMPATIBLE. CONSULT WITH PHARMACIST, IF AVAILABLE. WHEN INTRODUCING ADDITIVES, USE ASEPTIC TECHNIQUE, MIX THOROUGHLY AND DO NOT STORE. SINGLE-DOSE CONTAINER. FOR INTRAVENOUS USE. USUAL DOSE: SEE INSERT. STERILE, NONPYROGENIC. CAUTION: FEDERAL (USA) LAW PROHIBITS DISPENSING WITHOUT PRESCRIPTION. USE ONLY IF SOLUTION IS CLEAR AND CONTAINER IS UNDAMAGED. MUST NOT BE USED IN SERIES CONNECTIONS.
PATENT PENDING
©ABBOTT 1988   PRINTED IN USA
ABBOTT LABORATORIES, NORTH CHICAGO, IL60064, USA

D

1000 mL   NDC 0074-7926-09

5% Dextrose and 0.45% Sodium Chloride
Injection, USP

EACH 100 ML CONTAINS DEXTROSE, HYDROUS 5 G; SODIUM CHLORIDE 450 MG IN WATER FOR INJECTION.
ELECTROLYTES PER 1000 ML: SODIUM 77 mEq; CHLORIDE 77 mEq.
406 mOsmol/LITER (CALC). pH 4.3 (3.5 – 6.5)
ADDITIVES MAY BE INCOMPATIBLE. CONSULT WITH PHARMACIST, IF AVAILABLE. WHEN INTRODUCING ADDITIVES, USE ASEPTIC TECHNIQUE, MIX THOROUGHLY AND DO NOT STORE. SINGLE-DOSE CONTAINER. FOR INTRAVENOUS USE. USUAL DOSE: SEE INSERT. STERILE, NONPYROGENIC. CAUTION: FEDERAL (USA) LAW PROHIBITS DISPENSING WITHOUT PRESCRIPTION. USE ONLY IF SOLUTION IS CLEAR AND CONTAINER IS UNDAMAGED. MUST NOT BE USED IN SERIES CONNECTIONS.
PATENT PENDING
©ABBOTT 1989   PRINTED IN USA
ABBOTT LABORATORIES, NORTH CHICAGO, IL60064, USA

(A, B, C, & D Courtesy of Abbott Laboratories)

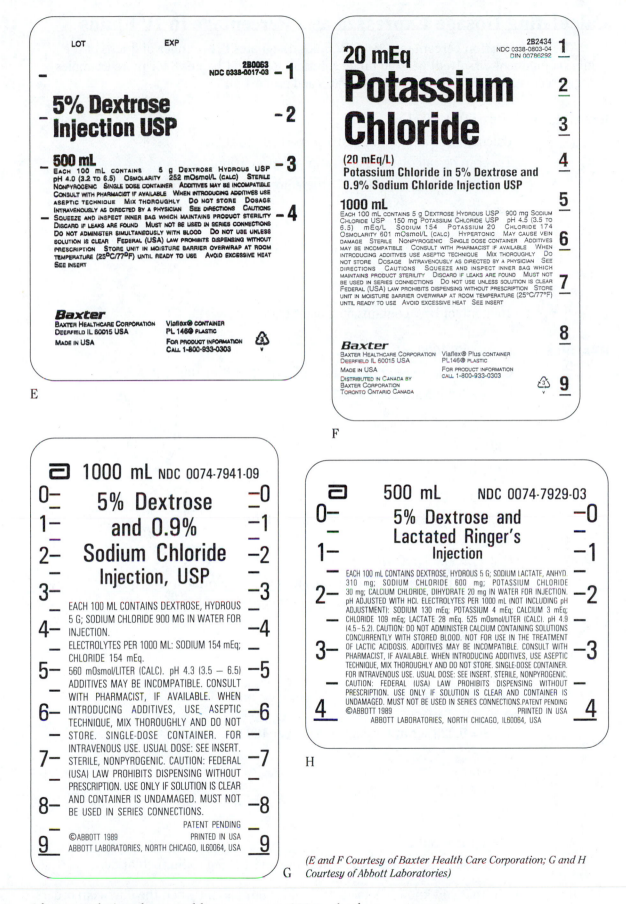

E

LOT   EXP

NDC 0338-0017-03   2B0063 —1

—2

5% Dextrose
Injection USP

500 mL —3

EACH 100 mL CONTAINS   5 g DEXTROSE HYDROUS USP
pH 4.0 (3.2 TO 6.5) OSMOLARITY 252 mOsmol/L (CALC) STERILE
NONPYROGENIC SINGLE DOSE CONTAINER ADDITIVES MAY BE INCOMPATIBLE
CONSULT WITH PHARMACIST IF AVAILABLE   WHEN INTRODUCING ADDITIVES USE
ASEPTIC TECHNIQUE   MIX THOROUGHLY   DO NOT STORE   DOSAGE —4
INTRAVENOUSLY AS DIRECTED BY A PHYSICIAN   SEE DIRECTIONS   CAUTIONS
SQUEEZE AND INSPECT INNER BAG WHICH MAINTAINS PRODUCT STERILITY
DISCARD IF LEAKS ARE FOUND   MUST NOT BE USED IN SERIES CONNECTIONS
DO NOT ADMINISTER SIMULTANEOUSLY WITH BLOOD   DO NOT USE UNLESS
SOLUTION IS CLEAR   FEDERAL (USA) LAW PROHIBITS DISPENSING WITHOUT
PRESCRIPTION   STORE UNIT IN MOISTURE BARRIER OVERWRAP AT ROOM
TEMPERATURE (25°C/77°F) UNTIL READY TO USE   AVOID EXCESSIVE HEAT
SEE INSERT

Baxter
BAXTER HEALTHCARE CORPORATION   VIAFLEX® CONTAINER
DEERFIELD IL 60015 USA   PL 146® PLASTIC
MADE IN USA   FOR PRODUCT INFORMATION
                                 CALL 1-800-933-0303

F

2B2434
NDC 0338-0803-04   1
DIN 00786292

20 mEq
Potassium
Chloride

(20 mEq/L)
Potassium Chloride in 5% Dextrose and
0.9% Sodium Chloride Injection USP

1000 mL

EACH 100 mL CONTAINS 5 g DEXTROSE HYDROUS USP   900 mg SODIUM
CHLORIDE USP   150 mg POTASSIUM CHLORIDE USP   pH 4.5 (3.5 TO
6.5)   mEq/L   SODIUM 154   POTASSIUM 20   CHLORIDE 174
OSMOLARITY 601 mOsmol/L (CALC)   HYPERTONIC   MAY CAUSE VEIN
DAMAGE STERILE NONPYROGENIC SINGLE DOSE CONTAINER ADDITIVES
MAY BE INCOMPATIBLE CONSULT WITH PHARMACIST IF AVAILABLE WHEN
INTRODUCING ADDITIVES USE ASEPTIC TECHNIQUE   MIX THOROUGHLY   DO
NOT STORE   DOSAGE   INTRAVENOUSLY AS DIRECTED BY A PHYSICIAN   SEE
DIRECTIONS   CAUTIONS   SQUEEZE AND INSPECT INNER BAG WHICH
MAINTAINS PRODUCT STERILITY   DISCARD IF LEAKS ARE FOUND   MUST NOT
BE USED IN SERIES CONNECTIONS   DO NOT USE UNLESS SOLUTION IS CLEAR
FEDERAL (USA) LAW PROHIBITS DISPENSING WITHOUT PRESCRIPTION   STORE
UNIT IN MOISTURE BARRIER OVERWRAP AT ROOM TEMPERATURE (25°C/77°F)
UNTIL READY TO USE   AVOID EXCESSIVE HEAT   SEE INSERT

2
3
4
5
6
7
8

Baxter
BAXTER HEALTHCARE CORPORATION   VIAFLEX® PLUS CONTAINER
DEERFIELD IL 60015 USA   PL146® PLASTIC
MADE IN USA   FOR PRODUCT INFORMATION
DISTRIBUTED IN CANADA BY   CALL 1-800-933-0303
BAXTER CORPORATION
TORONTO ONTARIO CANADA   9

G

⊃ 1000 mL NDC 0074-7941-09

0   —0
1   —1

5% Dextrose
and 0.9%
Sodium Chloride
Injection, USP

2   —2
3   —3

EACH 100 ML CONTAINS DEXTROSE, HYDROUS
5 G; SODIUM CHLORIDE 900 MG IN WATER FOR
INJECTION.
ELECTROLYTES PER 1000 ML: SODIUM 154 mEq;
CHLORIDE 154 mEq.
560 mOsmol/LITER (CALC). pH 4.3 (3.5 — 6.5)
ADDITIVES MAY BE INCOMPATIBLE. CONSULT
WITH PHARMACIST, IF AVAILABLE. WHEN
INTRODUCING ADDITIVES, USE ASEPTIC
TECHNIQUE, MIX THOROUGHLY AND DO NOT
STORE. SINGLE-DOSE CONTAINER. FOR
INTRAVENOUS USE. USUAL DOSE: SEE INSERT.
STERILE, NONPYROGENIC. CAUTION: FEDERAL
(USA) LAW PROHIBITS DISPENSING WITHOUT
PRESCRIPTION. USE ONLY IF SOLUTION IS CLEAR
AND CONTAINER IS UNDAMAGED. MUST NOT
BE USED IN SERIES CONNECTIONS.

4   —4
5   —5
6   —6
7   —7
8   —8

PATENT PENDING
©ABBOTT 1989   PRINTED IN USA
ABBOTT LABORATORIES, NORTH CHICAGO, IL60064, USA

9   —9

H

⊃   500 mL   NDC 0074-7929-03

0   —0

5% Dextrose and
Lactated Ringer's
Injection

1   —1

EACH 100 ML CONTAINS DEXTROSE, HYDROUS 5 G; SODIUM LACTATE, ANHYD.
310 mg; SODIUM CHLORIDE 600 mg; POTASSIUM CHLORIDE
30 mg; CALCIUM CHLORIDE, DIHYDRATE 20 mg IN WATER FOR INJECTION.
pH ADJUSTED WITH HCl. ELECTROLYTES PER 1000 mL (NOT INCLUDING pH
ADJUSTMENT): SODIUM 130 mEq; POTASSIUM 4 mEq; CALCIUM 3 mEq;
CHLORIDE 109 mEq; LACTATE 28 mEq. 525 mOsmol/LITER (CALC). pH 4.9
(4.5 – 5.2). CAUTION: DO NOT ADMINISTER CALCIUM CONTAINING SOLUTIONS
CONCURRENTLY WITH STORED BLOOD. NOT FOR USE IN THE TREATMENT
OF LACTIC ACIDOSIS. ADDITIVES MAY BE INCOMPATIBLE. CONSULT WITH
PHARMACIST, IF AVAILABLE. WHEN INTRODUCING ADDITIVES, USE ASEPTIC
TECHNIQUE, MIX THOROUGHLY AND DO NOT STORE. SINGLE-DOSE CONTAINER.
FOR INTRAVENOUS USE. USUAL DOSE: SEE INSERT. STERILE, NONPYROGENIC.
CAUTION: FEDERAL (USA) LAW PROHIBITS DISPENSING WITHOUT
PRESCRIPTION. USE ONLY IF SOLUTION IS CLEAR AND CONTAINER IS
UNDAMAGED. MUST NOT BE USED IN SERIES CONNECTIONS. PATENT PENDING
©ABBOTT 1989   PRINTED IN USA
ABBOTT LABORATORIES, NORTH CHICAGO, IL60064, USA

2   —2
3   —3
4   —4

*(E and F Courtesy of Baxter Health Care Corporation; G and H
Courtesy of Abbott Laboratories)*

After completing these problems, see page 308 to check your answers.

Calculating Dosage Expressed as a Percentage in IV Fluids

The concentration percentage (%) of IV fluids designates the number of grams of the solute (component dissolved) per 100 mL of solution. Refer to Chapter 8 for more examples using percentages and Chapter 9 to review ratio and proportion.

EXAMPLE 1:   Order: D_5W *1000 mL*

Calculate the amount of dextrose in 1000 mL D_5W.

This can be calculated using ratio and proportion.

Recall that % = g per 100 mL; therefore, 5% = 5 g dextrose per 100 mL.

$$\frac{5\ g}{100\ mL} \diagup\!\!\!\!\diagdown \frac{X\ g}{1000\ mL}$$

100X = 5000

$$\frac{100X}{100} = \frac{5000}{100}$$

X = 50 g

1000 mL of D_5W contains 50 g of dextrose.

EXAMPLE 2:   Order: *NS 1000 mL*

Calculate the amount of sodium chloride (NaCl) in 1000 mL NS.

0.9% = 0.9 g NaCl per 100 mL

$$\frac{0.9\ g}{100\ mL} \diagup\!\!\!\!\diagdown \frac{X\ g}{1000\ mL}$$

100X = 900

$$\frac{100X}{100} = \frac{900}{100}$$

X = 9 g NaCl

1000 mL of NS contains 9 g of sodium chloride.

EXAMPLE 3:   Order: $D_5\frac{1}{4}NS$ *500 mL*

Calculate the amount of dextrose and sodium chloride in 500 mL.

D_5 = Dextrose 5% = 5 g dextrose per 100 mL

$$\frac{5\ g}{100\ mL} \diagup\!\!\!\!\diagdown \frac{X\ g}{500\ mL}$$

100X = 2500

$$\frac{100X}{100} = \frac{2500}{100}$$

X = 25 g dextrose

$\frac{1}{4}$ NS = 0.225% NaCl = 0.225 g NaCl per 100 mL.

$$\frac{0.225\ g}{100\ mL} \diagup\!\!\!\!\diagdown \frac{X\ g}{500\ mL}$$

100X = 112.5

$$\frac{100X}{100} = \frac{112.5}{100}$$

X = 1.125 g NaCl

500 mL $D_5\frac{1}{4}$ NS contains 25 g dextrose and 1.125 g sodium chloride.

It is important that you know what you are giving your patient when the physician orders IV fluids, such as D_5W. Think, "I am hanging D_5W. Do I know what that fluid contains?" Now you can answer, "Yes."

review set 31

Calculate the amount of dextrose and/or sodium chloride in each of the following IV solutions.

1. 1000 mL of D_5NS

    dextrose   _____ g

    sodium chloride _____ g

2. 500 mL of $D_5\frac{1}{2}NS$

    dextrose   _____ g

    sodium chloride _____ g

3. 250 mL of $D_{10}W$

    dextrose   _____ g

4. 750 mL of 0.9%NS

    sodium chloride _____ g

After completing these problems, see pages 308 and 309 to check your answers.

IV Sites

IV fluids may be ordered via a *peripheral line*, such as a vein in the arm, scalp (for infants), or leg. They may also be ordered via a *central line*, in which a special catheter is inserted to access a large vein in the chest. The subclavian vein, for example, may be used for a central line. Central lines may be accessed either directly through the chest wall, or indirectly via a neck vein or peripheral vein in the arm. Larger veins can accommodate higher concentrations and faster rates of IV fluids. They are often utilized if the patient is expected to need IV therapy for an extended period of time.

Monitoring IVs

The nurse is responsible for monitoring the patient regularly during an IV infusion. Generally the IV site and infusion should be checked at least every hour (according to hospital policy) for remaining fluids, correct infusion rate, and signs of complications.

The major complications associated with IV therapy are phlebitis and infiltration. *Phlebitis* occurs when the vein becomes irritated, red, or painful. *Infiltration* is when the IV catheter becomes dislodged from the vein and IV fluid escapes into the subcutaneous tissue. Should phlebitis or infiltration occur, the IV is discontinued and another IV site chosen to restart the IV. The patient should be instructed to notify the nurse if he notices any pain or swelling.

Primary and Secondary IVs

Notice that Figure 11–1 shows *primary IV tubing* packaging. This IV set is used to set up a typical or *primary IV*. Primary IV tubing includes a drip chamber, injection port, and roller clamp, and is long enough to be attached to the hub of the IV catheter positioned in the patient's vein. The drip chamber is squeezed until it is half full of IV fluid. The nurse can either regulate the rate manually using the roller clamp (Figure 11–2a) or place the tubing in an electronic infusion pump.

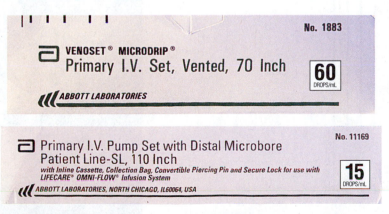

Fig. 11–1 Intravenous Infusion Tubing Packages:
Microdrop = 60 Drops/mL; Macrodrop = 15 Drops/mL

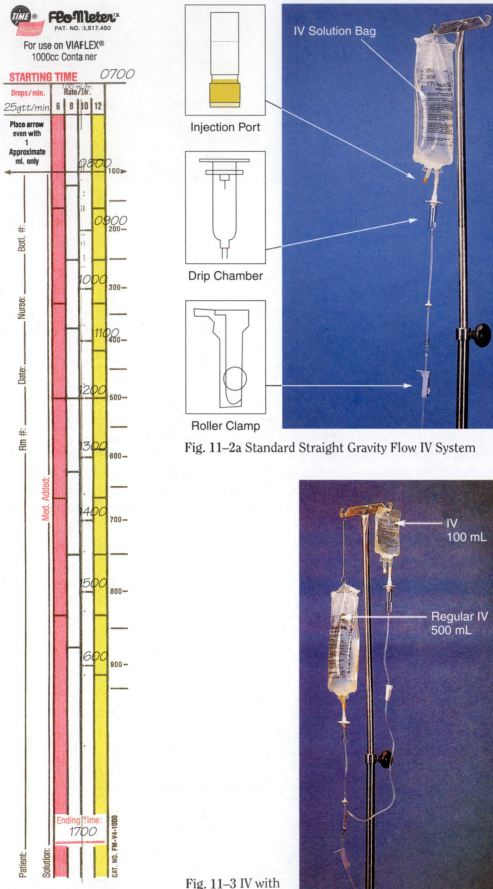

For use on VIAFLEX®
1000cc Container

STARTING TIME   *0700*

Drops/min.	100 ml./hr. Rate/hr.			
25gtt/min.	6	8	10	12

Place arrow
even with
1
Approximate
ml. only

0800 — 100►

Botl. #: _____

0900 — 200—

Nurse: _____

1000 — 300—

Date: _____

1100 — 400—

1200 — 500—

Rm #: _____

1300 — 600—

Med. Added:

1400 — 700—

1500 — 800—

1600 — 900—

Ending Time:
1700

Patient: _____

Solution: _____

CAT. NO. FM-V4-1000

Fig. 11–2b Infusion Label

Injection Port

Drip Chamber

Roller Clamp

IV Solution Bag

Fig. 11–2a Standard Straight Gravity Flow IV System

IV
100 mL

Regular IV
500 mL

Fig. 11–3 IV with
Piggyback (IV PB)

Secondary IV tubing is used when giving medications and is "piggybacked" into the primary line (Figure 11–3). This type of tubing (Figure 11–4) generally is shorter and also contains a drip chamber, injection port, and roller clamp. This gives access to the primary IV catheter without having to start another IV. You will notice that in this type of setup, the *secondary IV* set or *piggyback* is hung higher than the primary IV to allow the secondary set of medication to infuse first. When administering primary IV fluids, choose primary IV tubing; when hanging piggybacks, select secondary IV tubing. IV piggybacks are discussed further at the end of this chapter.

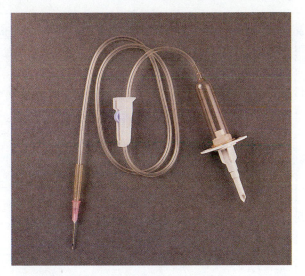

Fig. 11–4 Secondary IV Set

IV bags are often labeled with an infusion label (Figure 11–2b) that gives the nurse a visual check to monitor if the IV infusion is infusing on time as prescribed. These labels are attached to the IV bag and indicate the start and stop times of the infusion as well as how the IV should be progressing, such as at 100 mL/h.

IV Flow Rate

The *flow rate* of an intravenous (IV) infusion is ordered by the physician. It is the nurse's responsibility to regulate, monitor, and maintain this flow rate. Regulation of intravenous therapy is a critical skill in nursing. Since the fluids administered are infusing directly into the patient's circulatory system, careful monitoring is essential to be sure the patient does not receive too much or too little IV fluid and medication. It is important for the nurse to accurately set and maintain the flow rate to administer the prescribed volume of the IV solution within the specified time period. The IV fluids administered and IV flow rates are recorded on the IV administration record (IVAR), Figure 11–5.

IV solutions are usually ordered for a certain volume to run for a stated period of time, such as *125 mL/h or 1000 mL/8 h.* The nurse will use electronic or manual regulating equipment to monitor the flow rate. The calculations you must perform to set the flow rate will depend on the equipment used to administer the IV solutions.

Electronically Regulated IVs

Frequently IV solutions are regulated electronically by an infusion device, such as a controller or pump. The use of an electronic infusion device will be determined by the need to strictly regulate the IV. They can be set for a specific flow rate, and will alarm if this rate is interrupted.

Controllers depend on gravity to maintain the desired flow rate and do not force fluid into the system. They are often referred to as electronic flow clamps because they monitor the selected rate of infusion.

IV infusion pumps (Figure 11–6) do not rely on gravity but maintain the flow by adding pressure to the system to continue the flow at the preselected rate. Since pumps operate under pressure, they may continue to infuse, without alarming, in the presence of infiltration or phlebitis.

A *syringe pump* (Figure 11–7) is a type of electronic infusion pump. It is used to infuse fluids or medications directly from a syringe. It is most often used in pediatrics when a small volume of medication is being delivered, and in critical care when the drug cannot be mixed with other solutions or medications. Another advantage of the syringe pump is that a prescribed volume can be delivered over a prescribed time. This allows the fluid or medication to be given over less than one hour and is generally used when the desired time is 30 minutes or less.

Page:	of			DATE: 11/10/xx	through		
Correct	I.V. Order	Rate	Time	Initial	Site / Infusion Port	Pump / Other	Tubing Change
✓	D₅ ½ NS	100ml/hr	0900	GP	LH / PIV	☑	✓

CIRCULATORY ACCESS SITE

Time	Gauge	Length	Type	Site	# Attempts	Dressing Change	Site Condition	IV Lock	Initial	Time Catheter D/C Intact	Site Condition	Reason Code	Initial
0800	22	1½"	I	LH	1	✓	0	☐	GP				

Type:	Site:		Reason Code:	Infusion Port:	Site Condition:
I - Insyte	L - Left	A - Antecubital	1 - Infiltrate	PIV - Peripheral IV	0
B - Butterfly	R - Right	F - Femoral	2 - Physician Order	CVC - CVC	1+
C - Cathlon	H - Hand	J - Jugular	3 - Patient Removed	SG - Swan Ganz	2+
CVC - CVC	FA - Forearm	FT - Foot	4 - Clotted	D - Distal	3+
T - Tunnelled	UA - Upper Arm	S - Scalp	5 - Phlebitis	M - Middle	4+
IP - Implanted Port	SC - Subclavian	U - Umbilical	6 - Site Rotation	P - Proximal	5+
PICC - PICC	C - Chest	RA - Radial	7 - Leaking	R - Red	Tubing Change:
A - Arterial Line	Dressing Change:		8 - Positional	BL - Blue	P - Primary
SG - Swan Ganz	T - Transparent		9 - Not Patent	V - Venous	S - Secondary
DL - Dual Lumen Peripheral	A - Air Occlusive		10 - Family Refused	S - Sideport	E - Extension
UAC - UAC	B - Bandaid		Other:	AN - Access Needle	T - 3 Way Stopcock
UVC - UVC	PR - Pressure Dressing		D - Dial-a-flow	A - Arterial	H - Hemodynamic

ALLERGIES:

Initial / Signature - Circulatory Access Site(s) checked hourly.

GP / G. Pickar, R.N. _____ ____ / _____

____ / _____ ____ / _____

____ / _____ ____ / _____

Reconciled by: _____

IV ADMINISTRATION RECORD

602-0203 (2-94)dlg)MPC#32258)

Fig. 11–5 Intravenous Administration Record

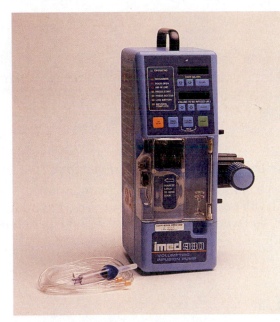

Fig. 11–6 IV Infusion Pump

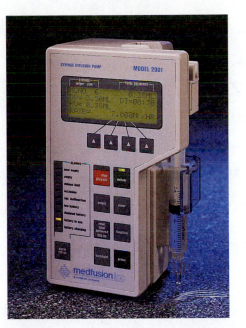

Fig. 11–7 Syringe Pump *(Photo courtesy of Medex Inc.)*

Patient controlled analgesia (PCA) pump (Figure 11–8) is used to allow the patient to self-administer IV medication to control pain. This type of device is often used for the patient to control postoperative pain and for cancer patients. A prefilled syringe of pain medication such as Demerol or morphine is inserted into the device, and the dosage and frequency of the medication are set as ordered by the physician. The patient presses the control button when in pain, and the medication is delivered and recorded by the PCA.

The device has a safety feature called the "lock-out" time period, which is set in the pump so the patient cannot receive an overdose. The pump also keeps a record of the number of times the patient pushed the button, which can be displayed for the nurse to document administration frequency.

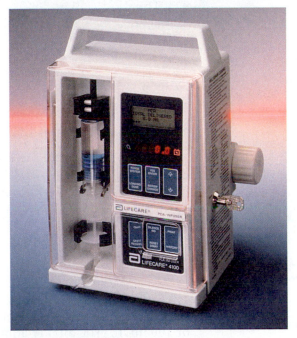

Fig. 11–8 PCA Pump *(Photo courtesy of Abbott Laboratories)*

Calculating Flow Rates for Electronic Regulators in mL/h

When an electronic infusion regulator is used, the flow rate is ordered by the physician and programmed by the nurse. The nurse sets the device for *milliliters per hour (mL/h).*

> **rule** To regulate an IV by electronic infusion pump or controller, calibrated in mL/h,
>
> $$\frac{\text{Total mL ordered}}{\text{Total h ordered}} = \text{mL/h (rounded to a whole number)}$$

Notice that this is actually a proportion of two equal ratios.

> **rule** To regulate an IV by an electronic infusion pump or controller calibrated in mL/h,
>
> $$\frac{\text{Total mL ordered}}{\text{Total h ordered}} = \frac{X \text{ mL}}{1 \text{ h}}$$

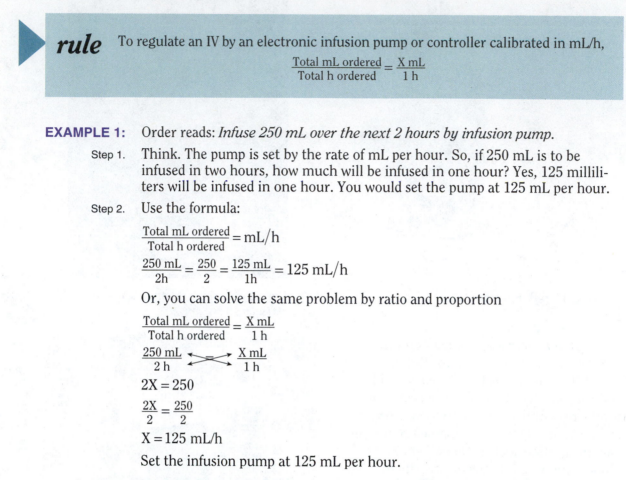

EXAMPLE 1: Order reads: *Infuse 250 mL over the next 2 hours by infusion pump.*

Step 1. Think. The pump is set by the rate of mL per hour. So, if 250 mL is to be infused in two hours, how much will be infused in one hour? Yes, 125 milliliters will be infused in one hour. You would set the pump at 125 mL per hour.

Step 2. Use the formula:

$$\frac{\text{Total mL ordered}}{\text{Total h ordered}} = \text{mL/h}$$

$$\frac{250 \text{ mL}}{2h} = \frac{250}{2} = \frac{125 \text{ mL}}{1h} = 125 \text{ mL/h}$$

Or, you can solve the same problem by ratio and proportion

$$\frac{\text{Total mL ordered}}{\text{Total h ordered}} = \frac{X \text{ mL}}{1 \text{ h}}$$

$$\frac{250 \text{ mL}}{2 \text{ h}} \quad \frac{X \text{ mL}}{1 \text{ h}}$$

$$2X = 250$$

$$\frac{2X}{2} = \frac{250}{2}$$

$$X = 125 \text{ mL/h}$$

Set the infusion pump at 125 mL per hour.

In most cases it is easy to calculate mL/h by simply dividing total mL by total h. However, an IV with medication added or a piggyback IV (IV PB) may be ordered to be administered by an electronic infusion device in *less than one hour*, but the pump or controller must still be set in mL/h. When the order is for an infusion of less than one hour (or less than 60 minutes), use ratio and proportion to find mL/h.

EXAMPLE 2: Order reads: *Ampicillin 500 mg IV in 50 mL $D_5 \frac{1}{2}$ NS in 30 min. by controller.*

Step 1. Think. The controller is set by the rate of mL per hour. If 50 mL is to be infused in 30 minutes, then set the controller at the rate of 100 mL per 60 min or 100 mL/h. (The total IV ampicillin will be infused within 30 minutes.)

Step 2. Use ratio-proportion:

Remember: 1 hour = 60 minutes.

$$\frac{50 \text{ mL}}{30 \text{ min}} \quad \frac{X \text{ mL}}{60 \text{ min}}$$

$$30X = 3000$$

$$\frac{30X}{30} = \frac{3000}{30}$$

$$X = 100 \text{ mL/h}$$

review set 32 _____

Calculate the flow rate you will program the electronic infusion regulator for the IVs ordered.

1. 1 L D_5W IV to infuse in 10 hours by infusion pump.
   _____ mL/h

2. 1800 mL Normal Saline IV to infuse in 15 hours by controller.
   _____ mL/h

3. 2000 mL D_5W IV in 24 hours by controller.
   _____ mL/h

4. 100 mL NS IV PB in 30 minutes by infusion pump.
   _____ mL/h

5. 30 mL antibiotic in D_5W IV in 15 minutes by infusion pump.
   _____ mL/h

6. 2.5 L NS IV in 20 hours by controller.
   _____ mL/h

After completing these problems, see page 309 to check your answers.

Manually Regulated IVs

When the electronic infusion device is not used, the nurse manually regulates the IV. To do this the nurse must calculate the number of drops the IV should flow per minute. The drop rate (gtt/min) is then set by adjusting the roller clamp and timed by counting the number of drops dripping per minute into the IV drip chamber (Figure 11–2a, page 210).

The number of drops per minute will depend partially upon the size of the drops delivered by the particular IV tubing used. This calibration is referred to as the *drop factor*, which is the number of drops per milliliter (gtt/mL). The drop factor varies according to the manufacturer of the IV equipment. Standard or *macrodrop* IV tubing sets have a drop factor of 10 gtt/mL, 15 gtt/mL, or 20 gtt/mL. All *microdrop* (or minidrip) IV tubing has a drop factor of 60 gtt/mL (Figure 11–9). The drop factor is stated on the package of the IV tubing (Figure 11–1, page 209).

▶ *rule*   Drop factor = gtt/mL

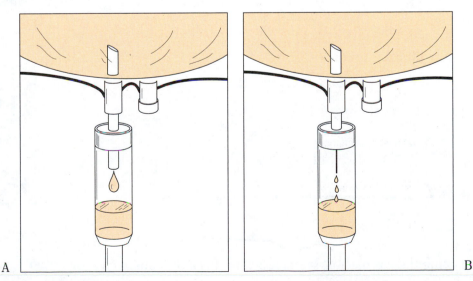

A   B

Fig. 11–9 Intravenous Drip Chambers: Comparison of (A) Macro and (B) Microdrops

review set 33

Identify the drop factor calibration of the primary IV tubing pictured.

No. 4967

ⓐ VENOSET® Piggyback
Primary I.V. Set, Vented, 80 Inch **15** DROPS/mL

ⓐ ABBOTT LABORATORIES, NORTH CHICAGO, IL60064, USA

1. _____ gtt/mL

No. 1871

ⓐ **Y-TYPE BLOOD SET**
WITH LATEX SLEEVE
For alternate administration from blood bag and I.V. solution container.

NONVENTED
78 INCH

20 DROPS/mL

ⓐ ABBOTT LABORATORIES, NORTH CHICAGO, IL60064, USA

2. _____ gtt/mL

2C5546 s
Baxter

**Continu-Flo®
Solution Set**
3 Injection Sites
Luer Lock Adapter

60

60 drops approx. 1 mL

2.7 m (108") long

*Sterile, nonpyrogenic fluid path

Caution: Federal (USA) law restricts this device
to sale by or on order of a physician.

3. _____ gtt/mL

2C5545 s
Baxter

**Continu-Flo®
Solution Set**
3 Injection Sites
Luer Lock Adapter

10

10 drops approx. 1 mL

2.7 m (105") long

*Sterile, nonpyrogenic fluid path

Caution: Federal (USA) law restricts this device
to sale by or on order of a physician.

No. 1883

ⓐ VENOSET® MICRODRIP®
Primary I.V. Set, Vented, 70 Inch **60** DROPS/mL

ⓐ ABBOTT LABORATORIES

4. _____ gtt/mL

5. _____ gtt/mL

After completing these problems, see page 309 to check your answers.

Calculating Flow Rates for Manually Regulated IVs in gtt/min

In this section you will learn two methods to calculate IV flow rate for manually regulated IVs: the formula method and the shortcut method.

IV Flow Rate Formula

The formula method can be used to determine the flow rate in drops per minute *(gtt/min)*.

▶ *rule*   The formula for IV flow rate is:

$$\frac{V}{T} \times C = R$$

In this formula:

V = Total VOLUME to be infused in mL
T = Total TIME in minutes
C = Drop factor CALIBRATION (gtt/mL)
R = RATE of flow (gtt/min)

NOTE: Carry calculations to two decimal places. Round gtt/min to the nearest whole number since you can only count whole drops.

Let's look at some examples.

EXAMPLE 1:   Calculate the IV flow rate for *1200 mL of Normal Saline to be infused in 6 hours*. The infusion set is calibrated for a drop factor of 15 gtt/mL.

Step 1.   Calculate total time in minutes.
$6 \times 60 = 360$ min

Step 2. $\frac{V}{T} \times C = R$: $\frac{1200}{360} \times 15 = 50$ gtt/min

EXAMPLE 2:   Calculate the IV flow rate for an *intravenous solution to infuse at the rate of 125 mL per hour*. The drop factor is 10 gtt/mL.

Step 1.   Calculate total time in minutes: 1 h = 60 min

Step 2. $\frac{V}{T} \times C = R$: $\frac{125}{60} \times 10 = 20.8 = 21$ gtt/min

EXAMPLE 3:   Calculate the IV flow rate for *200 cc of 0.9% NaCl IV over 2 hours*. The drop factor is 20 gtt/mL.

Step 1.   Calculate total time in minutes: 2 h = 120 min

Step 2. $\frac{V}{T} \times C = R$: $\frac{200}{120} \times 20 = 33.3 = 33$ gtt/min

EXAMPLE 4:   Calculate the IV flow rate for *400 mL 5% dextrose to run for 8 hours*. The drop factor is 60 gtt/mL.

Step 1.   Calculate total time in minutes.
$8 \times 60 = 480$ min

Step 2. $\frac{V}{T} \times C = R$: $\frac{400}{480} \times 60 = 50$ gtt/min

review set 34

1. State the formula used to calculate IV flow rate in gtt/min.

   _____

Calculate the IV flow rate in drops per minute (gtt/min) using the formula method.

2. Order: 3000 mL D$_5$W IV to run for 24 hours
   Drop factor: 10 gtt/mL
   _____ gtt/min

3. Order: 250 mL Lactated Ringer's IV to infuse in 5 hours
   Drop factor: 60 gtt/mL
   _____ gtt/min

4. Order: 100 mL NS antibiotic solution IV to infuse in 40 min
   Drop factor: 20 gtt/mL
   _____ gtt/min

5. Order: D$_5$ $\frac{1}{2}$ NS IV with 20 mEq KCl per liter to run at 25 mL/h
   Drop factor: 60 gtt/mL
   _____ gtt/min

6. Order: Two 500 mL units of whole blood IV to be infused in 4 hours
   Infusion set is calibrated to 20 drops per milliliter.
   _____ gtt/min

7. Hyperalimentation solution is ordered for 1240 mL to infuse in 12 hours using an infusion set with tubing calibrated for 20 gtt/mL
   _____ gtt/min

After completing these problems, see page 309 to check your answers.

Short Cut Method

By converting the volume and time in the formula method to mL/h (or mL/60 min), you can use a short cut to calculate flow rate. This short cut is derived from the drop factor (C) which cancels out each time and reduces the 60 minutes (T). You are left with the *drop factor constant*. Look at this example.

EXAMPLE 1:   Administer Normal Saline at 125 mL/h with a microdrop infusion set calibrated for *60 gtt/mL*. Use the formula $\frac{V}{T} \times C = R$.

$$\frac{125 \text{ mL}}{\underset{1}{\cancel{60} \text{ min}}} \times \overset{1}{\cancel{60}} \text{ gtt/mL} = \frac{125}{①} = 125 \text{ gtt/min}$$

The drop factor constant for an infusion set with 60 gtt/mL is 1. Therefore, to administer 125 mL/h, set the flow rate at 125 gtt/min.

Look at another example.

EXAMPLE 2:   Administer 125 mL/h IV with *20 gtt/mL* infusion set.

$$\frac{125 \text{ mL}}{\underset{3}{\cancel{60} \text{ min}}} \times \overset{1}{\cancel{20}} \text{ gtt/mL} = \frac{125}{③} = 41.7 = 42 \text{ gtt/min}$$

The drop factor constant is 3.
Therefore, each drop factor constant is obtained by dividing 60 minutes by the drop factor of the infusion set.

remember

Manufacturer	Drop Factor	Drop Factor Constant
Baxter-Travenol	10 gtt/mL	$6 = \frac{60}{10}$
Abbott	15 gtt/mL	$4 = \frac{60}{15}$
Armour	20 gtt/mL	$3 = \frac{60}{20}$
Any micro or minidrop	60 gtt/mL	$1 = \frac{60}{60}$

Since most hospitals consistently use infusion equipment manufactured by one company, you will become very familiar with the one used where you work; therefore, the shortcut method is very practical, quick, and simple to use.

rule   The short cut method to calculate IV flow rate is:

$$\frac{mL/h}{\text{Drop factor constant}} = gtt/min$$

Let's re-examine the previous four examples using the short cut method.

EXAMPLE 1:   Order: *1200 mL NS IV in 6 hours*
Drop factor: 15 gtt/mL
Drop factor constant: 4

Step 1. $mL/hr = \frac{1200}{6} = 200 \text{ mL/h}$

Step 2. $\frac{mL/h}{\text{Drop factor constant}} = \frac{200}{4} = 50 \text{ gtt/min}$

EXAMPLE 2:   Order: *125 mL D$_5$W IV in 1 hour*
Drop factor: 10 gtt/mL
Drop factor constant: 6

Step 1.   Done! 125 mL/h

Step 2. $\frac{125}{6} = 20.8 = 21 \text{ gtt/min}$

EXAMPLE 3.   Order: *200 cc 0.9% NaCl IV in 2 hours*
Drop factor: 20 gtt/mL
Drop factor constant: 3

Step 1. $\frac{200}{2} = 100 \text{ mL/h}$

Step 2. $\frac{100}{3} = 33.3 = 33 \text{ gtt/min}$

Chapter 11

EXAMPLE 4: Order: *400 mL 5% dextrose IV in 8 hours*
Drop factor: 60 gtt/mL
Drop factor constant: 1

Step 1. $\dfrac{400}{8} = 50$ mL/h

Step 2. $\dfrac{50}{1} = 50$ gtt/min

Easy! When the drop factor is 60, set the flow rate at the same gtt/min as the mL/h.

> **rule** When the drop factor is 60 gtt/mL, then mL/h = gtt/min.

review set 35

1. The drop factor <u>constant</u> is derived by dividing _____ by the drop factor calibration.

Determine the drop factor constant for each of the infusion sets.

2. 60 gtt/mL _____

3. 20 gtt/mL _____

4. 15 gtt/mL _____

5. 10 gtt/mL _____

6. State the rule for the short cut method to calculate the IV flow rate in gtt/min. _____

_____

Calculate the IV flow rate in drops per minute (gtt/min) using the short cut method.

7. Order: 1000 mL D$_5$W IV to infuse in 4 hours
Drop factor: 15 gtt/mL
_____ gtt/min

8. Order: 750 mL D$_5$W IV to infuse in 6 hours
Drop factor: 20 gtt/mL
_____ gtt/min

9. Order: 500 mL D$_5$W 0.45% Saline IV to infuse in 3 hours
Drop factor: 10 gtt/mL
_____ gtt/min

10. Order: 2 liters NS IV to infuse at 60 cc/h with microdrop infusion set of 60 gtt/mL
_____ gtt/min

After completing these problems, see page 310 to check your answers.

quick review

■ When regulating IV flow rate for an electronic infusion device, calculate mL/h.
■ When calculating IV flow rate to regulate an IV manually, find the drop factor and calculate gtt/min by using the:

Formula Method

$$\frac{V}{T} \times C = R$$

or Short Cut Method

$$\frac{mL/h}{\text{Drop factor constant}} = gtt/min$$

- Carefully monitor patients receiving intravenous fluids at least hourly.
- Check remaining IV fluids.
- Check IV flow rate.
- Observe IV site for complications.

review set 36

Calculate the IV flow rate.

1. Order: 3000 mL 0.45% NaCl IV for 24 hours
   Drop factor: 15 gtt/mL
   Flow rate: _____ gtt/min

2. Order: 200 mL D_5W IV to run for 2 hours
   Drop factor: Microdrop, 60 gtt/mL
   Flow rate: _____ gtt/min

3. Order: 800 cc $D_5 \frac{1}{3}$ NS IV for 8 hours
   Drop factor: 20 gtt/mL
   Flow rate: _____ gtt/min

4. Order: 1000 cc NS IV for 24 hours KVO (to keep the vein open)
   Drop factor: 60 gtt/mL
   Flow rate: _____ gtt/min

5. Order: 1500 mL D_5W IV for 12 hours
   Drop factor: 15 gtt/mL
   Flow rate: _____ gtt/min

6. Order: Aminophylline 0.5 g IV in 250 mL D_5W to run for 2 hours by infusion pump
   Flow rate: _____ mL/h

7. Order: 2500 mL D_5 0.45% NaCl IV for 24 hours
   Drop factor: 20 gtt/mL
   Flow rate: _____ gtt/min

8. Order: 500 mL D_5 0.45% NaCl IV for 3 hours
   Drop factor: 10 gtt/mL
   Flow rate: _____ gtt/min

9. Order: 1200 mL Normal Saline IV for 8 hours
   Drop factor: 10 gtt/mL
   Flow rate: _____ gtt/min

10. Order: 1000 cc D_5 0.45% NaCl IV to infuse over 8 hours
    Drop factor: On electronic infusion pump
    Flow rate: _____ mL/h

11. Order: 2000 cc D$_5$NS IV to infuse over 24 hours
     Drop factor: On electronic infusion controller
     Flow rate: _____ mL/h

12. Order: 500 cc Lactated Ringer's IV to infuse over 4 hours
     Drop factor: On electronic infusion controller
     Flow rate: _____ mL/h

After completing these problems, see page 310 to check your answers.

Adjusting IV Flow Rate

IV fluids, especially those with medicines added (called additives), are viewed as medications with specific dosages (rates of infusion, in this case). It is the responsibility of the nurse to maintain this rate of flow through careful calculations and **close observation** at regular intervals.

Various circumstances, such as gravity, condition, and movement of the patient can alter the set flow rate of an IV causing the IV to run ahead of or behind schedule. **It is not at the discretion of the nurse to arbitrarily speed up or slow down the flow rate in order to catch up the IV.** This practice can result in serious conditions of over or underhydration and electrolyte imbalance.

If during your regular monitoring of the IV, you find that the rate is not progressing as scheduled or is significantly ahead of or behind schedule, the physician may need to be notified as warranted by the patient's condition, hospital policy, or just good nursing judgment. *However, as allowed by hospital policy, the flow rate per minute may be adjusted by up to 25 percent more or less than the original rate depending on the condition of the patient.* In such cases, assess the patient, and if stable, recalculate the flow rate to administer the total milliliters remaining over the number of hours remaining of the original order.

> ### rule   To calculate IV percent changes:
>
> $$\frac{\text{New flow rate} - \text{Ordered flow rate}}{\text{Ordered flow rate}} = \text{Percent of variation}$$
>
> which will be (+) if administration is slow and needs to have administration rate increased, and (−) if being administered too fast, and rate needs to be decreased.

EXAMPLE: The order reads: *1000 mL D$_5$W/8 h.* The drop factor is 10 gtt/mL and the IV is correctly set at 21 gtt/min. You would expect that after 4 hours, one-half of the total or 500 mL of the solution would be infused. However, checking the IV bag the fourth hour after starting the IV, you find 600 milliliters remaining. You would compute a new flow rate for 600 milliliters to run for the remaining 4 hours.

Step 1.   4 h = 240 min

Step 2. $\frac{V}{T} \times C = R: \frac{600}{240} \times 10 = 25$ gtt/min

$$\frac{\text{New flow rate} - \text{Ordered flow rate}}{\text{Ordered flow rate}} = \text{Percent of variation}$$

$$\frac{25 - 21}{21} = \frac{4}{21} = 19\%$$

Compare 25 gtt/min (in the last example) with the start flow rate of 21 gtt/min. You can see that adjusting the total remaining volume over the total remaining hours changes the flow rate per minute very little (19%). Most patients can tolerate this small amount of increase per minute over several hours. However, trying to catch up the lost 100 milliliters in one hour can be very dangerous. To infuse an extra 100 milliliters in one hour, with a drop factor of 10, you would need to speed up the IV to a much faster rate.

$$\frac{V}{T} \times C = \frac{100}{60} \times \frac{10}{6} = 16.7 = 17 \text{ gtt/min}$$

To catch up the IV over the next hour, the flow rate would need to be 17 drops per minute faster than the original 21 drops per minute rate. The infusion would need to be set at 17 + 21 = 38 gtt/min for one hour and then slowed to the original rate. Such an increase would be $\frac{38-21}{21} = \frac{17}{21} = 81\%$, greater than the ordered rate. For a child or a seriously ill patient, this can present a serious problem. **Do not do it! If permitted by hospital policy, the flow rate must be recalculated when the IV is off schedule.**

Remember, a good rule of thumb is that the recalculated flow rate should not vary from the original rate by more than 25 percent. If the recalculated rate does vary from the original by more than 25 percent, contact your supervisor or the doctor for further instructions. The original order may need to be revised. Regular monitoring helps to prevent or minimize this problem.

Patients who require close monitoring for IV fluids will most likely have the IV regulated by an electronic infusion device. Because of the nature of their condition, "catching up" these IVs, if off schedule, is not recommended. If an IV regulated by an infusion pump or controller is off schedule or inaccurate, consider that the infusion pump may need recalibration. Consult with your supervisor, as needed.

quick review

- For manually regulated IVs, recalculate flow rate when off schedule, if permitted by the hospital policy: $\frac{\text{New flow rate} - \text{Ordered flow rate}}{\text{Ordered flow rate}} = \%$ Variation
- Recalculated flow rate must not vary from the original rate by more than 25 percent if allowed by hospital policy. Do not arbitrarily speed up or slow down to catch up.

review set 37

Compute the flow rate in drops per minute. Hospital policy permits recalculating IVs when off schedule with a maximum variation in rate of 25 percent.

1. Order: 1500 mL Lactated Ringer's for 12 hours
   Drop factor: 20 gtt/mL
   Flow rate: _____ gtt/min

   After six hours, there are 850 mL remaining; describe your action at this time. _____
   _____

2. Order: 1000 mL Lactated Ringer's for 6 hours
   Drop factor: 15 gtt/mL
   Flow rate: _____ gtt/min

   After 4 hours, there are 360 mL remaining; describe your action now. _____
   _____

3. Order: 1000 mL D₅W for 8 hours
   Drop factor: 20 gtt/mL
   Flow rate: _____ gtt/min

   After 4 hours, there are 800 mL remaining; describe your action now. _____
   _____

4. Order: 2000 mL NS for 12 hours
    Drop factor: 10 gtt/mL
    Flow rate: _____ gtt/min

    After 8 hours, there are 750 mL remaining; describe your action now. _____
    _____

5. Order: 100 mL NS for 4 hours
    Drop factor: 60 gtt/mL
    Flow rate: _____ gtt/min

    After $1\frac{1}{2}$ hours, there are 90 mL remaining; describe your action now. _____
    _____

After completing these problems, see pages 310 and 311 to check your answers.

IV Piggybacks

A medication may be ordered to be dissolved in a small amount of intravenous fluid (usually 50 to 100 mL) and run "piggyback" the regular intravenous fluids (Figure 11–3, page 210) Recall that the piggyback IV (or secondary IV) requires a secondary IV set (Figure 11–4, page 211).

The IV piggyback (IV PB) medication may come premixed by the manufacturer or pharmacy or may be the nurse's responsibility to properly prepare. Whichever the case, it is always the responsibility of the nurse to accurately administer the medication. The infusion time is usually less than 60 minutes.

Sometimes the physician's order for the IV PB medication will not include an infusion time or rate. It is understood, when this is the case, that the nurse will follow the manufacturer's guidelines for infusion rates, keeping in mind the amount of fluid accompanying the medication and any standing orders that limit fluid amounts or rates. Appropriate infusion times are readily available in many drug books, such as the *Hospital Formulary,* which is readily available on most nursing units, or you can consult with the hospital pharmacist.

EXAMPLE: Order: *Kefzol 0.5 g in 100 mL D₅W IV PB to run over 30 min*
Drop factor: 60 gtt/mL
What is the flow rate in gtt/min?
$$\frac{V}{T} \times C = R: \frac{100}{30} \times \frac{60}{1} = 200 \text{ gtt/min}$$

If an infusion pump or controller is used to administer the same order, remember that you would need to program the device in mL/h. If 100 mL will be administered in 30 minutes or one-half hour, then 200 mL will be administered in one hour or 60 minutes.

You can use ratio-proportion to calculate mL/h.

$$\frac{100 \text{ mL}}{30 \text{ min}} \diagdown\diagup \frac{X \text{ mL}}{60 \text{ min}} \quad (1 \text{ h} = 60 \text{ min})$$

$$30X = 6000$$

$$\frac{30X}{30} = \frac{6000}{30}$$

X = 200 mL/h

Set the electronic IV PB regulator to 200 mL/h

review set 38

Calculate the IV PB flow rate.

1. Order: Ancef 1 g in 100 cc D_5W IV PB to be infused over 45 minutes
   Drop factor: 60 gtt/mL
   Flow rate: _____ gtt/min

2. Order: Ancef 1 g in 100 cc D_5W IV PB to be administered by electronic infusion controller to infuse in 45 minutes
   Flow rate: _____ mL/h

3. Order: Geopen (carbenicillin disodium) 2 g IV PB diluted in 50 mL D_5W to infuse in 15 minutes
   Drop factor: 15 gtt/mL
   Flow rate: _____ gtt/min

4. Order: Geopen (carbenicillin disodium) 2 g IV PB diluted in 50 mL D_5W to infuse in 15 minutes, administered by an electronic infusion pump
   Flow rate: _____ mL/h

5. Order: 50 mL IV PB antibiotic solution to infuse in 30 minutes
   Drop factor: 60 gtt/mL
   Flow rate: _____ gtt/min

After completing these problems, see page 311 to check your answers.

Saline and Heparin IV Locks

Sometimes the patient needs to receive IV medications but does not need IV fluids. In this instance the physician may order a *saline* or *heparin lock*. IV locks can be attached to the hub of the IV catheter that is positioned in the vein. A small portion of extension tubing is attached to the IV catheter with a clamp. A sterile cap is then attached to the end. With this method, medications can be given via the IV route without IV fluids infusing at all times.

Medications can be given *IV push* or *bolus*, meaning to attach a syringe directly to the extension tubing and push in the medication. Or, the medication can be attached to an IV set up, such as a primary IV line, and manually regulated over a prescribed time or attached to an electronic regulator.

These IV locks may be referred to as saline locks, meaning saline is used to flush or maintain the line, or heparin locks if heparin is used to maintain the line. These lines must be flushed with saline or heparin at least twice a day or after each medication is given to keep the line patent. This is necessary because fluids are not infusing all the time. Refer to the policy at your hospital regarding the volume and concentration of saline or heparin to be used.

Make sure you are giving the correct dosage of heparin lock flush solution, usually 10 units/mL or 100 units/mL. This is a different solution than the commonly prescribed medication, heparin, which is available in much higher concentrations.

ADD-Vantage System

Another type of medication setup commonly used in hospitals is the ADD-Vantage system by Abbott Laboratories (Figure 11–10). In this system a specially designed IV bag with a medication vial port is used. The medication vial comes with the ordered dosage and medication prepared in a powder form. It is thoroughly mixed by the nurse in the IV fluid at the time of administration. The vial remains in the solution bag port throughout the infusion so the medication and dosage being delivered are clear.

Fig. 11–10 ADD-Vantage System: Medications Can Be Added to Another Solution Being Infused *(Reproduced with permission of Burroughs Wellcome Co.)*

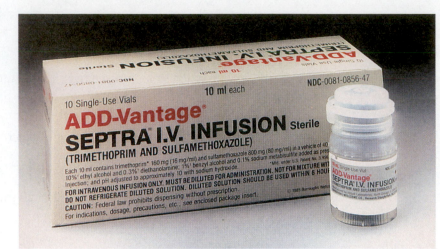

SEPTRA® I.V. INFUSION ADD-Vantage® Vials
(trimethoprim and sulfamethoxazole)

To Assemble ADD-Vantage® Vial and Flexible Diluent Container:

(Use Aseptic Technique)

1. Remove the protective covers from the top of the vial and the vial port on the diluent container as follows:

   a. To remove the breakaway vial cap, swing the pull ring over the top of the vial and pull down far enough to start the opening (see Figure 1), then pull straight up to remove the cap (see Figure 2). **NOTE:** Once the breakaway cap has been removed, do not access vial with syringe.

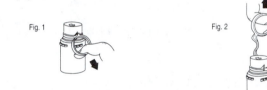

Fig. 1   Fig. 2

   b. To remove the vial port cover, grasp the tab on the pull ring, pull up to break the three tie strings, then pull back to remove the cover (see Figure 3).

2. Screw the vial into the vial port until it will go no further. THE VIAL MUST BE SCREWED IN TIGHTLY TO ASSURE A SEAL. This occurs approximately ½ turn (180°) after the first audible click (see Figure 4). The clicking sound does not assure a seal; the vial must be turned as far as it will go. **NOTE:** Once vial is seated, do not attempt to remove (see Figure 4).

3. Recheck the vial to assure that it is tight by trying to turn it further in the direction of assembly.

4. Label appropriately.

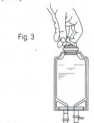   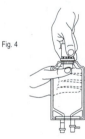

Fig. 3   Fig. 4

To Prepare Admixture:

1. Squeeze the bottom of the diluent container gently to inflate the portion of the container surrounding the end of the drug vial.

2. With the other hand, push the drug vial down into the container telescoping the walls of the container. Grasp the inner cap of the vial through the walls of the container (see Figure 5).

3. Pull the inner cap from the drug vial (see Figure 6). Verify that the rubber stopper has been pulled out, allowing the drug and diluent to mix.

4. Mix container contents thoroughly and use within the specified time.

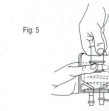   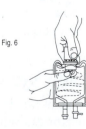

Fig. 5   Fig. 6

Preparation for Administration:

(Use Aseptic Technique)

1. Confirm the activation and admixture of vial contents.

2. Check for leaks by squeezing container firmly. If leaks are found, discard unit as sterility may be impaired.

3. Close flow control clamp of administration set.

4. Remove cover from outlet port at bottom of container.

Blood Transfusions

Blood transfusion or replacement is the IV administration of whole blood or a component such as packed red cells, plasma, or platelets. Transfusions are ordered when the patient has had blood loss following surgery, trauma, or hemorrhage. Blood products may be ordered for the patient with anemia or bone marrow depression from cancer. Plasma-clotting factors may be ordered for the patient with hemophilia.

Blood Typing and Cross Matching: The ABO System

Human blood is classified into four compatibility groups based on the ABO system. The four groups are A, B, O, and AB. Determination of blood group is based on the presence or absence of A and B red cell antigens. Individuals with A antigens, B antigens, or no antigens belong to groups A, B, and O, respectively. Likewise, the individual with A and B antigens has AB blood. Individuals with type A blood naturally produce anti-B antibodies in their plasma. Likewise, persons with type B blood naturally produce anti-A antibodies in their plasma. Type O individuals naturally produce both anti-A and anti-B antibodies, which is why persons with O type blood are considered universal donors. An individual with AB type blood produces neither antibody, which is why type AB individuals are considered universal recipients.

Another consideration when matching for blood transfusions is the Rh factor. The Rh factor refers to the presence of Rh antibodies on the surface of the red cell and is present in the majority of people. The blood of persons with the Rh factor is said to be Rh positive (+) whereas the blood of persons without the factor is said to be Rh negative (–). Persons with Rh negative blood should always receive Rh negative blood. Persons with Rh positive blood may receive either Rh positive or Rh negative blood.

Blood Administration

Administration of blood and blood products is a critical nursing skill that involves intensive monitoring of the patient before, during, and after the transfusion. Generally a consent form is signed prior to the administration of blood or blood products.

When the order for a blood transfusion is received a *type and cross match* is performed which involves drawing a blood sample for typing of the patient's blood and mixing some of the patient's blood with that of the donor to monitor for any hemolysis. A blood bank identification band is placed on the patient. When the transfusion is ready two nurses go to the bedside to identify the patient's blood bank number, blood type of donor, blood type of the patient, donor number, ordered components, and the expiration date. Once the identification process has occurred both nurses sign the blood tag.

Blood should be administered via a large-gauge IV catheter (18 or 19 gauge) to facilitate ease of blood flow due to the viscous nature of blood. Blood must be hung within 30 minutes after it is obtained from the blood bank. Blood is administered most often via a Y set infusion system (Figure 11–11) that contains two ports to allow normal saline to be infused to prime the IV line and to ensure all the blood has infused from the tubing. IV solutions containing Lactated Ringer's and dextrose are contraindicated for blood transfusions as they result in hemolysis of red blood cells. The Y set also contains a filter in the drip chamber to remove any debris or tiny clots from the blood.

Just prior to the blood transfusion the patient's vital signs are assessed. During the transfusion, vital signs are typically monitored 15 minutes after the initiation of the infusion and every 30 minutes during the infusion and 30 minutes after the infusion is completed. (See your institution's policy regarding frequency of vital signs). Generally speaking, blood must infuse within 4 hours of initiation. At any time during the infusion should the patient show any of the signs of a transfusion reaction (fever, chills, rash, urticaria, back pain, IV site pain, hematuria, dyspnea, changes in blood pressure, or increased pulse) the transfusion is stopped and the physician notified. However, the IV line is kept patent with saline.

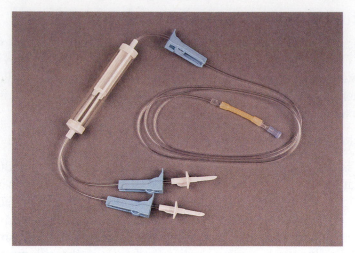

Fig. 11–11 Y-type Blood Administration Set

critical thinking skills

It is important to know the equipment you are using. Let's look at an example in which the nurse was unfamiliar with the IV piggyback setup.

■ error 1

Failing to follow manufacturer's directions when using a new IV piggyback system.

possible scenario

Suppose the physician ordered Rocephin 1 g IV q.12h for an elderly patient with streptococcus pneumonia. The medication was sent to the unit by pharmacy utilizing the ADD-Vantage system. Rocephin 1 gram was supplied in a powder form and attached to a 50 mL IV bag of D_5W. The directions for preparing the medication were attached to the label. The nurse, who was unfamiliar with the new ADD-Vantage system, hung the IV medication, calculated the drip rate, and infused the 50 mL of fluid. The nurse cared for the patient for three days. During walking rounds on the third day, the on-coming nurse noticed that the Rocephin powder remained in the vial and never was diluted in the IV bag. The nurse realized that the vial stopper inside of the IV bag was not open. Therefore the medication powder was not mixed in the IV fluid during this shift for the past three days.

potential outcome

The omission by the nurse resulted in the patient missing three doses of the ordered IV antibiotic. The delay in the medication administration could have serious consequences for the patient, such as worsening of the pneumonia, septicemia, and even death, especially in the elderly. The patient received only one-half of the daily dose ordered by the physician for three days. The physician would be notified of the error and likely order additional diagnostic studies, such as chest X ray, blood cultures, and an additional one-time dose of Rocephin.

prevention

This error could easily have been avoided had the nurse read the directions for preparing the medication or consulted with another nurse familiar with the system.

critical thinking skills

IV fluid calculations are just as critical as dosage calculations for specific medications. Calculation errors in IV fluid and medication administration pose an even greater threat to the patient because they infuse directly into the circulatory system. Let's look at an example in which the nurse assumed the drop factor of the IV setup without checking the IV set package to verify it.

■ error 2

Incorrectly calculating the IV drip rate by using the wrong drop factor.

possible scenario

Suppose the physician ordered D_5LR at 125 mL/h for an elderly patient just returning from the OR following abdominal surgery. The nurse gathered the IV solution and IV tubing, which had a drop factor of 20 gtt/mL. The nurse did not check the package for the drop factor and assumed it was 60 gtt/mL. The manual rate was calculated this way:

$$\frac{125 \text{ mL}}{60 \text{ min}} \times 60 \text{ gtt/mL} = 125 \text{ gtt/min} = 125 \text{ mL/h}$$

The nurse infused the D_5LR at 125 gtt/min for 8 hours. While giving report to the on-coming nurse, the patient called for the nurse complaining of shortness of breath. On further assessment the nurse heard crackles in the patient's lungs and noticed the patient's third 1000 mL bottle of D_5LR this shift was nearly empty again. At this point the nurse realized the IV rate was in error. The nurse was accustomed to using the 60 gtt/mL IV set up and therefore calculated the drip rate using the 60 gtt/mL (microdrip) drop factor. However, the tubing used delivered 20 gtt/mL (macrodrip) drop factor. The nurse never looked at the drop factor on the IV set package and assumed it was a 60 gtt/mL set.

potential outcome

The patient developed signs of fluid overload and possibly could have developed congestive heart failure due to the excessive IV rate. The physician would have been notified and likely ordered Lasix (a diuretic) to help eliminate the excess fluid. The patient likely would have been transferred to the ICU for closer monitoring.

prevention

This error could have been prevented had the nurse carefully inspected the IV tubing package to determine the drop factor. Every IV tubing set has the drop factor printed on the package, so it is not necessary to memorize or guess the drop factor. The IV calculation should have looked like this:

$$\frac{125 \text{ mL}}{60 \text{ min}} \times 20 \text{ gtt/mL} = 41.7 \text{ gtt/min} = 42 \text{ gtt/min}$$

With the infusion set of 20 gtt/mL, a flow rate of 42 gtt/min would infuse 125 mL/h. At the 125 gtt/min rate the nurse calculated, the patient received three times the IV fluid ordered hourly. Thus, the patient actually received 375 mL/h of IV fluid.

practice problems—chapter 11

Compute the flow rate in drops per minute or milliliters per hour as requested. Hospital policy permits recalculating IVs when off schedule with a maximum variation in rate of 25 percent.

1. Order: Ampicillin 500 mg dissolved in 200 mL D_5W IV to run for 2 hours
    Drop factor: 10 gtt/mL
    Flow rate: _____ gtt/min

2. Order: 1000 mL D_5W IV per 24h KVO (keep vein open)
    Drop factor: 60 gtt/mL
    Flow rate: _____ gtt/min

3. Order: 1500 mL D_5LR IV to run for 12 hours
    Drop factor: 20 gtt/mL
    Flow rate: _____ gtt/min

4. Order: 200 mL D_5RL IV to run KVO for 24 hours
    Drop factor: 60 gtt/mL
    Flow rate: _____ gtt/min

5. Order: 1 L $D_{10}W$ IV to run 1000 to 1800 hours
    Drop factor: On electronic infusion pump
    Flow rate: _____ mL/h

6. See No. 5. At 1100 there are 800 mL remaining. Describe your nursing action now.

    _____

7. Order: 1000 mL NS and 2000 mL D_5W IV to run for 24 hours
    Drop factor: 15 gtt/mL
    Flow rate: _____ gtt/min

8. Order: 2.5 L NS IV to infuse at 125 mL/h
    Drop factor: 20 gtt/mL
    Flow rate: _____ gtt/min

9. Order: 1000 mL D_5W IV for 6 hours
    Drop factor: 15 gtt/mL
    After 2 hours, 800 mL remain. Describe your nursing action now. _____

    _____

The IV tubing package below is the IV system available in your hospital for manually regulated, straight gravity flow IV administration with macrodrop of 15 gtt/mL. The patient has an order for 500 mL D_5W IV q.4h. The order was written at 1515 and you start the IV at 1530.

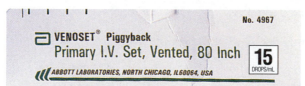

10. How much IV fluid will the patient receive in 24 hours? _____ mL

11. Who is the manufacturer of the IV infusion set tubing? _____

12. What is the drop factor calibration for the IV infusion set tubing? _____

13. What is the drop factor constant for the IV infusion set tubing? _____

14. Using the short cut (drop factor constant) method, calculate the flow rate of the IV as ordered. Show your work.
    Short cut method calculation: _____
    Flow rate: _____ gtt/min

15. Using the formula method, calculate the flow rate of the IV as ordered. Show your work.
    Formula method calculation: _____
    Flow rate: _____ gtt/min

16. At what time should you anticipate the first IV bag of 500 mL D_5W will be completely infused? _____ .

17. How much IV fluid should be infused by 1730? _____ mL

18. At 1730 you notice that the IV has 210 mL remaining. After assessing your patient and confirming that his or her condition is stable, what should you do? _____
    _____

19. At 1800 the IV is significantly behind schedule, after consulting the physician you decide to use an electronic controller to better regulate the flow rate. The physician orders that the controller be set to infuse 500 mL per 4 hours. You should set the controller for
    _____ .

20. The next day the physician adds the order Amoxicillin 250 mg in 50 mL D_5W IV PB to infuse in 30 min. q.i.d. The patient is still on the IV controller. To infuse the IV PB, set the controller for _____ .

21. List the components and concentration strengths of the fluid $D_{2.5}\frac{1}{2}NS$.
    _____

22. Calculate the amount of dextrose and sodium chloride in D_5NS 500 mL.
    dextrose _____
    NaCl _____

23. Define a central line. _____
    _____

24. Define a primary line. _____
    _____

25. Describe the purpose of a saline or heparin lock. _____
    _____

26. Potassium chloride is ordered in the _____ unit of measurement.

27. Describe the purpose of the PCA pump. _____
    _____

28. Identify two advantages of the syringe pump. _____
    _____

29. List two complications of IV sites. _____
    _____

30. How often should the IV site be monitored? _____
    _____

31. Identify three instances where blood transfusions may be indicated. _____
    _____

32. Name the four blood types. _____
    _____

33. Describe the identification process prior to the initiation of blood transfusions.

_____

_____

34. Describe the purpose of the Y-set IV system. _____

35. State the rationale for frequent assessment of the patient during blood transfusions.

_____

_____

Upon completion of these problems, see pages 329 and 330 to check your answers.

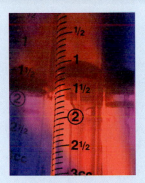

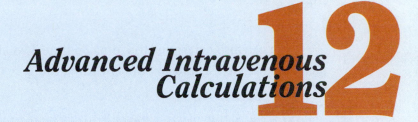

Advanced Intravenous Calculations

12

objectives

Upon mastery of Chapter 12, you will be able to perform advanced intravenous calculations. To accomplish this you will also be able to:

- Calculate infusion time.
- Calculate infusion volume.
- Calculate pediatric intermittent IV medications administered with infusion control sets, like Buretrol.
- Mix proportionate IV additive medications using pediatric volume IV solutions.
- Calculate the minimal dilution in which an IV medication can be safely prepared and delivered to a child, such as via a syringe pump.
- Calculate pediatric IV maintenance fluids.
- Calculate hourly heparin dosages.
- Assess safe hourly heparin dosages.
- Calculate heparin IV flow rates.
- Calculate the flow rate and assess safe dosages for critical care IV medication to be administered over a specified time period, such as mg/min.
- Calculate the flow rate for primary IV and IV PB solutions for patients with restricted fluid intake.

Calculating IV Infusion Time

Sometimes the physician will order intravenous solutions to be administered at a prescribed number of milliliters per hour, such as *1000 mL Lactated Ringer's IV to run at 125 mL per hour*. You may need to calculate the total infusion time in order to anticipate when to add a new bag or bottle, or discontinue the IV.

> **rule** To calculate IV infusion time:
> $$\frac{\text{TOTAL volume}}{\text{mL/h}} = \text{TOTAL hours}$$

EXAMPLE 1: *1000 mL Lactated Ringer's IV to run at 125 mL/h.* How long will this IV last?

$$\frac{1000 \text{ mL}}{125 \text{ mL/h}} = 8 \text{ hours}$$

EXAMPLE 2: *1000 mL D_5W IV to infuse at 60 mL/h to begin at 0600 hours.* At what time will this IV be complete?

$$\frac{1000 \text{ mL}}{60 \text{ mL/h}} = 16.67 \text{ hours} = 16\frac{2}{3} \text{ hours} = 16 \text{ hours and } 40 \text{ minutes}$$

The IV will be complete at 0600 + 1640 = 2240 hours

You can also determine the infusion time if you know the volume, flow rate, and drop factor. Calculate the infusion time by using the $\frac{V}{T} \times C = R$ formula, T is unknown.

> ▶ **rule** Use the flow rate formula to calculate time:
>
> $$\frac{V}{T} \times C = R$$
>
> "T" is the unknown.

EXAMPLE: *80 mL D₅W IV at 20 microdrops/min*
The drop factor is 60 gtt/mL. Calculate the infusion time.

Step 1. $\frac{V}{T} \times C = R$

$\frac{80 \text{ mL}}{T \text{ min}} \times 60 \text{ gtt/mL} = 20 \text{ gtt/min}$

$\frac{80}{T} \times \frac{60}{1} = 20$

$\frac{4800}{T} \hspace{1cm} \frac{20}{1}$

$20T = 4800$

$\frac{20T}{20} = \frac{4800}{20}$

$T = \frac{4800}{20} = 240 \text{ minutes}$

Step 2.   Convert: minutes to hours; 1 hr = 60 min

$\frac{240}{60} = 4 \text{ hours}$

Calculating IV Fluid Volumes

If you have an IV that is regulated at a particular flow rate (gtt/min) and you know the drop factor (gtt/mL) and the amount of time, you can determine the volume to be infused.
Apply the flow rate formula; V (volume) is unknown.

> ▶ **rule** To calculate IV volume:
>
> $$\frac{V}{T} \times C = R$$
>
> "V" is the unknown.

EXAMPLE: When you start your shift at 7 AM, there is an IV bag of *D₅W infusing at the rate of 25 gtt/min*. The infusion set is calibrated for a drop factor of *15 gtt/mL*. How much can you anticipate the patient will receive during your 8-hour shift?

8 h × 60 min/h = 480 min

$\frac{V}{T} \times C = R = \frac{V \text{ mL}}{480 \text{ min}} \times \frac{15 \text{ gtt/mL}}{1} = 25 \text{ gtt/min}$

$\frac{15 V}{480} \hspace{1cm} \frac{25}{1}$

$15 V = 12,000$

$\frac{15V}{15} = \frac{12,000}{15}$

V = 800 mL; delivered over 480 min or 800 mL/8h

quick review

■ The formula to calculate IV infusion time, when mL/h is known:

$$\frac{\text{TOTAL volume}}{\text{mL/h}} = \text{TOTAL hours}$$

■ The formula to calculate IV infusion time, when flow rate (gtt/min) and drop factor (gtt/mL) are known:

$$\frac{V}{T} \times C = R$$

"T" is the unknown.

■ The formula to calculate IV volume, when flow rate (gtt/min), drop factor (gtt/mL), and time are known:

$$\frac{V}{T} \times C = R$$

"V" is the unknown.

review set 39

Calculate the infusion time and rate (as requested) for the following IV orders:

1. Order: 500 mL D$_5$W at 30 gtt/min
   Drop factor: 20 gtt/mL
   Time: _____

2. Order: 1000 mL Lactated Ringer's at 25 gtt/min
   Drop factor: 10 gtt/mL
   Time: _____

3. Order: 800 mL D$_5$ Lactated Ringer's at 25 gtt/min
   Drop factor: 15 gtt/mL
   Time: _____

4. Order: 120 mL Normal Saline to run at 20 mL/h
   Drop factor: 60 microdrops/mL
   Time: _____
   Flow rate: _____ gtt/min

5. Order: 80 mL D$_5$W to run at 20 mL/h
   Drop factor: 60 microdrops/mL
   Time: _____
   Flow rate: _____ gtt/min

Calculate the completion time for the following IVs.

6. At 1600 hours the nurse started an IV of 1200 mL D$_5$W at 27 gtt/min. The infusion set used is calibrated for a drop factor of 15 gtt/mL. _____

7. At 1530 hours the nurse starts 2000 mL of D$_5$W to run at 125 mL/h. The infusion set used is calibrated for a drop factor of 10 gtt/mL. The IV rate should be set at _____ gtt/min, and the IV should be completed at _____.

Calculate the total volume (mL) per 24 hours to be infused.

8. A 1000 mL bag of D$_5$ Lactated Ringer's is infusing at 42 gtt/min. The infusion set is calibrated for a drop factor of 60 gtt/mL.
    mL/24h = _____

9. An IV is flowing at 12 gtt/min and the infusion set has a drop factor of 15 gtt/mL.
    mL/24h = _____

10. IV: D$_5$W
    Flow rate: 21 gtt/min
    Drop factor: 10 gtt/mL
    mL/24h = _____

After completing these problems, see pages 311 and 312 to check your answers.

Pediatric Infusion Control Sets

Infusion control sets, Figure 12–1, are most frequently used to administer intermittent IV medications to children. They are usually referred to by their trade names, Buretrol, Volutrol, or Soluset. The fluid chamber will hold 100–150 milliliters of fluid to be infused in a specified

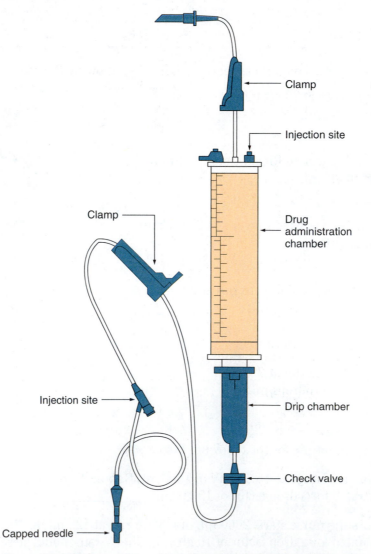

Figure 12–1 Volume Control Set (Buretrol, Volutrol, or Soluset)

time period as ordered, usually 60 minutes or less. The medication is added to the IV fluid in the chamber for a prescribed dilution volume.

Since the volume of fluid in the chamber is controlled, the patient is protected from receiving more volume than the chamber will hold. This is especially important for children who can tolerate only a narrow range of fluid volume. Volume control sets like Buretrol may also be used to administer intermittent IV medications to adults with fluid restrictions, such as heart or kidney patients. An electronic controller or pump may also be used to regulate the flow rate. When used, the electronic device will alarm when the Buretrol chamber empties.

After the Buretrol has emptied and the medication has infused, a flush of IV fluid is given to be sure all the medication has cleared the tubing. The standard is 15 mL flush for peripheral lines and 20 mL flush for central lines. To calculate the IV flow rate for the Buretrol, you must consider the total fluid volume of the medication and the IV fluid used for dilution, plus the volume of IV flush fluid. Volume control sets are microdrip sets with a drop factor of 60 gtt/mL.

EXAMPLE: Order: *Kefzol 250 mg q.8h in 50 mL $D_5 \frac{1}{4}$ NS to infuse in 60 minutes followed by a 15 mL flush*

Supply: Kefzol is reconstituted to 125 mg/mL.

Step 1.   Calculate the total volume of the intermittent IV medication and the IV flush.
50 mL + 15 mL = 65 mL

Step 2.   Calculate the flow rate of the IV medication and IV flush. Remember: the drop factor is 60 gtt/mL.

$$\frac{V}{T} \times C = R$$

$$\frac{65}{60} \times 60 = 65 \text{ gtt/min}$$

Step 3.   Calculate the volume of the medication to be administered.

$$\frac{125 \text{ mg}}{1 \text{ mL}} \diagdown \diagup \frac{250 \text{ mg}}{X \text{ mL}}$$

$$125X = 250$$

$$\frac{125X}{125} = \frac{250}{125}$$

$$X = 2 \text{ mL}$$

Step 4.   Calculate the volume of IV fluid needed to add to the Buretrol chamber for a dilution volume of 50 mL. 50 − 2 = 48 mL. Run a total of 48 mL 0.9% NaCl into the Buretrol chamber and add 2 mL of Kefzol. This provides the prescribed volume of 50 mL in the chamber.

Step 5.   Set the flow rate of the 50 mL of intermittent IV medication for 65 gtt/min. Follow with the 15 mL flush also set at 65 gtt/min. When complete, resume the regular IV as ordered.

The patient may also have an intermittent medication ordered as part of a continuous infusion at a prescribed IV volume per hour. In such cases the patient is to receive the same fluid volume each hour, regardless of the addition of intermittent medications.

EXAMPLE: Order: *D_5W IV at 30 mL/h for continuous infusion. Ancef 125 mg IV q.6h.*
Supply: Ancef 125 mg/mL with instructions to "add to Buretrol and infuse over 30 minutes"
An infusion controller is in use with the Buretrol.

Step 1.   Use ratio-proportion to determine the dilution volume required to administer the Ancef at the prescribed continuous flow rate of 30 mL/h.

$$\frac{30\ mL}{60\ min} = \frac{X\ mL}{30\ min}$$

$$60X = 900$$

$$\frac{60X}{60} = \frac{900}{60}$$

$$X = 15\ mL$$

Therefore, the IV fluid dilution volume required to administer 125 mg of Ancef in 30 minutes is 15 mL to maintain the prescribed, continuous infusion rate of 30 mL/h.

Step 2. Determine the volume of Ancef and IV fluid to add to the Buretrol. 125 mg/mL Ancef available and 125 mg ordered. Add 14 mL D_5W and 1 mL Ancef for a total volume of 15 mL.

Step 3. Set the controller to 30 mL/h to deliver 15 mL of intermittent IV Ancef solution in 30 minutes. Resume the regular IV which will also flush out the tubing. The continuous flow rate will remain at 30 mL/h.

quick review

- Volume control sets have a drop factor of 60 gtt/mL.
- The total volume of the medication, IV dilution fluid, and the IV flush fluid must be considered to calculate flow rates when using sets like Buretrol.
- Use ratio-proportion to calculate flow rates for intermittent medications when a continuous IV rate in mL/h is prescribed.

review set 40 _____

Calculate the IV flow rate to administer the following IV medications by Buretrol and determine the amount of IV fluid to be added to the Buretrol.

1. Order: Antibiotic X 60 mg IV q.8h in 50 mL D_5W over 45 minutes. Flush with 15 mL.
   Available: Antibiotic X 60 mg/2 mL
   Flow rate: _____ gtt/min
   Add _____ mL IV fluid.

2. Order: Medication Y 75 mg IV q.6h in 60 mL D_5W over 60 minutes. Flush with 15 mL.
   Available: Medication Y 75 mg/3 mL
   Flow rate: _____ gtt/min
   Add _____ mL IV fluid.

3. Order: Antibiotic Z 15 mg IV b.i.d. in 25 mL 0.9% NaCl over 20 minutes. Flush with 15 mL.
   Available: Antibiotic Z 15 mg/3 mL
   Flow rate: _____ gtt/min
   Add _____ mL IV fluid.

Calculate the amount of IV fluid to be added to the Buretrol.

4. Order: 0.9% NaCl at 50 mL/h for continuous infusion with Ancef 250 mg IV q.8h to be infused over 30 minutes by Buretrol.
   Available: Ancef 125 mg/mL
   Add _____ mL IV fluid.

5. Order: D_5W at 30 mL/h for continuous infusion with Medication X 60 mg q.6h to be infused over 20 minutes by Buretrol.

Available: Medication X 60 mg/2 mL

Add _____ mL IV fluid.

After completing these problems, see page 313 to check your answers.

Preparing Pediatric IVs

The physician may order a medication such as potassium chloride (KCl) to be added to an IV fluid for continuous infusion. The volume of the IV solution bag selected for children is usually smaller than that for adults, since the total volume required per 24 hours is less. Therefore, the amount of medication to be added must be adjusted proportionately to the total volume of the IV bag. Use ratio-proportion to determine the appropriate amount of medication to add for the prescribed dilution.

EXAMPLE 1:   Order: $D_5\frac{1}{2}$ NS IV $\bar{c}$ 20 mEq KCl/L to infuse at 30 mL/h

At the rate of 30 mL/h, the child would receive only 720 mL in 24 hours, so you choose a 500 mL bag of $D_5\frac{1}{2}$ NS rather than a one liter or 1000 mL bag. How many mEq of KCl should you add to the 500 mL bag?

Convert: 1 L to 1000 mL

Think: 500 mL is half of 1000 mL, so you would need half of the 20 mEq of KCl or 10 mEq.

Calculate: $\dfrac{20\ mEq}{1000\ mL} \diagdown\!\!\!\!\diagup \dfrac{X\ mEq}{500\ mL}$

1000X = 10,000

$\dfrac{1000X}{1000} = \dfrac{10,000}{1000}$

X = 10 mEq

Potassium chloride is available in 2 mEq per mL. How much KCl should you add to the 500 mL IV bag?

$\dfrac{2\ mEq}{1\ mL} \diagdown\!\!\!\!\diagup \dfrac{10\ mEq}{X\ mL}$

2X = 10

$\dfrac{2X}{2} = \dfrac{10}{2}$

X = 5 mL

EXAMPLE 2:   Order: D_5W with aminophylline 1 g/L at 30 mL/h

Supply: aminophylline 500 mg/20 mL and a 500-mL bag of D_5W

Child is 9 years old and weighs 66 pounds.

Step 1.   How many mg aminophylline should be added to the 500 mL bag?

Convert: 1 g = 1000 mg

1 L = 1000 mL

Think: 1000 to 1000 is the same as 500 to 500. You want 500 mg.

Calculate: $\dfrac{1000\ mg}{1000\ mL} = \dfrac{X\ mg}{500\ mL}$

1000X = 500,000

$\dfrac{1000X}{1000} = \dfrac{500,000}{1000}$

X = 500 mg

Step 2. How many mL aminophylline should be added to the 500 mL bag?

Convert: No conversion is necessary.

Think: The answer is obvious. There are 500 mg/20 mL; you need 20 mL.

Calculate: $\dfrac{500\ mg}{20\ mL} \Large\diagdown\hspace{-1.2em}\diagup\normalsize \dfrac{500\ mg}{X\ mL}$

$500X = 10,000$

$\dfrac{500X}{500} = \dfrac{10,000}{500}$

$X = 20\ mL$

Step 3. How many mg of aminophylline will the child receive per hour?

Convert: No conversion is necessary.

Think: 500 is to 500 as 30 is to 30. You want to give 30 mg/h.

Calculate: $\dfrac{500\ mg}{500\ mL} = \dfrac{X\ mg/h}{30\ mL/h}$

$500\ X = 15,000$

$\dfrac{500X}{500} = \dfrac{15,000}{500}$

$X = 30\ mg/h$

Step 4. The recommended maintenance dosage of aminophylline for children 1–9 years is 1 mg/kg/h. Based on the recommended maintenance dosage, how many mg/h of aminophylline should this child receive?

Convert: lb to kg

$\dfrac{1\ kg}{2.2\ lb} \Large\diagdown\hspace{-1.2em}\diagup\normalsize \dfrac{X\ kg}{66\ lb}$

$2.2X = 66$

$\dfrac{2.2X}{2.2} = \dfrac{60}{2.2}$

$X = 30\ kg$

Think: 1 is to 1 as 30 is to 30. It is obvious that the child should receive 30 mg/h, which is the same dosage to be infused at the ordered rate of 30 mL/h. Therefore, the dose ordered is safe.

Calculate: per hour dosage

$\dfrac{1\ mg/h}{1\ kg} \Large\diagdown\hspace{-1.2em}\diagup\normalsize \dfrac{X\ mg/h}{30\ kg}$

$X = 30\ mg/h$

Is the dosage ordered safe and reasonable? Yes, the child can safely receive 30 mg/h and that is the dose ordered.

review set 41

Order: $D_5W \frac{1}{2}$ NS IV $\bar{c}$ 20 mEq KCl per L to infuse at 15 mL/h
Supply: 250 mL $D_5W \frac{1}{2}$ NS and KCl 2 mEq/mL

Answer questions 1–3.

1. How many mEq KCl should be added to the 250 mL bag? _____ mEq

2. How many mL KCl should be added to the 250 mL bag? _____ mL

3. How many mEq of KCl will the child receive per hour? _____ mEq/h

Order: D$_5$W IV c̄ aminophylline 1 g per L at 20 mL/h
Supply: Aminophylline 500 mg/20 mL and 250 mL bag of D$_5$W
Child is 8 years old and weighs 19 kg.

Answer questions 4–8.

4. How many mg aminophylline should be added to the 250 mL bag? _____ mg

5. How many mL aminophylline should be added to the 250 mL bag? _____ mL

6. How many mg of aminophylline will the child receive per hour? _____ mg/h

7. The recommended maintenance dosage of aminophylline for children 1–9 years old is 1 mg/kg/h. Based on the recommended maintenance dosage, how many mg per hour of aminophylline should this child receive? _____ mg/h

8. Is the dosage ordered safe and reasonable? _____

After completing these problems, see page 313 to check your answers.

Minimal Dilutions for IV Medications

Intravenous medications in infants and young children (or adults on limited fluids) are often ordered to be given in the smallest volume or maximal safe concentration to prevent fluid overload. Consult a pediatric reference, the hospital formulary, or drug insert to assist you in problem-solving. These types of medications are usually given via a syringe pump.

> ▶ **rule** Ratio for recommended drug dilution equals ratio for desired drug dilution.

EXAMPLE: The physician orders 40 mg of Vancocin IV for an infant who weighs 4000 g. What is the minimal amount of IV fluid in which the vancomycin can be safely diluted? The package insert is provided for your reference. Notice that a "concentration of no more than 10 mg/mL is recommended."

$$\frac{10 \text{ mg}}{1 \text{ mL}} \diagdown\!\!\!\!\diagup \frac{40 \text{ mg}}{X \text{ mL}}$$

$$10X = 40$$

$$\frac{10X}{10} = \frac{40}{10}$$

$$X = 4 \text{ mL}$$

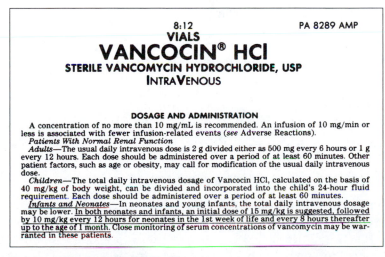

8:12
VIALS   PA 8289 AMP
VANCOCIN® HCl
STERILE VANCOMYCIN HYDROCHLORIDE, USP
INTRAVENOUS

DOSAGE AND ADMINISTRATION
A concentration of no more than 10 mg/mL is recommended. An infusion of 10 mg/min or less is associated with fewer infusion-related events (*see* Adverse Reactions).
Patients With Normal Renal Function
Adults—The usual daily intravenous dose is 2 g divided either as 500 mg every 6 hours or 1 g every 12 hours. Each dose should be administered over a period of at least 60 minutes. Other patient factors, such as age or obesity, may call for modification of the usual daily intravenous dose.
Children—The total daily intravenous dosage of Vancocin HCl, calculated on the basis of 40 mg/kg of body weight, can be divided and incorporated into the child's 24-hour fluid requirement. Each dose should be administered over a period of at least 60 minutes.
Infants and Neonates—In neonates and young infants, the total daily intravenous dosage may be lower. In both neonates and infants, an initial dose of 15 mg/kg is suggested, followed by 10 mg/kg every 12 hours for neonates in the 1st week of life and every 8 hours thereafter up to the age of 1 month. Close monitoring of serum concentrations of vancomycin may be warranted in these patients.

Portion of Vancocin Package Insert

Calculation of Daily Rate for Maintenance Fluids

Another common pediatric IV calculation is to calculate maintenance IV fluids for children. The following formula is used to calculate IV fluid rates for children.

> **rule** Use this formula to calculate the daily rate of pediatric maintenance IV fluids.
>
> 100 mL per kg per day for first 10 kg of body weight
> 50 mL per kg per day for next 10 kg of body weight
> 20 mL per kg per day for each kg of body weight above 20

Let's look at the daily rate of maintenance fluids and the hourly flow rate for the children in the following examples.

EXAMPLE 1:   6-kg child

$$\frac{100 \text{ mL}}{1 \text{ kg}} \diagdown \frac{X \text{ mL}}{6 \text{ kg}}$$

X = 600 mL

Total = 600 mL/24h

$$\frac{600 \text{ mL}}{24 \text{ h}} = 25 \text{ mL/h}$$

EXAMPLE 2:   12-kg child

For the first 10 kg, at 100 mL/kg/day

$$\frac{100 \text{ mL}}{1 \text{ kg}} = \frac{X \text{ mL}}{10 \text{ kg}}$$

X = 10 × 100 = 10.00. = 1000 mL/day for first 10 kg

12 kg − 10 kg = 2 kg

For the remaining 2 kg, at 50 mL/kg/day

$$\frac{50 \text{ mL}}{1 \text{ kg}} \diagdown \frac{X \text{ mL}}{2 \text{ kg}}$$

X = 50 × 2

X = 100 mL/day for next 2 kg

1000 mL + 100 mL = 1100 mL

Total = 1100 mL/24h

$$\frac{1100 \text{ mL}}{24 \text{ h}} = 45.8 \text{ or } 46 \text{ mL/h}$$

EXAMPLE 3:   24-kg child

For the first 10 kg, at 100 mL/kg/day

$$\frac{100 \text{ mL}}{1 \text{ kg}} \diagdown \frac{X \text{ mL}}{10 \text{ kg}}$$

X = 10 × 100 = 10.00. = 1000 for first 10 kg

For the next 10 kg, at 50 mL/kg/day

$$\frac{50 \text{ mL}}{1 \text{ kg}} \diagdown \frac{X \text{ mL}}{10 \text{ kg}}$$

X = 50 × 10 = 50.0. = 500 mL/day for next 10 kg

24 kg − 20 kg = 4 kg remaining

For the last 4 kg, at 20 mL/kg/day

$$\frac{20 \text{ mL}}{1 \text{ kg}} \xrightarrow{\hspace{1cm}} \frac{X \text{ mL}}{4 \text{ kg}}$$

$X = 20 \times 4$

$X = 80$ mL for the last 4 kg

1000 mL + 500 mL + 80 mL = 1580 mL

Total = 1580 mL/24h

$$\frac{1580 \text{ mL}}{24 \text{ h}} = 65.8 \text{ or } 66 \text{ mL/h}$$

review set 42

1. If a child is receiving Claforan 400 mg IV q.6h and the minimal dilution is 100 mg/mL, what is the least volume of fluid in which the medication can be safely diluted? _____mL

2. If a child is receiving Gentamicin 25 mg IV q.8h and the minimal dilution is 4 mg/mL, what is the least volume of fluid in which the medication can be safely diluted? _____mL

3. Calculate the hourly IV flow rate for a 25-kg child receiving maintenance IV fluids. _____mL/h

4. Calculate the hourly IV flow rate for a 13-kg child receiving maintenance IV fluids. _____mL/h

After completing these problems, see page 314 to check your answers.

IV Heparin

Heparin is an anticoagulant for the prevention of clot formation. It is measured in USP units (Figure 12–2). Intravenous heparin should be administered by an electronic infusion device. Because of the potential for hemorrhage or clots with incorrect dosage, careful monitoring of patients receiving heparin is a critical nursing skill. The nurse is responsible for administering correct dosage and for assuring that the dosage is safe.

▶ *rule* The normal adult heparinizing dosage is 20,000–40,000 units per 24 hours.

Intravenous heparin is frequently ordered in units per hour. Based on the normal heparinizing dosage, the nurse must determine if the order is safe and effective.

EXAMPLE 1: Order: *Heparin IV to infuse at 1000 U/h*

Is this dosage safe?

Normal adult range = 20,000–40,000 U/24h

$$\frac{1000 \text{ U}}{1 \text{ h}} \xrightarrow{\hspace{1cm}} \frac{X \text{ U}}{24 \text{ h}}$$

$X = 24 \times 1000 = 24.000. = 24,000$ U/24h

Yes, 1000 U/h is safe.

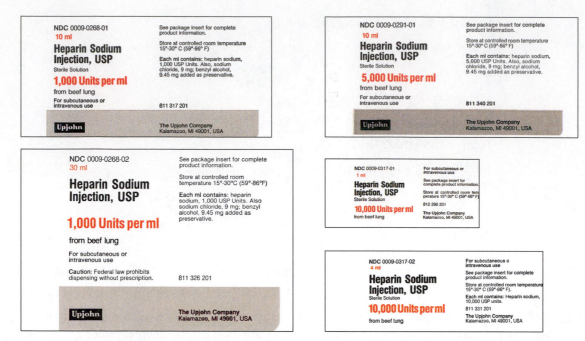

Fig. 12–2 Various Heparin Dosage Strengths

EXAMPLE 2:   Order: *Heparin IV to infuse at 850 U/h*

Is this dosage safe?

$$\frac{850 \text{ U}}{1 \text{ h}} \quad \diagdown\!\!\!\diagup \quad \frac{\text{X U}}{24 \text{ h}}$$

X = 20,400 U/24h

Yes, 850 U/h is safe.

EXAMPLE 3:   Order: *Heparin 2000 U/h*

Is this dosage safe?

$$\frac{2000 \text{ U}}{1 \text{ h}} \quad \diagdown\!\!\!\diagup \quad \frac{\text{X U}}{24 \text{ h}}$$

X = 48,000 U/24h

No, this dosage is not within the recommended range. Notify the physician.

When heparin is ordered in U/h, use ratio-proportion to calculate the flow rate in mL/h.

EXAMPLE 1:   Order: *Heparin IV to infuse at 1000 U/h*

Available: 500 mL bag of D₅W with 25,000 U heparin added. What is the flow rate in mL/h?

Calculate the flow rate in mL/h which will administer 1000 U/h.

$$\frac{25,000 \text{ U}}{500 \text{ mL}} \quad \diagdown\!\!\!\diagup \quad \frac{1000 \text{ U}}{\text{X mL}}$$

25,000X = 500,000

$$\frac{25,000\text{X}}{25,000} = \frac{500,000}{25,000}$$

X = 20 mL/h

EXAMPLE 2:   Order: *Heparin IV to infuse at 850 U/h*

Available: 500 mL bag of D_5W with 25,000 U heparin added.

Calculate mL/h:

$$\frac{25,000\ U}{500\ mL} \diagup\!\!\!\!\diagdown \frac{850\ U/h}{X\ mL/h}$$

$$25,000X = 425,000$$

$$\frac{25,000X}{25,000} = \frac{425,000}{25,000}$$

$$X = 17\ mL/h$$

Heparin may also be ordered by the physician to infuse at a predetermined flow rate in milliliters per hour. The nurse must determine the hourly unit dosage to verify that the dosage is within the safe and effective range of 20,000–40,000 U/24h.

EXAMPLE 1:   Order: *1L D_5W IV c̄ heparin 40,000 U to infuse at 30 mL/h*

What is the hourly heparin dosage?

$$\frac{40,000\ U}{1000\ mL} \diagup\!\!\!\!\diagdown \frac{X\ U/h}{30\ mL/h}$$

$$1000X = 1,200,000$$

$$\frac{1000X}{1000} = \frac{1,200,000}{1000}$$

$$X = 1200\ U/h$$

Is this hourly dosage safe?

$$\frac{1200\ U}{1\ h} \diagup\!\!\!\!\diagdown \frac{X\ U}{24\ h}$$

$$X = 28,800\ U/24h$$

Yes, it is safe. The dosage is within the normal range.

EXAMPLE 2:   Order: *1000 mL D_5W IV c̄ 40,000 U heparin to infuse at 40 mL/h*

What is the hourly heparin dosage?

$$\frac{40,000\ U}{1000\ mL} \diagup\!\!\!\!\diagdown \frac{X\ U/h}{40\ mL/h}$$

$$1000X = 1,600,000$$

$$\frac{1000X}{1000} = \frac{1,600,000}{1000}$$

$$X = 1600\ U/h$$

Is this hourly dosage safe?

$$\frac{1600\ U}{1\ h} \diagup\!\!\!\!\diagdown \frac{X\ U}{24\ h}$$

$$X = 38,400\ U/24h$$

Yes, the dosage is within the normal range.

EXAMPLE 3:   The patient has *500 mL D₅NS with 5000 U heparin added infusing at 80 mL/h.*

What is the hourly heparin dosage?

$$\frac{5000 \text{ U}}{500 \text{ mL}} \underset{\longleftarrow}{\overset{\longrightarrow}{\times}} \frac{\text{X U/h}}{80 \text{ mL/h}}$$

$$500\text{X} = 400,000$$

$$\frac{500\text{X}}{500} = \frac{400,000}{500}$$

$$\text{X} = 800 \text{ U/h}$$

Is this hourly dosage safe?

$$\frac{800 \text{ U}}{1 \text{ h}} \underset{\longleftarrow}{\overset{\longrightarrow}{\times}} \frac{\text{X U}}{24 \text{ h}}$$

$$\text{X} = 19,200 \text{ U/24h}$$

No, this dosage is not within the normal therapeutic range; therefore, it is not safe to proceed. The order should be reviewed and the physician notified.

quick review

- Normal adult heparinizing dosage = 20,000–40,000 U/24h.
- Use ratio-proportion to calculate mL/h when you know U/h and U/mL.
- Use ratio-proportion to calculate U/h when you know mL/h and U/mL.

review set 43

Calculate the flow rate and indicate whether the heparin dosage is safe.

1. Order: 1000 mL 0.45% NS with 25,000 U heparin to infuse at 1000 U/h.
   Flow rate: _____ mL/h
   Safe? _____

2. Order: 500 mL D₅W IV c̄ 40,000 U heparin to infuse at 1100 U/h.
   Flow rate: _____ mL/h
   Safe? _____

3. Order 500 mL 0.45% NS IV c̄ 25,000 U heparin to infuse at 500 U/h.
   Flow rate: _____ mL/h
   Safe? _____

4. Order 500 mL D₅W IV c̄ 40,000 U heparin to infuse at 2500 U/h.
   On infusion pump with a setting 31 mL/h
   Is the setting accurate and is the hourly dosage safe? _____
   If not, what should you do? _____

5. Order 25,000 U heparin IV per liter D₅W. On rounds, you assess the patient and observe that the infusion pump is set at 120 mL/h.
   Is the hourly dosage of heparin safe? _____

6. Order: 500 mL 0.45% NS IV c̄ 30,000 U heparin to infuse at 25 mL/h.
   Is the hourly dosage safe? _____

7. Order 1 L D$_5$W IV c̄ 40,000 U heparin to infuse at 80 mL/h.
   Is the hourly dosage safe? _____

8. Order: 1000 mL D$_5$W IV c̄ 20,000 U heparin to infuse at 60 mL/h.
   Is the hourly dosage safe? _____

9. The patient is receiving 500 mL D$_5$W IV with 30,000 U heparin. The IV is infusing at 96 mL/h.
   Is the hourly dosage safe? _____

10. Order: 1000 mL D$_5$ $\frac{1}{2}$ NS IV c̄ 10,000 U heparin at 80 mL/h.
    Is the hourly dosage safe? _____

The same method can be used to calculate flow rates for other medications ordered similarly. Try the next two problems.

11. Order: 500 mL 0.9% NaCl IV c̄ 500 U insulin to infuse at 10 U/h by electronic infusion pump.
    Flow rate: _____ mL/h

12. Order: 1 L D$_5$W IV c̄ 40 mEq KCl to infuse at 2 mEq/h by electronic infusion controller.
    Set the electronic infusion controller at _____ mL/h.

After completing these problems, see pages 314 and 315 to check your answers.

Critical Care IV Calculations: Calculating Flow Rate of an IV Medication to Be Given over a Specified Time Period

With increasing frequency, medications are ordered for patients in critical care situations as a prescribed amount to be administered in a specified time period such as X mg per minute. Such medications are usually administered by electronic infusion devices, programmed in mL/h.

> **rule** To calculate the flow rate (mL/h) for IV medications ordered in mg/min:
> Step 1. Calculate dosage in (mL/min)
> Step 2. Calculate the quantity to administer in mL/h

EXAMPLE 1: Order: *Lidocaine 2 g IV in 500 mL D$_5$W at 2 mg/min via infusion pump.*
You must prepare and hang 500 mL of D$_5$W IV solution that has 2 grams of Lidocaine added to it. Then, you must regulate the flow rate so the patient receives 2 milligrams of the Lidocaine every minute. To determine the flow rate (mL/h):

Step 1. Determine mL/min

Convert: 2 g to 2000 mg

Think: The order is for 2 mg/min. If you calculate how many mL contain 2 mg, you will know the mL needed to infuse per minute.

Calculate: $\dfrac{2000 \text{ mg}}{500 \text{ mL}} \underset{\longleftarrow}{\overset{\longrightarrow}{\times}} \dfrac{2 \text{ mg/min}}{X \text{ mL/min}}$

$2000X = 1000$

$\dfrac{2000X}{2000} = \dfrac{1000}{2000}$

$X = 0.5 \text{ mL/min}$

Step 2.   Determine the flow rate (mL/h)

Convert: 1 h to 60 min. You must set up the proportion to compare like measurements.

Think: 0.5 is half of 1, and 30 is half of 60.

Calculate: $\dfrac{0.5 \text{ mL}}{1 \text{ min}} \bowtie \dfrac{X \text{ mL}}{60 \text{ min}}$

X = 30 mL/60 min or 30 mL/h

Set the flow rate to 30 mL/h

EXAMPLE 2:   Order: *Aminophylline 500 mg IV in 200 mL D$_5$W to infuse at 15 mg/min*
Calculate the flow rate in mL/h to program the infusion pump.

Step 1.   Determine the mL/min

Convert: No conversion necessary

Think: The order is for 15 mg per min. If you calculate how many mL contain 15 mg, you will know the mL needed to infuse per minute.

Calculate: $\dfrac{500 \text{ mg}}{200 \text{ mL}} \bowtie \dfrac{15 \text{ mg/min}}{X \text{ mL/min}}$

500X = 3000

$\dfrac{500X}{500} = \dfrac{3000}{500}$

X = 6 mL/min

Step 2.   Determine mL/h

Convert: 1 hr to 60 min

Think: If there are 6 mL per 1 min, then there are 6 times 60 mL or 360 mL per 60 min.

Calculate: $\dfrac{6 \text{ mL}}{1 \text{ min}} = \dfrac{X \text{ mL}}{60 \text{ min}}$

X = 360 mL/60 min = 360 mL/h

The physician may also order the amount of medication in an IV solution that a patient should receive in a specified time period per kilogram of body weight. An electronic infusion device is usually used to administer these orders.

EXAMPLE 3:   Order: *Add 225 mg of a medication to 250 mL of IV solution and administer 3 mcg/kg/min via infusion pump for a person who weighs 110 lb.*
To determine the flow rate (mL/h):

Step 1.   Convert the weight in lb to kg

$\dfrac{1 \text{ kg}}{2.2 \text{ lb}} \bowtie \dfrac{X \text{ kg}}{110 \text{ lb}}$

2.2X = 110

$\dfrac{2.2X}{2.2} = \dfrac{110}{2.2}$

X = 50 kg

Step 2.   Calculate the desired dosage of medication.

$\dfrac{3 \text{ mcg/min}}{1 \text{ kg}} \bowtie \dfrac{X \text{ mcg/min}}{50 \text{ kg}}$

X = 150 mcg/min

Step 3.   Convert to like units (mcg to mg).

$$\frac{1 \text{ mg}}{1000 \text{ mcg}} \xrightleftharpoons{} \frac{X \text{ mg}}{150 \text{ mcg}}$$

$$1000X = 150$$

$$\frac{1000X}{1000} = \frac{150}{1000}$$

$$X = .150. = 0.150 = 0.15 \text{ mg}$$

Step 4.   Determine the dosage in mL/min.

$$\frac{225 \text{ mg}}{250 \text{ mL}} \xrightleftharpoons{} \frac{0.15 \text{ mg/min}}{X \text{ mL/min}}$$

$$225X = 37.5$$

$$\frac{225X}{225} = \frac{37.5}{225}$$

$$X = 0.17 \text{ mL/min}$$

Step 5.   Determine the flow rate (mL/h).

$$\frac{0.17 \text{ mL}}{1 \text{ min}} \xrightleftharpoons{} \frac{X \text{ mL}}{60 \text{ min}}$$

$$X = 60 \times 0.17 = 10.2 = 10 \text{ mL/60 min} = 10 \text{ mL/h}$$

Regulate the flow rate at 10 mL/h to deliver 150 mcg/min.

Varying IV Medication Dosage and Infusion Time

Sometimes IV medications may be ordered to be administered at an initial dosage over a specified time period and then continued at a different dosage and time. These situations are common in obstetrics. Remember that IV medications administered over a specified time period are regulated by electronic infusion pumps calibrated in mL/h.

rule   An alternate method to calculate flow rate (mL/h) for IV medications ordered over a specified time period is:

Step 1: Calculate mg (or g)/mL

Step 2: Calculate mL/h

EXAMPLE :   Order: Add magnesium sulfate 20 g to LR 1000 mL IV. Start with bolus of 4 g/30 min, then maintain a continuous infusion at 2 g/h.

What is the flow rate in mL/h for the bolus order?

Step 1:   Calculate: The bolus rate in g/mL

There are 20 g in 1000 mL; how many mL are necessary to infuse 4 g?

$$\frac{20 \text{ g}}{1000 \text{ mL}} \xrightleftharpoons{} \frac{4 \text{ g}}{X \text{ mL}}$$

$$20X = 4000$$

$$\frac{20X}{20} = \frac{4000}{20}$$

$$X = 200 \text{ mL}$$

There are 4 g in 200 mL to be administered over 30 minutes.

Step 2:   Calculate: The bolus rate in mL/h

What is the flow rate in mL/h to infuse 200 mL (which contain 4 g of magnesium sulfate)? Remember 1 h = 60 min.

$$\frac{200 \text{ mL}}{30 \text{ min}} \underset{\longleftarrow}{\overset{\longrightarrow}{\times}} \frac{X \text{ mL}}{60 \text{ min}}$$

$$30X = 12{,}000$$

$$\frac{30X}{30} = \frac{12{,}000}{30}$$

$$X = 400 \text{ mL}/60 \text{ min} = 400 \text{ mL/h}$$

Set the infusion pump at 400 mL/h to deliver the bolus as ordered at 4 g/30 min.

Calculate: The continuous IV rate in mL/h

What is the flow rate in mL/h for the continuous infusion of magnesium sulfate of 2 g/h? You can use ratio and proportion again to determine how many mL contain 2 g.

$$\frac{20 \text{ g}}{1000 \text{ mL}} \underset{\longleftarrow}{\overset{\longrightarrow}{\times}} \frac{2 \text{ g/h}}{X \text{ mL/h}}$$

$$20X = 2000$$

$$\frac{20X}{20} = \frac{2000}{20}$$

$$X = 100 \text{ mL}$$

Because there are 2 g in 100 mL, reset the infusion pump to 100 mL/h to deliver 2 g/h.

Titrated IV Medications

Some medications, such as dopamine, Isuprel, and Pitocin, are ordered to be *titrated*, or *regulated*, to obtain a measurable response. Sometimes they may be ordered by milliunits (mU). Recall from chapter 2, that 1 U = 1000 mU. For example, Pitocin may be ordered beginning at 1 milliunit (mU) per minute, then increased by 1 mU per minute every 15–30 minutes to a maximum of 20 mU/min until adequate labor is reached. Dosage will be titrated or adjusted until the desired effect is obtained. The lowest dosage is set first and increased or decreased as needed. The upper limit is not exceeded unless a new order is received. An electronic infusion pump is used and it is set in mL/h. Let's look at an example demonstrating titration using Pitocin.

EXAMPLE :   A physician's order is written to induce labor as follows: *Add Pitocin 20 U to LR 1000 mL IV. Begin a continuous infusion @ 1 mU/min, increase by 1 mU/min q.15–30 min to a maximum of 20 mU/min.*

What is the flow rate in mL/h to deliver 1 mU/min?

In this example the medication is measured in units and milliunits (instead of grams or mg).

Step 1:   Convert U to mU.

Equivalent: 1 U = 1000 mU

$$\frac{1 \text{ mU}}{1000 \text{ mU}} \underset{\longleftarrow}{\overset{\longrightarrow}{\times}} \frac{20 \text{ U}}{X \text{ mU}}$$

$$X = 20 \times 1000 = 20.000. = 20{,}000 \text{ mU}$$

Step 2:   Calculate mL/min.

$$\frac{20{,}000 \text{ mU}}{1000 \text{ mL}} \underset{\longleftarrow}{\overset{\longrightarrow}{\times}} \frac{1 \text{ mU/min}}{X \text{ mL/min}}$$

$$20{,}000X = 1000$$

$$\frac{20{,}000X}{20{,}000} = \frac{1000}{20{,}000}$$

$$X = 0.05 \text{ mL/min}$$

Therefore, 1 mU is infused at the rate of 0.05 mL/min.

Step 3:   What is the flow rate in mL/h to infuse 0.05 mL/min (that contains 1 mU Pitocin)?

$$\frac{0.05 \text{ mL}}{1 \text{ min}} \diagup\diagdown \frac{X \text{ mL}}{60 \text{ min}}$$

X = 3 mL/60 min 3 mL/h

Set the infusion pump at 3 mL/h to infuse the order of Pitocin 1 mU/min.

What is the maximum flow rate in mL/h that the Pitocin infusion can be set for the titration as ordered? Notice that the standard and the order allow a maximum of 20 mU/min.

You know that 1 mU/min is infused at 3 mL/h. Calculate the mL/h to infuse 20 mU/min.

$$\frac{3 \text{ mL/h}}{1 \text{ mU/min}} \diagup\diagdown \frac{X \text{ mL/h}}{20 \text{ mU/min}}$$

X = 60 mL/h

Verifying Safe Dosage

It is also a critical nursing skill to be sure that patients are receiving safe dosages of medications. Occasionally safe dosages may be recommended in mg/min. Therefore, you must also be able to convert critical care IVs with additive medications to **mg/h** or **mg/min** to check safe or normal dosage ranges.

> *rule*   To check safe dosage of IV medications ordered in mL/h:
>
> Step 1. Calculate mg/h
>
> Step 2. Convert mg/h to mg/min

EXAMPLE: The *Hospital Formulary* states that the normal dosage of Lidocaine is 1–4 mg/min. The patient has an order for *500 mL D₅W IV c̄ Lidocaine 1 g to infuse at 30 mL/h.* Is the Lidocaine dosage within the normal range? (1 g = 1000 mg.)

Step 1.   Calculate mg/h

$$\frac{1000 \text{ mg}}{500 \text{ mL}} \diagup\diagdown \frac{X \text{ mg/h}}{30 \text{ mL/h}}$$

500X = 30,000

$$\frac{500X}{500} = \frac{30,000}{500}$$

X = 60 mg/h

60 mg are administered when the infusion rate is 30 mL/h. Therefore, 60 mg/h are being administered.

Step 2.   Convert mg/h to mg/min

$$\frac{60 \text{ mg}}{60 \text{ min}} = \frac{X \text{ mg}}{1 \text{ min}}$$

60X = 60

$$\frac{60X}{60} = \frac{60}{60}$$

X = 1 mg/min

Therefore, 1 mg/min is within the safe, normal range of 1–4 mg/min.

quick review

- For IV flow rate for medications ordered in mg/min, calculate:
    1. mL/min
    2. mL/h
  or calculate:
    1. mg (or g, U, or mU)/mL
    2. mL/h
- To check safe dosages of IV medications ordered in mL/h, calculate:
    1. mg/h
    2. mg/min

review set 44

Compute the flow rate in mL/h for each of these medications administered by infusion pump.

1. Order: Lidocaine 2 g IV per 1000 mL D$_5$W at 4 mg/min
   Rate: _____ mL/h

2. Order: Pronestyl 0.5 g IV per 250 mL D$_5$W at 2 mg/min
   Rate: _____ mL/h

3. Order: Isuprel 2 mg IV per 500 cc D$_5$W at 5 mcg/min
   Rate: _____ mL/h

4. Order: Medication "X" 450 mg IV per 500 mL NS at 4 mcg/kg/min
   Weight: 198 lb
   Rate: _____ mL/h

5. Order: Dopamine 800 mg in 500 mL NS IV at 15 mcg/kg/min
   Weight: 70 kg
   Rate: _____ mL/h

Order: 500 mL D$_5$W IV c̄ Dobutrex 500 mg to infuse at 15 mL/h. The patient weighs 125 pounds. Normal range: 2.5–10 mcg/kg/min

Answer questions 6–10.

6. What range in mcg/min of Dobutrex should the patient receive? _____ mcg/min

7. What range in mg/min of Dobutrex should the patient receive? _____ mg/min

8. Is the Dobutrex as ordered within the safe range? _____

Order: 500 mL D$_5$W IV c̄ 2 g Pronestyl to infuse at 60 mL/h. Normal range: 2–6 mg/min

9. How many mg/min is the patient receiving? _____ mg/min

10. Is the dosage within the normal range? _____

11. Order: Add magnesium sulfate 20 g to LR 500 mL. Start with a bolus of 2 g to infuse over 30 min. Then maintain a continuous infusion at 1 g/h.
    Rate: _____ mL/h for bolus
          _____ mL/h for continuous infusion

12. A physician's order is written to induce labor as follows:
    Add Pitocin 15 U to LR 250 mL. Begin a continuous infusion at the rate of 1 mU/min.
    Rate: _____ mL/h

After completing these problems, see pages 315–317 to check your answers.

Limiting Infusion Volumes

Calculating IV rates to include the IV PB volume is occasionally necessary to limit the total volume of IV fluid a patient receives. In order to do this you must calculate the flow rate for both the regular IV and the piggyback IV. In such instances of restricted fluids, the piggyback IVs are to be included as part of the total prescribed IV volume and time.

> ▶ *rule* Follow these six steps to calculate the flow rate of an IV that includes IV PB. Calculate:
>
> 1. IV PB flow rate
> 2. Total IV PB time
> 3. Total IV PB volume
> 4. Total regular IV volume
> 5. Total regular IV time
> 6. Regular IV flow rate

EXAMPLE 1:   Order: *3000 mL 5% dextrose in Lactated Ringer's for 24h with Kefzol 1 g IV PB/100 mL D$_5$W q.6h to run 1 hour. Limit total fluids to 3000 mL q.d. The drop factor is 10 gtt/mL.*

NOTE: The order intends that the patient will receive a maximum of 3000 mL in 24 hours. Remember, when fluids are restricted, the piggybacks are to be *included* in the total 24-hour intake, not in addition to it.

Step 1.   Calculate the flow rate of the IV PB.

$$\frac{V}{T} \times C = R: \frac{100 \text{ mL}}{60 \text{ min}} \times 10 \text{ gtt/mL} =$$

$$\frac{100}{6} = 16.7 = 17 \text{ gtt/min}$$

or, $\dfrac{\text{mL/h}}{\text{Drop factor constant}} = \dfrac{100}{6}$

$$\frac{100}{6} = 16.7 = 17 \text{ gtt/min}$$

Set the flow rate for the IV PB at 17 gtt/min to infuse 1 g Kefzol in 100 mL over 1 hour or 60 min.

Step 2.   Determine the total time the IV PB will be administered.
Kefzol 1 g q.6h to run 1 h = Kefzol 1 g 4 times/24h = Kefzol 1 g to run 4h/24h.

Step 3.   Determine the total volume of the IV PB.
Kefzol 1 g q.6h dissolved in 100 mL = 400 mL IV PB per 24 hours.

Step 4.   Determine the volume of the regular IV fluids to be administered between IV PB. Total volume of regular IV minus total volume of IV PB = 3000 − 400 = 2600 mL.

Step 5.   Determine the total regular IV time or the time between IV PB. Total IV time minus total IV PB time = 24h − 4h = 20 h

Step 6.   Compute the flow rate of the regular IV.

$$\frac{V}{T} \times C = R$$

$$\frac{2600 \text{ mL}}{1200 \text{ min}} \times 10 \text{ gtt/mL} = 21.7 = 22 \text{ gtt/min}$$

or, $\dfrac{\text{mL/h}}{\text{Drop factor constant}} = R$

$$\text{mL/h} = \frac{2600 \text{ mL}}{20 \text{ h}} = 130 \text{ mL/h}; \text{ drop factor constant is 6.}$$

$$\frac{130}{6} = 21.7 = 22 \text{ gtt/min}$$

Set the regular IV of 5% dextrose in Lactated Ringer's at the flow rate of 22 gtt/min. Then after 5 hours, switch to the Kefzol IV PB at the flow rate of 17 gtt/min for one hour.

EXAMPLE 2:   Order: *2000 mL Normal Saline IV for 24h with 80 mg gentamycin in 80 mL IV PB q.8h to run for 30 min. Limit fluid intake to 2000 mL q.d.*

Drop factor: 15 gtt/mL

Calculate the flow rate for the regular IV and for the IV PB.

Step 1.   IV PB flow rate $= \frac{V}{T} \times C = R$: $\frac{80 \text{ mL}}{30 \text{ min}} \times 15 \text{ gtt/mL} = \frac{80}{2} = 40$ gtt/min

Step 2.   Total IV PB time = q.8h = 3 times/24h = 3×30 min = 90 min = $1\frac{1}{2}$h

Step 3.   Total IV PB volume = 80 mL $\times$ 3 = 240 mL

Step 4.   Total regular IV volume = 2000 mL – 240 mL = 1760 mL

Step 5.   Total regular IV time = 24h – $1\frac{1}{2}$h = $22\frac{1}{2}$h = 1350 min

Step 6.   Regular IV flow rate $= \frac{V}{T} \times C = R$

$\frac{1760 \text{ mL}}{1350 \text{ min}} \times 15 \text{ gtt/mL} = 19.56 = 20$ gtt/min

or, $\frac{\text{mL/h}}{\text{Drop factor constant}} = R$

mL/h $= \frac{1760 \text{ mL}}{22.5 \text{ h}} = 78$ mL/h; drop factor constant is 4.

$\frac{78}{4} = 19.5 = 20$ gtt/min

Set the regular IV of normal saline at the flow rate of 20 gtt/min. After $7\frac{1}{2}$ hours, switch to the gentamycin IV PB at the flow rate of 40 gtt/min for 30 minutes.

Patients receiving a primary IV at a specific rate via an infusion controller or pump may require that the infusion rate be altered when a secondary (piggyback) medication is being administered. To do this, calculate the flow rate of the secondary medication in mL/h as you would for the primary IV and reset the infusion device.

Some infusion controllers or pumps allow you to set the flow rate for the secondary IV independent of the primary IV; then upon completion of the secondary infusion, the infusion device automatically returns to the original flow rate. If this is not the case, be sure to manually readjust the primary flow rate after the completion of the secondary set.

review set 45

Calculate the flow rates for the IV ordered and the IV PB ordered. These patients are on limited fluid volume (restricted fluids).

1.   Order: 3000 mL Normal Saline IV for 24h
      Penicillin G 1,000,000 U IV PB q.4h in 100 mL
      Normal Saline to run for 30 minutes
      Drop factor: 10 gtt/mL
      IV PB flow rate: _____ gtt/min
      IV flow rate: _____ gtt/min

2.   Order: 1000 mL D₅W IV for 24h
      Garamycin 40 mg q.i.d. in 40 mL IV PB to run 1 hour
      Drop factor: 60 gtt/mL
      IV PB flow rate: _____ gtt/min
      IV flow rate: _____ gtt/min

3. Order: 3000 mL D_5 Lactated Ringer's IV for 24h
    Ampicillin 0.5 g q.6h IV PB in 50 mL D_5W to run 30 min
    Drop factor: 15 gtt/mL
    IV PB flow rate: _____ gtt/min
    IV flow rate: _____ gtt/min

4. Order: 2000 mL $\frac{1}{2}$ Normal Saline IV for 24h
    Chloromycetin 500 mg/50 mL Normal Saline IV PB q.6h to run 1 hour
    Drop factor: 60 gtt/mL
    IV PB flow rate: _____ gtt/min
    IV flow rate: _____ gtt/min

5. Order: 1000 mL Lactated Ringer's IV for 24h
    Kefzol 250 mg IV PB/50 mL D_5W q.8h to run 1 hour
    Drop factor: 60 gtt/mL
    IV PB flow rate: _____ gtt/min
    IV flow rate: _____ gtt/min

6. Order: 2400 cc of D_5 Lactated Ringer's for 24h
    Ancef 1 g IV PB q.6h in 50 cc D_5W to run in over 30 min
    Drop factor: On infusion pump
    IV PB flow rate: _____ mL/h
    IV flow rate: _____ mL/h

7. Order: 2000 cc NS for 24h
    Garamycin 100 mg IV PB q.8h in 100 cc D_5W to run in over 30 min
    Drop factor: On infusion controller
    IV PB flow rate: _____ mL/h
    IV flow rate: _____ mL/h

8. Order: 3000 cc D_5 and 0.45% NS to run over 24h
    Zantac 50 mg q.6h in 50 cc D_5W to infuse over 15 min
    Drop factor: On infusion pump
    IV PB flow rate: _____ mL/h
    IV flow rate: _____ mL/h

After completing these problems, see pages 317 and 318 to check your answers.

critical thinking skills

The importance of knowing the therapeutic dose of a given medication is a critical nursing skill. Let's look at an example in which the order was unclear and the nurse did not verify the safe dosage.

■ error 1

Failing to clarify an order and failing to recognize a dosage that was unsafe.

possible scenario

Suppose the physician ordered a heparin drip for a patient with thrombophlebitis. The order was written this way:

Heparin 20,000 units in 500 mL of D_5W at 30 mL/h

The nurse, unsure if the order was for 30 mL/h or 80 mL/h, asked a coworker what the order meant. The coworker stated "It looks like 80 mL/h to me, but I'm not sure." The nurse set up the heparin drip and decided to run the rate at 80 mL/h as the coworker suggested. The patient received the heparin for 24 hours when he began to bleed from his IV site, had blood in his urine, and developed tachycardia and hypotension. When notified, the physician asked, "What is the rate of the heparin drip?" The nurse replied, "80 milliliters per hour," to which the physician stated, "I ordered the drip at 30 mL/h not 80 mL/h; 80 mL/h is an unsafe dosage."

potential outcome

The physician would likely have discontinued the heparin, ordered a stat PTT to evaluate the patient's clotting times, and ordered protamine sulfate, the antidote for heparin. Whether the interventions would have occurred in time to help this patient are unknown.

prevention

The nurse had several opportunities to correct this potentially fatal error. First, had the nurse clarified the unclear order with the physician who ordered the medication, this error would not have occurred. Second, had the nurse calculated the hourly dosage of heparin at 80 mL/h, the unsafe dosage would have been discovered and the nurse would have known to question the order. Let's look at the calculations. First, what the nurse gave:

$$\frac{20,000\ U}{500\ mL} = \frac{X\ U}{80\ mL}$$

$$500X = 1,600,000$$

$$\frac{500X}{500} = \frac{1,600,000}{500}$$

X = 3200 units of heparin per hour

$$\frac{3200\ U}{1\ h} = \frac{X\ U}{24\ h}$$

X = 76,800 U/24h

You recall that the therapeutic dose of heparin is 20,000–40,000 units per 24 hours. This dosage (76,800 U/24 h) exceeds the recommended daily dose by almost two times.

Now let's look at what the physician intended for the patient to receive.

$$\frac{20,000\ U}{500\ mL} = \frac{X\ U}{30\ mL}$$

$$500X = 600,000$$

$$\frac{500X}{500} = \frac{600,000}{500}$$

X = 1200 units per hour

$1200 \times 24 = 28,800$ units in 24 hours, a safe dosage.

The nurse had two opportunities to prevent this error. Whenever an order is unclear, clarify with the writer. Also, as part of the professional staff we are accountable for our actions and inactions. The nurse should have calculated the hourly heparin dosage to verify what dosage to administer to the patient and to determine its safety. Remember if you administer it, you are legally responsible.

critical thinking skills

Let's look at an example in which the nurse *prevents* a medication error by calculating the safe dosage of a medication before administering the drug to a child.

■ error 2

Dosage that is too high for a child.

possible scenario

Suppose a physician ordered aminophylline 500 mg IV to be diluted in 500 mL of D_5W to run at a rate of 22 mL/h. The child weighed 22 pounds. The nurse looked up aminophylline in her pediatric reference guide and noted that the safe dosage of aminophylline is 1 mg/kg/h. The nurse calculated the child's weight in kilograms and the mg/h dosage:

The nurse calculated the child's weight in kg.

$$\frac{1 \text{ kg}}{2.2 \text{ lb}} = \frac{X \text{ kg}}{22 \text{ lb}}$$

$$2.2X = 22$$

$$\frac{2.2X}{2.2} = \frac{22}{2.2}$$

$$X = 10 \text{ kg}$$

Then the nurse calculated the mg/h dosage.

$$\frac{1 \text{ mg}}{1 \text{ kg}} = \frac{X \text{ mg}}{10 \text{ kg}}$$

$$X = 10 \text{ mg/h is the safe dosage for this child.}$$

The nurse calculated that the 10-kilogram child should receive 10 mL per hour of aminophylline because if there are 500 mg in 500 mL, then there is 1 mg/mL of aminophylline being delivered. At a rate of 22 mL/h, the child would have received 22 mg of aminophylline. It occurred to the nurse that possibly the physician ordered the dose based on the child's weight in pounds not kilograms. The nurse notified the physician and questioned the order. The physician responded, "Thank you. You are correct. I did order the dose based on the child's weight in pounds. This was my error. I'm glad you caught it." The physician then decreased the rate of the aminophylline drip to 10 mL/h.

potential outcome

If the nurse had not questioned the order, the child would have received the dosage of 22 mg of aminophylline every hour. The child likely would have developed signs of toxicity beginning with irritability, tachycardia, and progressing to nausea, vomiting, and possibly cardiac arrhythmia and seizures. The severity of the symptoms would be directly related to how long the infusion occurred at double the therapeutic rate.

prevention

This is an instance in which the nurse prevented a medication error by checking the safe dosage and notifying the physician before administering the infusion. Let this be you!

practice problems—chapter 12 _____

You are working on the day shift 0700–1500 hours. You observe that one of the patients assigned to you has an intravenous infusion with a Buretrol volume control set. The patient's orders include:

1. D_5W IV @ 50 mL/h for continuous infusion

2. Pipracil 1 g IV q.6h

The pharmacy supplies the Pipracil in a prefilled syringe labeled 1 g per 5 mL with instructions to "add Pipracil to Buretrol and infuse over 30 minutes." Answer questions 1–5.

1. What is the drop factor of the Buretrol? _____ gtt/mL

2. What amount of Pipracil will you add to the Buretrol? _____ mL

3. How much D_5W IV fluid will you add to the Buretrol with the Pipracil? _____ mL

4. To maintain the flow rate at 50 mL/h, you will time the IV Pipracil to infuse at _____ gtt/min.

5. The medication administration record indicates that the patient received his last dose of IV Pipracil at 0600. How many doses of Pipracil will you administer during your shift? _____

6. Order: Heparin drip–25,000 U heparin in 250 mL 0.45% NS IV to infuse at 1200 U/h
   Drop factor: On infusion pump
   Flow rate: _____ mL/h
   Is this order safe? _____

7. Order: Aminophylline 0.5 g in 250 mL D_5W IV to infuse at 30 mg/h
   Drop factor: On infusion pump
   Flow rate: _____ mL/h

8. Order: 20 mEq KCl/L D_5W IV continuous infusion at 20 mL/h
   Supply: Since this is a child, you choose a 250 mL bag of D_5W. The KCl is available in a solution strength of 2 mEq/mL.
   Add _____ mL KCl to the 250 mL bag of D_5W.

9. You monitor a patient's IV of 1 L D_5W with 40,000 U heparin infusing at 100 mL/h on an infusion pump. The patient is receiving _____ U/h of heparin. Is the hourly heparin dosage safe? _____

10. At the rate of 4 cc/min, how long will it take to administer 1.5 L of IV fluid? _____

11. Order: Lidocaine drip IV to run at 4 mg/min
    Supply: 500 mL D_5W with Lidocaine 2 g added
    Drop factor: On infusion pump
    Flow rate: _____ mL/h

12. Order: Xylocaine 1 g IV in 250 mL D_5W IV at 3 mg/min
    Drop factor: On infusion controller
    Flow rate: _____ mL/h

13. Order: Procainamide 1 g in 500 cc D_5W IV to infuse at 2 mg/min
    Drop factor: On infusion pump
    Flow rate: _____ mL/h

14. Order: Dobutamine 250 mg in 250 cc D_5W IV to infuse at 5 mcg/kg/min
    Weight: 80 kg
    Drop factor: On infusion controller
    Flow rate: _____ mL/h

15. Your patient has 1 L D_5W IV with 2 g Lidocaine added infusing at 75 mL/h. The normal continuous IV dosage of Lidocaine is 1–4 mg/min. Is this dosage safe? _____

16. Order: Restricted fluids: 3000 mL D_5 NS IV for 24 hours
    Chloromycetin 1 g IV PB in 100 mL NS q.6h to run 1 hour
    Drop factor: 10 gtt/mL
    Flow rate: _____ gtt/min IV PB and _____ gtt/min primary IV

17. Order: Restricted fluids: 3000 mL D_5W IV for 24 hours
    Ampicillin 500 mg in 50 mL D_5W IV PB q.i.d. for 30 min
    Drop factor: 60 gtt/mL
    Flow rate: _____ gtt/min IV PB and _____ gtt/min primary IV

18. Order: 50 mg Nitropress IV in 500 mL D_5W to infuse at 3 mcg/kg/min
    Weight: 125 lb
    Drop factor: On infusion pump
    Flow rate: _____ mL/h

19. Order: KCl 40 mEq to each liter IV fluid
    Situation: IV discontinued with 800 mL remaining
    How much KCl infused? _____

20. The IV infusion rate is 125 mL/h. Calculate mL/min. _____

21. You find 250 mL of IV fluid remaining. The flow rate is 25 gtt/min. The drop factor is 10 gtt/mL. Calculate the time remaining. _____

22. It is 1630 hours and you find 100 mL of an IV running at a flow rate of 33 gtt/min. The drop factor is 60 gtt/mL. At what time will this 100 mL be completed? _____

23. An IV has a flow rate of 48 gtt/min. The infusion set has a drop factor of 15 gtt/mL. How much IV fluid will be infused in 8 hours? _____

24. Order: 1500 mL $\frac{1}{2}$ NS IV to run at 100 mL/h. Calculate the infusion time. _____

Baxter Continu-Flo® Set   2.7 m (108") long Luer Lock   **60** drops/mL   3 Inj Sites

Use the infusion set above to calculate the information requested for items 25 and 26.

25. Order: KCl 40 mEq/L D_5W IV to infuse at 2 mEq/h
    Rate: _____ mL/h
    Rate: _____ gtt/min

26. Order: Heparin 50,000 U/L D_5W IV to infuse at 3750 U/h
    Rate: _____ mL/h
    Is this dosage safe? _____

27. If the minimal dilution for Tobramycin is 5 mg/mL and you are giving 37 mg, what is the least amount of IV fluid in which you could safely dilute the dose? _____

28. Calculate the hourly IV rate for an 8-kg child receiving maintenance IV fluids. You may use the following formula for your calculations based on body weight.

   1st 10 kg   = 100 mL/kg/day
   2nd 10 kg   = 50 mL/kg/day
   each additional kg = 20 mL/kg/day
   Rate: _____ mL/h

29. Order: Add magnesium sulfate 20 g to 500 mL of LR IV solution. Start with a bolus of 3 g to infuse over 30 min. Then maintain a continuous infusion at 2 g/h.
   You will use an electronic infusion pump.
   Rate: _____ mL/h for bolus
   Rate: _____ mL/h for continuous infusion

30. Order: Add Pitocin 15 U to 500 mL of LR IV solution. Infuse at 1 mU/min.
   You will use an electronic infusion pump.
   Rate: _____ mL/h

After completing these problems, see pages 330–333 to check your answers.

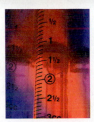

Posttest 1

Use proper metric, apothecaries', and medical notation.

1. The abbreviation for *both eyes* is _____ .

2. The abbreviation for *when necessary* is _____ .

3. The abbreviation *q.i.d.* means _____ .

4. The abbreviation *h.s.* means _____ .

5. The abbreviation *IV PB* means _____ .

6. 99°F = _____ °C

7. 39°C = _____ °F

Record the amount needed to administer one dose of the following orders. Assume that all tablets are scored in half. Indicate parenteral dosages that should be divided.

8. Order: Inderal 30 mg p.o. b.i.d.
   Supply: Inderal 60 mg tablets
   Give: _____ tablet(s)

9. Order: Orinase 250 mg p.o. b.i.d.
   Supply: Orinase 0.5 g tablets
   Give: _____ tablet(s)

10. Order: Levothroid 0.3 mg p.o.
    Supply: Levothroid 150 mcg tablets
    Give: _____ tablet(s)

11. Order: Sudafed 60 mg p.o. q.i.d.
    Supply: Sudafed 30 mg tablets
    Give: _____ tablet(s)

12. Order: Pen Vee K 600,000 U p.o. q.8h
    Supply: Pen Vee K 250 mg (400,000 U)
      per 5 mL
    Give: _____ mL

13. Order: Rimactane 0.6 g p.o. q.d.
    Supply: Rimactane 300 mg capsules
    Give: _____ capsule(s)

14. Order: Codeine gr ss p.o. q.4h p.r.n.,
      pain
    Supply: Codeine 30 mg tablets
    Give: _____ tablet(s)

15. Order: Arlidin gr $\frac{1}{5}$
    Supply: Arlidin (nylidrin HCl) 12 mg
      tablets
    Give: _____ tablet(s)

16. Order: Ceclor 175 mg p.o. q.8h
    Supply: Ceclor 250 mg per 5 mL
    Give _____ mL

17. Order: Synthroid 150 mcg p.o. q.d.
    Supply: Synthroid 0.05 mg tablets
    Give: _____ tablet(s)

18. Order: Erythromycin oral suspension
    600 mg p.o. q.6h
    Supply: E-Mycin E (Erythromycin)
    Liquid 400 mg/5 mL
    Give: _____ mL
    State the discharge instructions you
    should give; include dosage in house-
    hold measure, route, and frequency.

    _____

    _____

    _____

19. Order: Amoxicillin 0.5 g p.o. q.8h
    Supply: Amoxicillin 250 mg tabs
    Give: _____ tablet(s)

20. Order: Morphine sulfate 12 mg IM q. 4h
      p.r.n., pain
    Supply: Morphine sulfate gr $\frac{1}{4}$ per mL
    Give: _____ mL

21. Order: Atropine 0.4 mg IM on call to O.R.
    Supply: Atropine gr $\frac{1}{150}$ per mL
    Give: _____ mL

22. Order: Demerol 65 mg IM on call to O.R.
    Supply: Demerol 75 mg per 1.5 mL
    Give: _____ mL

23. Order: Vistaril 35 mg IM q.3–4h p.r.n.,
      nausea
    Supply: Vistaril 50 mg/cc
    Give: _____ mL

24. Order: Vistaril 25 mg IM stat
    Supply: Hydroxyzine (Vistaril) 100 mg
       per 2 cc
    Give: _____ mL

25. Order: Thorazine 15 mg IM q.4h p.r.n.,
       agitation
    Supply: Thorazine 25 mg/mL
    Give: _____ mL

26. Order: Cleocin 0.3 g IM q.i.d.
    Supply: Cleocin 300 mg per 2 mL
    Give: _____ mL

27. Order: Vitamin B_{12} 0.5 mg IM today
    Supply: Vitamin B_{12} 1000 mcg/mL
    Give: _____ mL

28. Order: Garamycin 50 mg IM q.8h
    Supply: Garamycin 40 mg/mL
    Give: _____ mL

29. Order: Compazine 4 mg IM q.3–4h
       p.r.n., nausea
    Supply: Compazine 5 mg/mL
    Give: _____ mL

30. Order: Heparin 8000 U SC q.8h
    Supply: Heparin 10,000 U/mL
    Give: _____ mL

31. Order: Meperidine hydrochloride 20 mg
       IM q.3–4h p.r.n., pain
    Supply: Demerol (meperidine hydro-
       chloride) 25 mg/0.5 mL
    Give: _____ mL

32. Order: Cefizox 1 g IM q.6h
    Supply: Cefizox 2 g vial
    Directions: Add 6 mL of sterile water to
       provide two 1 g doses of 3.7 mL each.
    Give: _____ mL

33. Order: Carbenicillin 1.5 g IM q.6h
    Supply: 5 g Geopen (carbenicillin)
    Reconstitution directions: "Add 9.5 mL
       sterile water to provide 1 g in 2.5 mL."
    Give: _____ mL

34. Order: Isuprel 1 mg IV diluted in 500
       mL D_5W
    Supply: Isuprel 1: 5000
    Amount of Isuprel needed to prepare IV
    dosage: _____ mL

35. Order: Chloromycetin 25 mg/kg/day IV
       in four equally divided doses
    Infant's weight: 3000 g
    Supply: Chloromycetin 100 mg/mL
    Give: _____ mL

36. Order: Elixophyllin 3 mg/kg p.o. q.6h.
    Patient's weight: 88 pounds
    Supply: Elixophyllin 80 mg per 15 mL
    Give: _____ mL

37. Order: Ceclor oral suspension 20 mg/kg/
       day p.o. in three equally divided doses
    Child's weight: 20 lb
    Supply: Ceclor 125 mg per 5 mL
    Discharge instructions: "Give
       _____ t three times a day"

Calculate the IV information as requested.

38. Your patient is to receive 2000 mL of IV fluids over the next 24 hours. The IV tubing is
    calibrated for a drop factor of 15 gtt/mL. What is the flow rate? _____ gtt/min

39. You have a new order for 10,000 U heparin in 500 mL NS IV to infuse at 750 U/h on an
    infusion pump. What is the flow rate? _____ mL/h

40. Your patient returns from the delivery room at 1530 hours with 400 mL D_5 Lactated
    Ringer's infusing at 24 gtt/min. The drop factor is 15 gtt/mL. Her postpartum orders
    include "discontinue IV when complete." At what time should you anticipate discontinu-
    ing this IV? _____

41. Your patient has orders for restricted fluids of 1500 mL per day. Medication orders are
    1500 mL NS IV per 24h with 300,000 U penicillin G potassium added IV PB q.4h to 100
    mL NS. The IV PB is to run for 30 minutes each. The drop factor is 60 gtt/mL. What is
    the flow rate for the IV PB? _____ gtt/min   regular IV? _____ gtt/min

42. (See No. 41) You have available penicillin G potassium reconstituted to 250,000 U per mL.
    How much should you add to the IV PB fluids to administer 300,000 U? _____ mL

43. You start your shift at 3:00 PM. On your nursing assessment rounds you find that Mr.
    Johnston has an IV of D_5W infusing at 32 gtt/min. The IV tubing is calibrated for

15 gtt/mL. How many total mL will Mr. Johnston receive during your 8 hour shift? _____ mL

For 44–49, use the medication labels that follow to calculate the following medication orders.

44. Morphine sulfate gr $\frac{1}{8}$ SC q.3–4h p.r.n., pain Give: _____ mL

45. Ilosone 50 mg/kg/day p.o. given in two equally divided doses q.12h. The child weighs 33 lb. Give: _____ mL

46. Kefzol 250 mg IV q.8h Give: _____ mL

47. Heparin 6000 U SC q.8h Give: _____ mL

48. Potassium chloride 20 mEq p.o. q.d. Give: _____ mL

49. Oncovin 2 mg/m² (BSA) IV today. The child is of normal height and weighs 44 lb. Give: _____ mL (West's Nomogram follows item 50.)

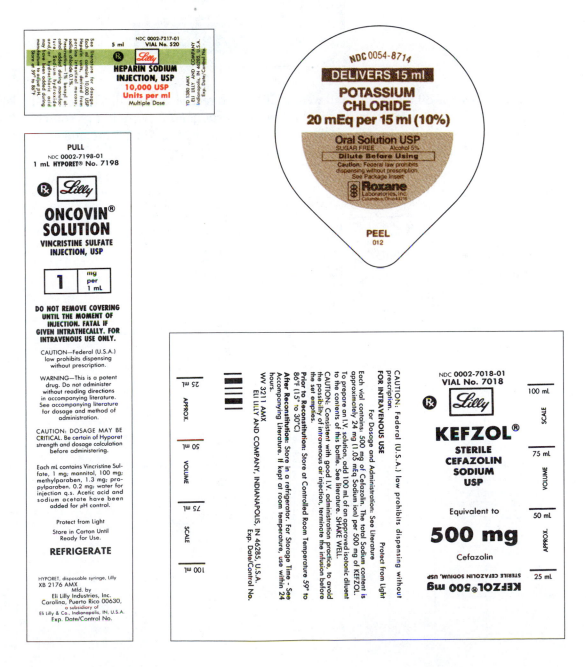

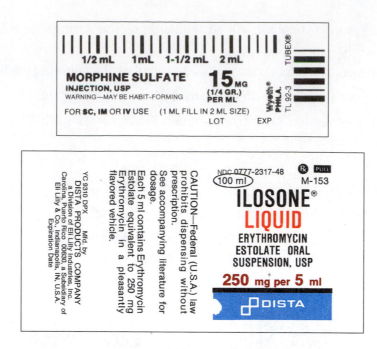

50. A child who is 30 inches tall and weighs 26 lb is to receive Staphcillin IM q.6h calculated by BSA. The usual adult dose according to the *Hospital Formulary* is 1 g. You have available Staphcillin 1 g. The reconstitution directions state add 1.5 mL and each 1 mL will contain 500 mg. You will give the child _____ mL.

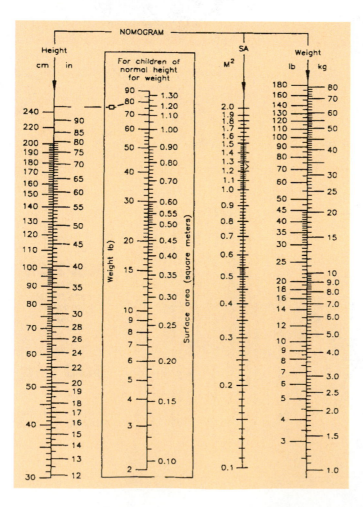

(Reprinted with permission from Behrman, R. E. and Vaughan, V. C. *Nelson Textbook of Pediatrics,* 15th ed., 1996, W. B. Saunders Company, Philadelphia, PA 19105.)

51. Order: 1 L D₅W IV c̄ 25 mg nitroglycerin to infuse at 5 mcg/min. Set the infusion controller to administer _____ mL/h.

52. Order: KCl 40 mEq/L D₅W IV to infuse at 2 mEq/h. Using a microdrip infusion set, the flow rate is _____ gtt/min.

Draw an arrow to demonstrate the correct measurement of the dosages given.

53. 1.33 mL

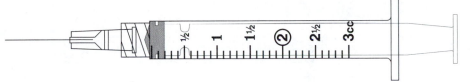

54. 2.5 mL

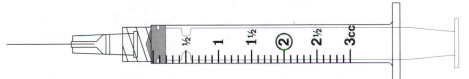

55. 0.33 mL

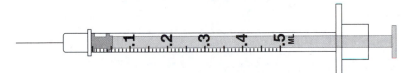

56. 70 U of U-100 insulin

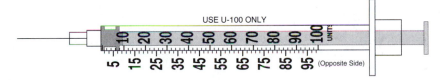

57. 37 U of U-100 insulin

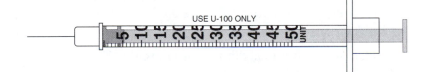

58. 15 mL

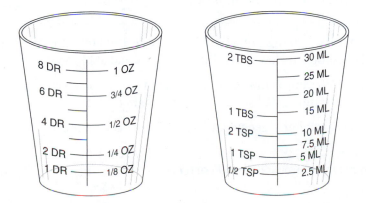

59. Select the one best choice of the following two syringes to be used to measure 0.45 mL of medication for a child. Draw an arrow on that syringe to demonstrate the correct measurement.

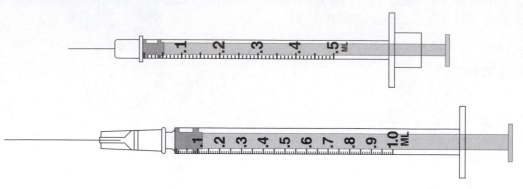

60. Select the one best choice of the following three syringes to be used to measure 36 units of U-100 insulin. Draw an arrow on that syringe to demonstrate the correct measurement.

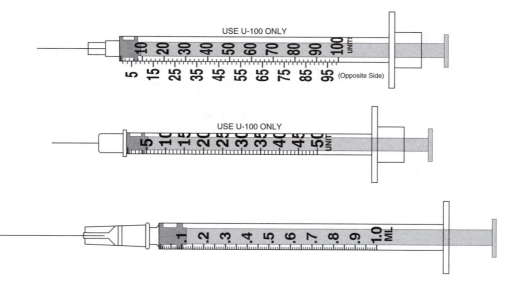

61. Order: Ticarcillin 750 mg IV q.6h. Calculate the safe daily dosage range of Ticarcillin for a child weighing 15 kg. The pediatric reference guide states the safe dosage of Ticarcillin is 200–300 mg/kg/day. _____

62. Refer to #61. Calculate the minimal dilution of Ticarcillin. The minimal dilution recommended is 100 mg/mL. _____

63. Interpret this order: D_5NS c̄ 20 mEq KCl/L IV @ 100mL/h. _____
_____

64. The physician orders 20 mEq of KCl to be added to 1000 mL of IV fluid. You are hanging a 500-mL bag of solution. How much KCl should be added to the IV bag? _____

65. Refer to #64. If potassium chloride is available in a solution strength of 2 mEq/mL and you need 10 mEq, how much KCl should you prepare to add to the IV bag? _____

After completing these problems, see pages 333–337 to check your answers.

Perfect Score = 100%   My score = _____
Minimum mastery score = 90% (59 correct)

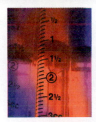

Posttest 2

Donna Smith, a 46-year-old patient of Dr. J. Physician, has been admitted to the Progressive Care Unit (PCU) with complaints of an irregular heartbeat, shortness of breath, and chest pain relieved by nitroglycerin. Items #1–14 refer to the admitting orders on page 268 for Mrs. Smith. The labels shown represent available medications and infusion set.

1. How much furosemide will you give Mrs. Smith for her first dose? Draw an arrow on the appropriate syringe to indicate how much you will prepare.

   Give: _____ mL

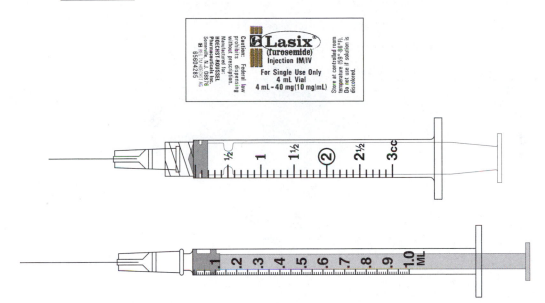

2. After the initial dose of furosemide, how much will you administer for the subsequent doses?

   Give: _____ tablet(s)

3. How many capsules of nitroglycerin will you give Mrs. Smith?

   Give: _____
   capsules

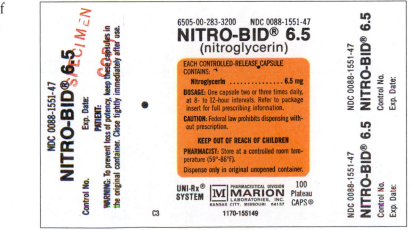

		ENTERED	FILLED	CHECKED	VERIFIED

NOTE: A NON-PROPRIETARY DRUG OF EQUAL QUALITY MAY BE DISPENSED - IF THIS COLUMN IS NOT CHECKED!

DATE	TIME WRITTEN	PLEASE USE BALL POINT - PRESS FIRMLY	✓	TIME NOTED	NURSES SIGNATURE
9/3/xx	1600	Admit to PCU, monitored bed	✓		
		Bedrest c̄ bathroom privileges	✓		
		Nitro-Bid 13 mg p.o. q.8h	✓		
		Lasix 20 mg IV stat, then 20 mg p.o. b.i.d.	✓		
		Digoxin 0.25 mg IV stat, repeat in 4 hours,	✓	1610 GP	
		then 0.125 mg p.o. qd			
		KCl 10 mEq per L D$_5$ ½ NS IV @ 80 cc/h	✓		
		Acetaminophen 650 mg p.r.n headache	✓		
		Labwork: Electrolytes and CBC in am	✓		
		Soft diet, advance as tolerated	✓		
		Dr. J. Physician			

AUTO STOP ORDERS: UNLESS REORDERED, FOLLOWING WILL BE D/C'D AT 0800 ON:

DATE	ORDER		
		☐ CONT ☐ D/C	PHYSICIAN SIGNATURE
		☐ CONT ☐ D/C	PHYSICIAN SIGNATURE
		☐ CONT ☐ D/C	PHYSICIAN SIGNATURE

CHECK WHEN ANTIBIOTICS ORDERED   ☐ Prophylactic   ☐ Empiric   ☐ Therapeutic

Allergies: None Known

Chest Pain

PATIENT DIAGNOSIS

HEIGHT 5' 6"   WEIGHT 110 lb.

FORM 959-708 (6-90)   **PHYSICIANS ORDER**   Reynolds + Reynolds LITHO IN U.S.A. K41814 (7-90) D339360

Smith, Donna
ID #257-226-3

①

4. Sometimes nitroglycerin is ordered by the SL route. "SL" is the medical abbreviation for: _____ Explain: _____

5. How much IV digoxin will you give on admission?
   Draw an arrow on the syringe to indicate how much you will prepare.
   Give: _____ mL

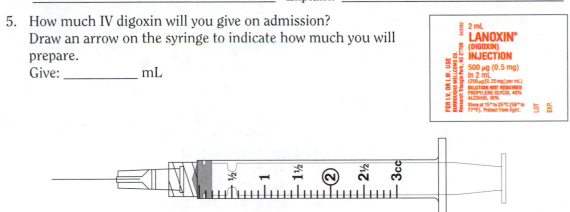

6. How many digoxin tablets will you need for a 24-hour supply of the p.o. order?
   24-hour supply equals _____ tablet(s).

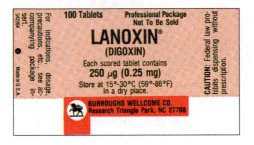

7. Calculate the drip rate for the IV fluid ordered. _____ gtt/min

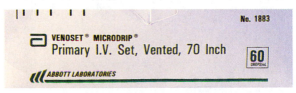

8. The KCl is available in a solution strength of 30 mEq per 15 mL. How much KCl will you add to the IV? Draw an arrow on the appropriate syringe to indicate the amount.
   Add: _____ mL

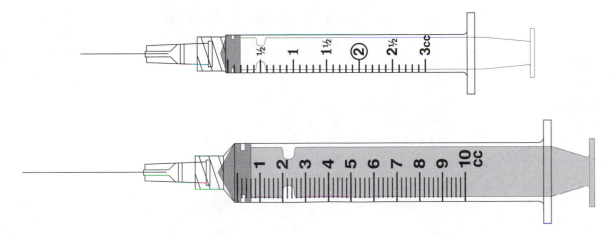

9. How many mEq KCl will Mrs. Smith receive per hour? _____ mEq

10. At the present infusion rate, how much $D_5 \frac{1}{2}$ NS will Mrs. Smith receive in a 24-hour period? _____ mL

11. The IV is started at 1630. Estimate the date and time that you should plan to hang the next liter of $D_5 \frac{1}{2}$ NS. _____ hours _____ date

12. Mrs. Smith has a headache. How much acetaminophen will you give her?
    Give: _____ tablet(s)

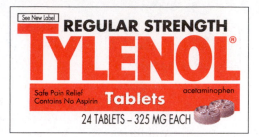

13. You have located an infusion controller for Mrs. Smith's IV. At what rate will you set the controller? _____ mL/hr

14. Which of Mrs. Smith's medications are ordered by their generic names? _____
    _____

Despite your excellent care, Mrs. Smith's condition worsens. She is transferred into the coronary care unit (CCU) with the medical orders noted on page 271. Items #15–20 refer to these orders. She weighs 110 pounds.

15. How much lidocaine will you give for the bolus? You have lidocaine 10 mg/mL available. Draw an arrow on the appropriate syringe to indicate the amount you will give.
    Give: _____ mL

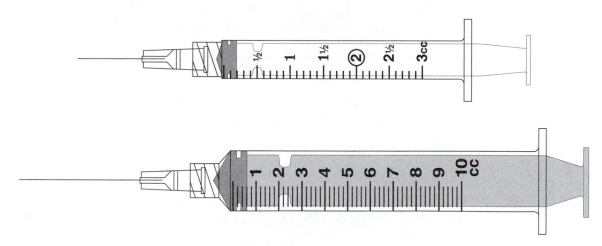

16. The infusion pump is calibrated to administer mL/h. At what rate will you initially set the infusion pump for the lidocaine drip? _____ mL/h

		ENTERED	FILLED	CHECKED	VERIFIED

NOTE: A NON-PROPRIETARY DRUG OF EQUAL QUALITY MAY BE DISPENSED - IF THIS COLUMN IS NOT CHECKED!

DATE	TIME WRITTEN	PLEASE USE BALL POINT - PRESS FIRMLY	✓	TIME NOTED	NURSES SIGNATURE
9/4/xx	2230	Transfer to CCU	✓		
		NPO	✓		
		Discontinue Nitro-Bid	✓		
		Lidocaine bolus 50 mg IV stat, then begin	✓		
		lidocaine drip 2 g in 500 cc D_5W			
		@ 2 mg/min by infusion pump			
		Increase lidocaine to 4 mg/min if PVCs	✓		
		(premature ventricular contractions)			
		persist		2235 MS	
		Dopamine 400 mg IV PB in 250 cc D_5W	✓		
		@ 10 mcg/kg/min by infusion pump			
		Increase KCl to 20 mEq per L D_5W	✓		
		$\frac{1}{2}$ NS IV @ 50 cc/h			
		Increase Lasix to 40 mg IV q. 12h	✓		
		O_2 @ 30% p̄ ABGs (arterial blood gases)	✓		
		Labwork: Electrolytes stat and in am and	✓		
		ABGs stat & p.r.n.			
		Dr. J. Physician			

AUTO STOP ORDERS: UNLESS REORDERED, FOLLOWING WILL BE D/C'D AT 0800 ON:

DATE	ORDER		PHYSICIAN SIGNATURE
		☐ CONT ☐ D/C	
		☐ CONT ☐ D/C	PHYSICIAN SIGNATURE
		☐ CONT ☐ D/C	PHYSICIAN SIGNATURE

CHECK WHEN ANTIBIOTICS ORDERED   ☐ Prophylactic   ☐ Empiric   ☐ Therapeutic

Allergies:
   None Known

   Chest Pain

PATIENT DIAGNOSIS

HEIGHT 5' 6"   WEIGHT 110 lb.

Smith, Donna
ID #257-226-3

FORM 959-708 (8-90) **PHYSICIANS ORDER** Reynolds + Reynolds LITHO IN U.S.A. K41814 (7-90) D339360

①

17. How much dopamine will you add to mix the dopamine drip? You have dopamine 80 mg/mL available. Draw an arrow on the appropriate syringe to indicate the amount you will add.
    Add: _____ mL

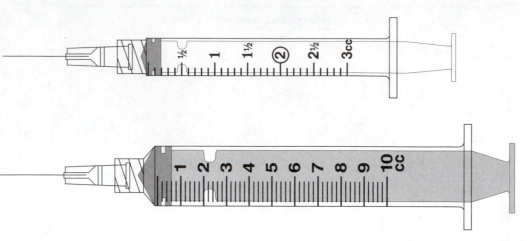

18. Calculate the rate for the infusion pump for the dopamine drip.
    _____ mL/h

19. How many mEq KCl will Mrs. Smith now receive per hour?
    _____ mEq/h

20. Mrs. Smith is having increasing amounts of PVCs. To increase her lidocaine drip to 4 mg/min you will now change your IV infusion pump setting to _____ mL/hr.

You are assigned to give "Team Medications" on a busy Adult Medical Unit. The following medications are in your medication cart. Calculate the amount you will administer for one dose. Assume all tablets are scored. Draw an arrow on the appropriate syringe to indicate how much you will prepare for parenteral medications.

21. Order: Dilantin 50 mg IV q.8h
    Give: _____ mL

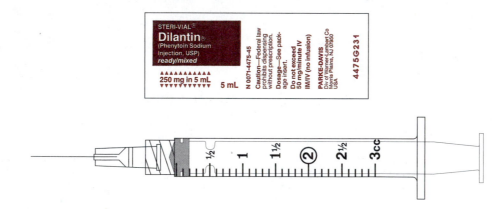

22. Order: Phenergan 12.5 mg IM q.3–4h p.r.n. nausea
    Give: _____ mL

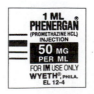

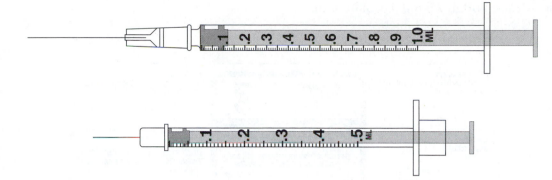

23. Order: Thorazine 35 mg IM stat
    Give: _____ mL

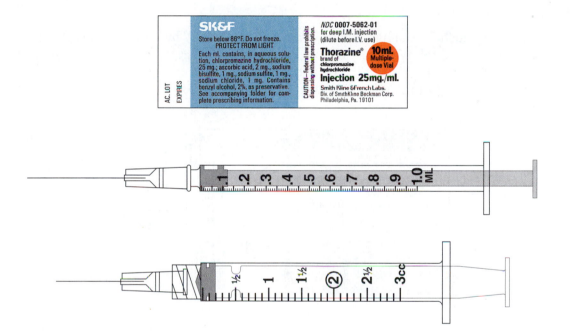

24. Order: Tagamet 400 mg p.o. h.s.
    Give: _____ tablet(s)

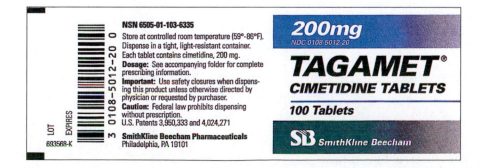

25. Order: Lortab 7.5 mg p.o. q.3h p.r.n.
     Give: _____ tablet(s)

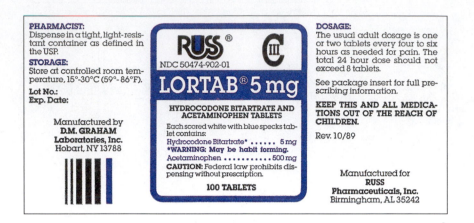

26. Order: IV flush Prostaphlin 500 mg q.6h in 50 mL D$_5$W IV by Buretrol over 60 min.
     Follow with 15 mL IV flush.
     Reconstitute with _____ mL diluent.
     Add _____ mL Prostaphlin and _____ mL D$_5$W to Buretrol.

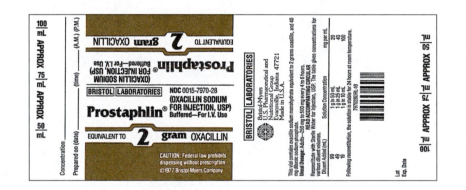

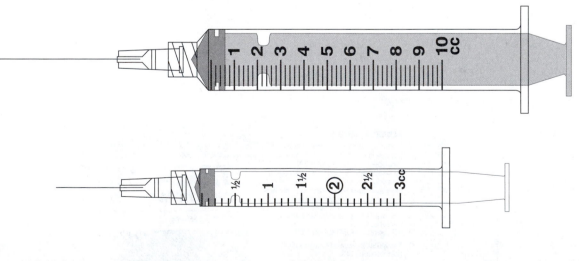

Set the Buretrol flow rate at _____ gtt/min.

27.   Order: Lanoxin 0.125 mg IV q.d.
      Give: _____ mL

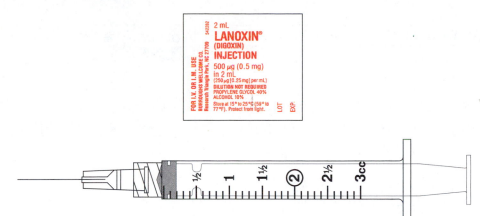

28.   Order: Phenobarbital gr $\frac{1}{8}$ p.o. q.i.d.
      Give: _____ tablet(s)

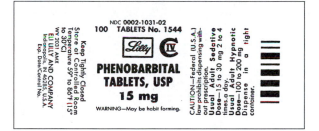

29.   Order: Kantrex 350 mg IM b.i.d.
      Supply: 500 mg per 2 mL
      Give: _____ mL

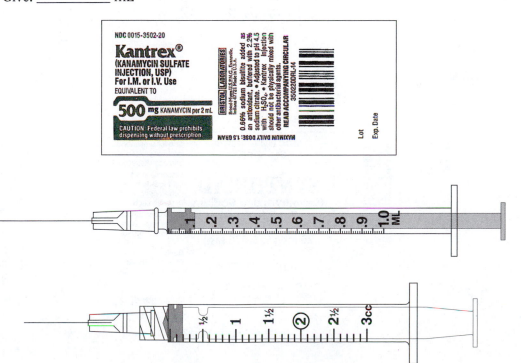

30. Order: Novolin R Regular U-100 insulin SC ac per sliding scale and blood sugar (BS) level. The patient's blood sugar at 1730 is 238.

SLIDING SCALE		INSULIN DOSAGE
BS:	0 – 150	0 U
BS:	151 – 250	8 U
BS:	251 – 350	13 U
BS:	351 – 400	18 U
BS:	> 400	Call M.D.

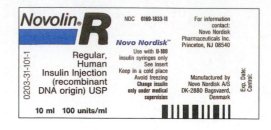

Give: _____ U which equals _____ mL.

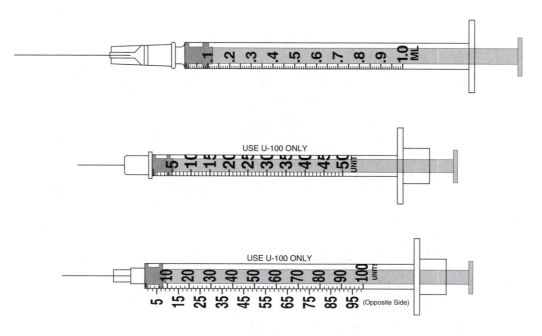

31. Order: Synthroid 0.05 mg p.o. q. AM
     Give: _____ tablet(s)

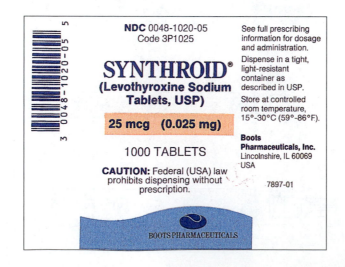

32. Order: Calan 40 mg p.o. t.i.d.
     Give: _____ tablet(s)

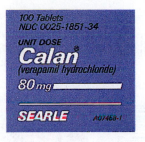

33. Order: Naprosyn 375 mg p.o. b.i.d.
     Give: _____ tablet(s)

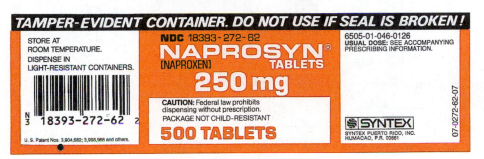

34. Order: Phenergan 40 mg IM stat
     Give: _____ mL

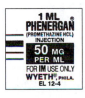

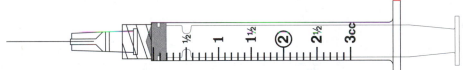

35. Order: Stadol 3 mg IM stat
     Supply: 2 mg per mL
     Give: _____ mL

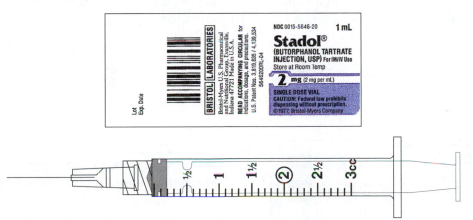

36. Order: Betapen-VK 100 mg p.o. q.6h
    Give: _____ mL

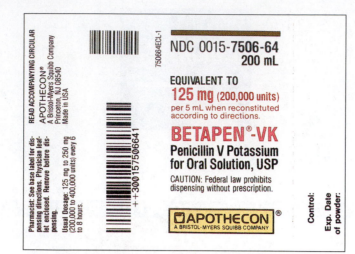

37. Order: Atropine gr $\frac{1}{100}$ IM stat
    Give: _____ mL

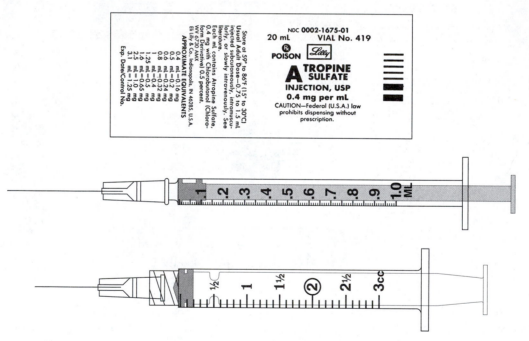

38. Order: Ampicillin 0.5 g in 50 mL normal saline IV PB over 30 min. Add _____ mL ampicillin to the normal saline and set the flow rate to _____ gtt/min.

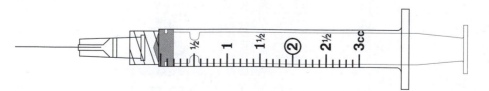

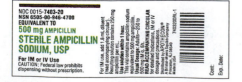

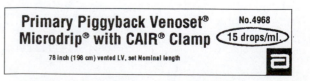

39. Order: Heparin 10,000 U in 500 cc D$_5$W to infuse at 1200 U/h.
    Add _____ mL heparin to the IV solution.
    Set the flow rate to _____ mL/h.

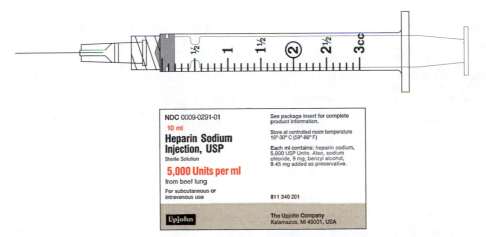

40. Order: Lente human insulin 46 U $\bar{c}$ regular human insulin 22 U.

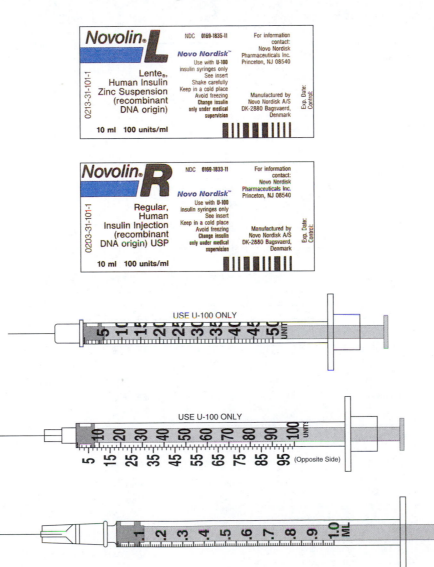

09/11/xx
06:26 PM
CHECKED BY: — — — — — — — — — — —

2ND   241
  217A   532729
     Smedley, Betty

MEDICATION ADMINISTRATION RECORD

PAGE: 1
REPT: PHR20B

DIAGNOSIS: 71590
ALLERGIES: NKA

NOTES:

DX: OSTEOARTHROS NOS-UNSPEC

DIET: Regular

ADMIT: 09/11/xx
WT: 154 lbs.

	ADMINISTRATION PERIOD:	07:30	09/12/xx	TO	07:29	09/13/xx	

ORDER # DRUG NAME, STRENGTH, DOSAGE FORM DOSE RATE ROUTE SCHEDULE	START	STOP	TIME PERIOD 07:30 TO 15:29	TIME PERIOD 15:30 TO 23:29	TIME PERIOD 23:30 TO 07:29
NURSE:					
• • • PRN's FOLLOW • • • • • • PRN's FOLLOW • • •					
264077 TYLENOL 325MG TABLET PRN **2 TABS** ORAL Q4H/PRN FOR TEMP > 101 F	09:30 09/11/xx				

264147   TORADOL   60MG   SYRINGE
PRN   **60 MG**   IM   PRN
    GIVE 60MG FOR BREAKTHROUGH PAIN X1 DOSE
    THEN 30MG Q6H/PRN
	15:00
	
	09/11/xx				

264148   TORADOL   60MG   SYRINGE
PRN   **30 MG**   IM   Q6H/PRN
    GIVE 6 HOURS AFTER 60MG DOSE FOR BREAK-
    THROUGH PAIN.
	15:00
	
	09/11/xx				

264151   INAPSINE   2.5MG/ML   AMPULE
PRN   **SEE NOTE**   IV   Q6H/PRN
    SAME AS DROPERIDOL; DOSE IS 0.625MG TO
    1.25MG (0.5-1.0 ML) FOR NAUSEA
	15:00
	
	09/11/xx				

264152 NUBAIN 10MG/ML AMPULE PRN **2 MG** IV Q4H/PRN FOR ITCHING	15:00 09/11/xx				
264153 NARCAN 0.4MG/ML AMPULE PRN **0.4 MG** IV PRN FOR RR< 8 AND IF PT. IS UNAROUSABLE	15:00 09/11/xx				
NURSE:					
NURSE:					

INITIALS	SIGNATURE	INITIALS	SIGNATURE	NOTES

             1500   0100

PHYSICIAN: J. Physician, MD

217A   Betty Smedley   AGE: 73   SEX: F

Mrs. Betty Smedley in Room 217A is assigned to your team. She is hospitalized with osteoarthritis. Refer to her MAR (on page 280) to answer questions 41–45. The medications available from the pharmacy are noted on the MAR.

41. Mrs. Smedley had her last dose of Tylenol at 2110 hours. It is now 0215 hours and her temperature is 39° C. Is Tylenol indicated? _____

    Explain: _____

    _____

42. How many tablets of Tylenol should she receive for each dose? _____

    Each dose is equivalent to _____ mg Tylenol.

43. Mrs. Smedley had 60 mg of Toradol at 1500 hours. At 2130 hours she is complaining of severe pain again. How much Toradol in the prefilled syringe will you give her now? Give _____ of the syringe amount.

44. Mrs. Smedley is complaining of itching. What p.r.n. medication would you select and how much will you add to the IV? Select _____ and give _____ mL.

    Draw an arrow on the appropriate syringe to indicate how much you will give.

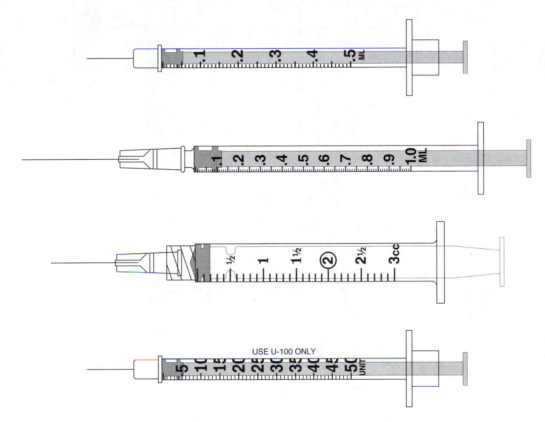

45. Mrs. Smedley's respiratory rate (R.R.) is 7 and she is difficult to arouse. What medication is indicated? _____ Draw an arrow on the syringe to indicate how much of this medication you will give.

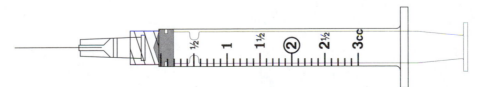

PAGE _____ of _____

MEDICATION ADMINISTRATION RECORD

ORIGINAL ORDER DATE	DATE STARTED / RENEWED	MEDICATION - DOSAGE	ROUTE	SCHEDULE 11-7	7-3	3-11	DATE 3-10-xx 11-7	7-3	3-11	DATE 3-11-xx 11-7	7-3	3-11	DATE 3-12-xx 11-7	7-3	3-11	DATE 3-14-xx 11-7	7-3	3-11
	3-10	Aminophylline 150 mg in 50 ml D₅W x 30 min q.6h	IV PB	12 6	12	6		GP 12	MS 6	JJ12 JJ6								
	3-10	SoluMedrol 125 mg q.6h	IV	12 6	12	6		GP 12	MS 6	JJ12 JJ6								
	3-10	Carafate 1 g 15 min ac & hs	PO	6:45	11:45 9:45	5:45		GP 11:45	MS5:45 MS9:45	JJ6:45								
	3-10	Novulin R Regular U-100 insulin ac	SC					GP7:30 GP11:30	MS5:50									
		per sliding scale:																
		Blood sugar _Units_																
		0-150 0 U																
		151-250 8 U																
		251-350 13 U																
		351-400 18 U																
		>400 Call M.D.																

PRN

INJECTION SITES

B - RIGHT ARM	D - RIGHT ANTERIOR THIGH	H - LEFT ABDOMEN	L - LEFT BUTTOCKS
C - RIGHT ABDOMEN	G - LEFT ARM	J - LEFT ANTERIOR THIGH	M - RIGHT BUTTOCKS

DATE GIVEN	TIME	INT.	ONE - TIME MEDICATION - DOSAGE	RT.	SCHEDULE 11-7	7-3	3-11	DATE 11-7	7-3	3-11	DATE 11-7	7-3	3-11	DATE 11-7	7-3	3-11	DATE 11-7	7-3	3-11

SIGNATURE OF NURSE ADMINISTERING MEDICATIONS

11-7		
7-3	JJ J.Jones LPN	
3-11	GP. G.Pickar,RN	

DATE GIVEN	TIME	INT.	MEDICATION-DOSAGE-CONT.	RT.
			MS. M.Smith,RN	
RECOPIED BY:				
CHECKED BY:				

Beck, John
ID #76834-21

ALLERGIES:

602-31 (7-92) (MPC# 1355)

LITHO IN U.S.A. K6508 (7-92) D395538

1
ORIGINAL COPY

John Beck, 19 years old, is diabetic. He is admitted to the medical unit with asthma. You are administering his medications. The MAR on page 282 is in the medication notebook on your medication cart. The labels represent the medications in his medication cart drawer. Items #46–50 refer to John.

46. Aminophylline is available in a solution strength of 250 mg/10 mL. How much aminophylline will you add to the 50 mL D$_5$W IV PB? Add _____ mL. Set the flow rate at _____ gtt/min.

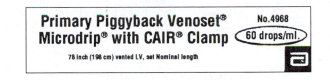

47. An infusion pump becomes available and you decide to use it for John's IV. It is calibrated in mL/h. To administer the aminophylline by infusion pump, set the pump at _____ mL/h.

48. Reconstitute the Solu-Medrol with _____ mL diluent and give _____ mL.

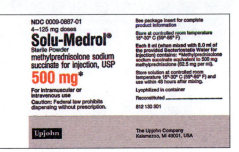

49. Mealtimes and bedtime are 8 AM, 12 N, 6 PM, and 10 PM. Using 24-hour time, give _____ tablet(s) of Carafate per dose each day at _____, _____, _____, and _____ hours.

50. At 0730 John's blood sugar is 360. You will give him _____ U of insulin. Draw an arrow on the appropriate syringe to indicate the correct dosage.

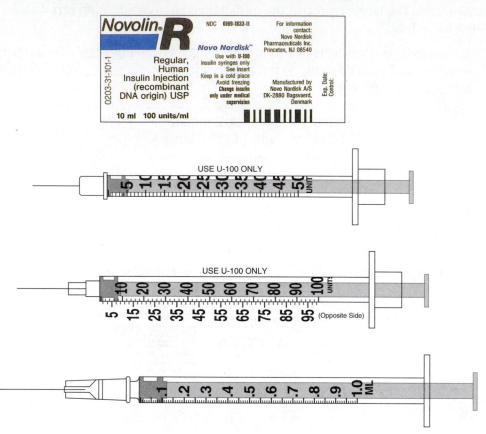

You are now administering medications to children.

51. Julie Thomas is a six-year-old pediatric patient who weighs 32 pounds. She is in the hospital for fever of unknown origin. Julie complains of burning on urination and her urinalysis shows E. Coli bacterial infection. The doctor prescribes Kantrex 15 mg/kg/day to be administered by Buretrol in three equal doses in 25 mL D_5W $\frac{1}{2}$ NS IV over 1 hour followed by 15 mL flush. Calculate one dose of Julie's Kantrex.
Add _____ mL Kantrex and _____ mL D_5W to the Buretrol and set the flow rate for _____ gtt/min.

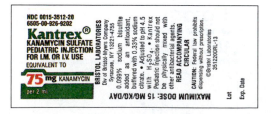

Jane Short is a 10-year-old with asthma. She weighs 56 pounds. Items #52 and 53 refer to Jane.

52. Jane has an order for aminophylline 25 mg/h by continuous IV drip. You are using an IV pump and an IV preparation of D_5W 250 mL with 250 mg aminophylline added. Set the pump to _____ mL/h.

53. The recommended maintenance dosage of aminophylline is 1 mg/kg/h. Is Jane's order safe and reasonable? _____

Jimmy Bryan is brought to the pediatric clinic by his mother. He is a 15-pound baby with an ear infection. Items #54–57 refer to Jimmy.

54. The doctor orders amoxicillin 50 mg p.o. q.8h for Jimmy. To reconstitute the amoxicillin, add _____ mL water.

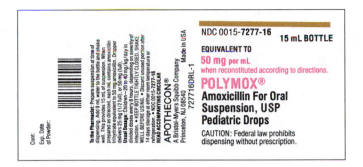

55. Is Jimmy's amoxicillin order safe and reasonable? _____ Explain: _____
_____

56. The doctor asks you to give Jimmy one dose of the amoxicillin stat. You will give Jimmy _____ mL.

57. The doctor also asks you to instruct Jimmy's mother about administering the medication at home. Tell Jimmy's mother to give the baby _____ droppersful for each dose. How often? _____

Items #58 and 59 refer to this situation.

You are preparing IV fluids for a young child according to the following order:

$$\text{KCl 20 mEq per L } D_5 \tfrac{1}{2} \text{ NS IV at 30 cc/hr.}$$

58. You have chosen to use a 250 mL bag of $D_5 \tfrac{1}{2}$ NS. How many mEq KCl will you add? _____ mEq

59. Your supply of KCl is 2 mEq/mL. How much KCl will you add to the 250-mL bag? _____ mL

60. Jill Jones is a 16-year-old, 110-pound teenager with a duodenal ulcer and abdominal pain. She has an order for cimetidine 5 mg/kg in 50 mL D_5W IV PB to be infused in 20 minutes. Available is Tagamet for injection, 300 mg/2 mL. The label represents the infusion set available.
Add: _____ mL cimetidine and set the flow rate at _____ gtt/min.

Jamie Smith is hospitalized with a staphlococcal bone infection. He weighs 35 pounds. Items #61–65 refer to Jamie.

Orders: D_5W $\tfrac{1}{2}$ NS IV at 50 mL/h for continuous infusion.
Vancocin 20 mg/kg IV b.i.d.

Available: Vancocin 500 mg/10 mL with instructions to "add to Buretrol and infuse over 60 min"

61. How much Vancocin will you add to the Buretrol? _____ mL

62. How much IV fluid will you add to the Buretrol with the Vancocin? _____ mL

63. At what flow rate will you set the Buretrol? _____ gtt/min

64. At what flow rate will you set the primary IV? _____ gtt/min

65. The doctor writes a new order for strict intake and output assessment for Jamie. During your eight-hour shift, in addition to his IV fluids, he consumed the following oral fluids:

    gelatin - ℥ iv

    water - ℥ iii × 2

    apple juice - pt i

    What is his total fluid intake during your shift?_____ mL

After completing these problems, see pages 337–344 to check your answers.

Perfect Score = 100

Minimum mastery score = 90 (59 correct)   My score = _____

Answers

Mathematics Diagnostic Test from pages 1–3.

1. 1517.63	11. 36	21. $1\frac{1}{4}$	31. 4	41. $\frac{1}{5}$
2. 27	12. 2500	22. $6\frac{13}{24}$	32. 0.09	42. 1:50
3. 100.66	13. XI	23. $1\frac{11}{18}$	33. 0.22	43. 5
4. $323.72	14. 6.25	24. $\frac{3}{5}$	34. 0.31	44. $\frac{1}{4}$
5. 46.11	15. $\frac{4}{5}$	25. $14\frac{7}{8}$	35. 4	45. 30
6. 754.5	16. 40%	26. $\frac{1}{100}$	36. 0.75	46. 3.3
7. VIII	17. 0.4%	27. 0.009	37. 3	47. 6.67
8. 19,494.7	18. 0.05	28. 320	38. 500	48. 5
9. $173.04	19. 1:3	29. 3	39. 18.24	49. 90%
10. 403.26	20. 0.02	30. 0.05	40. 2.4	50. 5:1

Solutions—Mathematics Diagnostic Test

3.
```
    9.50
   17.06
   32.00
   41.11
    0.99
  ------
  100.66
```

6.
```
   1005.0
 −  250.5
  -------
    754.5
```

10.
```
     17.16
  ×  23.5
  -------
    8580
   5148
  3432
  ----------
  403.260 = 403.26
```

12.
$$0.001\overline{)2.500} = 2500$$ (quotient 2500.)

19. $33\frac{1}{3}\% = 0.333 = \frac{1}{3} = 1:3$

23.
$$1\frac{5}{6} = 1\frac{15}{18}$$
$$-\frac{2}{9} = \frac{4}{18}$$
$$\overline{1\frac{11}{18}}$$

25. $4\frac{1}{4} \times 3\frac{1}{2} = \frac{17}{4} \times \frac{7}{2} = \frac{119}{8} = 14\frac{7}{8}$

29. $\frac{0.02 + 0.16}{0.4 - 0.34} = \frac{0.02}{+0.16} \; \frac{0.40}{-0.34} = 0.06\overline{)0.18} = 3$

32. $\frac{1}{2}\% = 0.005$
```
      18
  ×0.005
  ------
  0.090 = 0.09
```

34.
$$\frac{500}{125} \times \frac{1.25}{X}$$
$$500X = 125 \times 1.25$$
$$500X = 156.25$$
$$\frac{500X}{500} = \frac{156.25}{500}$$
$$X = 0.3125$$
$$X = 0.31$$

36.
$$\frac{5}{1.5} \times \frac{2.5}{X}$$
$$5X = 2.5 \times 1.5$$
$$5X = 3.75$$
$$\frac{5X}{5} = \frac{3.75}{5}$$
$$X = 0.75$$

38.
$$\frac{1.7}{X} \times \frac{0.51}{150}$$
$$0.51X = 1.7 \times 150$$
$$0.51X = 255$$
$$\frac{0.51X}{0.51} = \frac{255}{0.51}$$
$$X = 500$$

40.
$$\frac{\frac{1}{300}}{1.2} \times \frac{\frac{1}{150}}{X}$$
$$\frac{1X}{300} = \frac{1}{150} \times 1.2$$
$$\frac{1X}{300} \times \frac{300}{1} = \frac{1.2}{150} \times \frac{300}{1}$$
$$X = \frac{1.2}{\cancel{150}_1} \times \frac{\cancel{300}^2}{1}$$
$$X = 2.4$$

45. $\frac{66}{2.2} = 30$ or $\frac{2.2 \text{ lb.}}{1 \text{ kilogram}} \diagup\!\!\!\!\!\diagdown \frac{66 \text{ lb.}}{X \text{ kilograms}}$

$2.2X = 66$

$X = \frac{66}{2.2} = 30$ kilograms

49. $\begin{array}{r} 50 \\ -\ \ 5 \\ \hline 45 \end{array}$ $\frac{45}{50} = \frac{9}{10} = 90\%$

50. $\frac{\text{Female}}{\text{Male}} = \frac{5}{1}$ or $5:1$

Review Sets

Review Set 1 from page 5.

1. XXVIII
2. XIII
3. XVII
4. XV
5. IX
6. 30
7. 23
8. 5
9. 24
10. 4
11. XX
12. XXX
13. IV
14. V
15. XXIV

Review Set 2 from pages 8–10.

1. $\frac{6}{6}$, $\frac{7}{5}$
2. $\frac{1}{100}$ $\frac{1}{150}$
3. $\frac{1}{4}$, $\frac{1}{14}$, $\frac{1\frac{1}{4}}{14}$
4. $1\frac{2}{9}$, $1\frac{1}{4}$, $5\frac{7}{8}$
5. $\frac{3}{4} = \frac{6}{8}$, $\frac{1}{5} = \frac{2}{10}$, $\frac{3}{9} = \frac{1}{3}$
6. $\frac{13}{2}$
7. $\frac{6}{5}$
8. $\frac{32}{3}$
9. $\frac{47}{6}$
10. $\frac{411}{4}$
11. 2
12. 1
13. $3\frac{1}{3}$
14. $1\frac{1}{3}$
15. $2\frac{3}{4}$
16. $\frac{6}{8}$
17. $\frac{4}{16}$
18. $\frac{8}{12}$
19. $\frac{4}{10}$
20. $\frac{6}{9}$
21. $\frac{1}{100}$
22. $\frac{1}{10,000}$
23. $\frac{5}{9}$
24. $\frac{3}{10}$
25. $\frac{1}{8}$
26. 2 bottles; $1\frac{1}{2}$ bottles will be used
27. $\frac{1}{20}$
28. $\frac{9}{10}$
29. $\frac{1}{2}$ dose
30. $\frac{1}{2}$ teaspoon

Solutions—Review Set 2

8. $10\frac{2}{3} = \frac{(3 \times 10) + 2}{3} = \frac{32}{3}$

14. $\frac{100}{75} = 1\frac{25}{75} = 1\frac{1}{3}$

18. $\frac{2}{3} \times \frac{4}{4} = \frac{8}{12}$

25.

$\frac{1}{2}$ of $\frac{1}{4} = \frac{1}{2} \times \frac{1}{4} = \frac{1}{8}$

27. $\begin{array}{r} 57 \\ +\ \ 3 \\ \hline 60 \end{array}$ people in class

The men represent $\frac{3}{60}$ or $\frac{1}{20}$ of the class.

29. $\frac{80}{160} = \frac{1}{2}$ of a dose

30. $\frac{1}{2}$ of 1 teaspoon $= \frac{1}{2}$ teaspoon

Review Set 3 from pages 14 and 15.

1. $\frac{1}{40}$
2. $\frac{36}{125}$
3. $\frac{35}{48}$
4. $\frac{3}{100}$
5. 3
6. $1\frac{2}{3}$
7. $\frac{4}{5}$
8. $8\frac{7}{15}$
9. $1\frac{5}{12}$
10. $17\frac{5}{24}$
11. $1\frac{1}{24}$
12. $32\frac{5}{6}$
13. $\frac{1}{2}$
14. $4\frac{5}{6}$
15. $\frac{1}{24}$
16. $66\frac{23}{33}$
17. $299\frac{4}{5}$
18. $\frac{1}{30}$
19. $3\frac{1}{3}$
20. $\frac{3}{20}$
21. $\frac{1}{3}$
22. $1\frac{1}{3}$
23. $1\frac{1}{9}$
24. 60 calories
25. 560 seconds
26. $\frac{2}{3}$ unshaded
27. 40 doses
28. $31\frac{1}{2}$ tablets

Solutions—Review Set 3

3. $\frac{5}{8} \times 1\frac{1}{6} = \frac{5}{8} \times \frac{7}{6} = \frac{35}{48}$

5. $\frac{\overset{1}{\cancel{6}}}{\underset{4}{\cancel{6}}} \times \frac{3}{\underset{3}{\cancel{2}}} = \left(\frac{1}{6} \times \frac{4}{1}\right) \times \left(\frac{3}{1} \times \frac{3}{2}\right) = \frac{4}{6} \times \frac{9}{2} =$

$\frac{\overset{1}{\cancel{2}}}{\underset{1}{\cancel{3}}} \times \frac{\overset{3}{\cancel{9}}}{\underset{1}{\cancel{2}}} = 3$

10. $4\frac{2}{3} + 5\frac{1}{24} + 7\frac{1}{2} = 4\frac{16}{24}$

$5\frac{1}{24}$

$+ 7\frac{12}{24}$

$16\frac{29}{24} = 17\frac{5}{24}$

16. $\begin{array}{r} 100\frac{1}{33} \\ - 33\frac{1}{3} \\ \hline \end{array} = \begin{array}{r} 99\frac{34}{33} \\ - 33\frac{11}{33} \\ \hline 66\frac{23}{33} \end{array}$

19. $2\frac{1}{2} \div \frac{3}{4} = \frac{5}{2} \div \frac{3}{4} = \frac{5}{\cancel{2}} \times \frac{\overset{2}{\cancel{4}}}{3} = \frac{10}{3} = 3\frac{1}{3}$

22. $\dfrac{\frac{3}{4}}{\frac{7}{8}} \div \dfrac{1\frac{1}{2}}{2\frac{1}{3}} = \left(\frac{3}{4} \times \frac{\overset{2}{\cancel{8}}}{7}\right) \div \left(\frac{3}{2} \times \frac{3}{7}\right) =$

$\frac{\overset{2}{\cancel{6}}}{7} \div \frac{9}{14} = \frac{\overset{2}{\cancel{6}}}{\cancel{7}} \times \frac{\overset{2}{\cancel{14}}}{\cancel{9}} = \frac{4}{3} = 1\frac{1}{3}$

26. $12 - 4 = 8$

$\frac{8}{12} = \frac{2}{3}$ unshaded

28. $3 \times 7 = 21$ doses

$21 \times \frac{3}{2} = \frac{63}{2} = 31\frac{1}{2}$

Review Set 4 from pages 16 and 17.

1. 0.2, two-tenths

2. $\frac{17}{20}$, 0.85

3. $1\frac{1}{20}$, one and five-hundredths

4. $\frac{3}{500}$, six-thousandths

5. 10.015, ten and fifteen-thousandths

6. $1\frac{9}{10}$, one and nine-tenths

7. $5\frac{1}{10}$, 5.1

8. 0.8, eight-tenths

9. $250\frac{1}{2}$, two hundred fifty and five-tenths

10. 33.03, thirty-three and three-hundredths

11. $\frac{19}{20}$, ninety-five hundredths

12. 2.75, two and seventy-five hundredths

13. $7\frac{1}{200}$, 7.005

14. 0.084, eighty-four thousandths

15. $12\frac{1}{8}$, twelve and one hundred twenty-five thousandths

16. $20\frac{9}{100}$, twenty and nine-hundredths

17. $22\frac{11}{500}$, 22.022

18. $\frac{3}{20}$, fifteen-hundredths

19. 1000.005, one thousand and five-thousandths

20. $4085\frac{3}{40}$, 4085.075

Solutions—Review Set 4

4. $\frac{6}{1000} = \frac{3}{500}$

8. $\frac{4}{5} = 5\overline{)4.0}^{\,0.8}$

14. $\frac{21}{250} = 250\overline{)21.000}^{\,0.084}$
$\underline{20\ 00}$
$1\ 000$
$\underline{1\ 000}$

15. $12.125 = 12\frac{125}{1000} = 12\frac{1}{8}$

18. $0.15 = \frac{15}{100} = \frac{3}{20}$

Review Set 5 from page 18.

1. 22.585	5. 175.199	9. $18.91	13. 4.15	17. 374.35
2. 44.177	6. 25.007	10. $22.71	14. 1.51	18. 604.42
3. 12.309	7. 0.518	11. 6.403	15. 10.25	19. 27.449
4. 11.3	8. $9.48	12. 0.27	16. 2.517	20. 23.619

Solutions—Review Set 5

2. $\begin{array}{r} 7.517 \\ 3.200 \\ 0.160 \\ 33.300 \\ \hline 44.177 \end{array}$

9. $\begin{array}{r} \scriptstyle 8\ 9\ 10 \\ \$1\cancel{9.00} \\ - 0.09 \\ \hline \$18.91 \end{array}$

Review Set 6 from page 22.

1. 5.83
2. 2.2
3. 42.75
4. 0.15
5. 403.14
6. 75,100.75
7. 32.86
8. 2.78
9. 348.58
10. 0.02
11. 400
12. 3.74
13. 5
14. 2.98
15. 4120
16. 5.45
17. 272.67
18. 1.5
19. 50,020
20. 300
21. 562.50. = 56,250
22. 16.0. = 160
23. .025. = 0.025
24. .032.005 = 0.032005
25. .00.125 = 0.00125
26. 23.2.5 = 232.5
27. 71.7.717 = 71.7717
28. 83.1.6 = 831.6
29. 0.33. = 33
30. 14.106. = 14,106

Solutions—Review Set 6

10. $1.14 \times 0.014 = 0.01596 = 0.02$

14. $45.5 \div 15.25 = 2.983 = 2.98$

Review Set 7 from page 23.

1. 0.4, 40%, 2:5
2. $\frac{1}{20}$, 5%, 1:20
3. 0.17, $\frac{17}{100}$, 17:100
4. 0.25, $\frac{1}{4}$, 25%
5. 0.06, $\frac{3}{50}$, 3:50
6. 0.17, 17%, 1:6
7. 0.5, $\frac{1}{2}$, 1:2
8. 0.01, $\frac{1}{100}$, 1%
9. $\frac{9}{100}$, 9%, 9:100
10. 0.38, 38%, 3:8
11. 0.67, $\frac{2}{3}$, 67%
12. 0.33, 33%, 1:3
13. $\frac{13}{25}$, 52%, 13:25
14. 0.45, $\frac{9}{20}$, 45%
15. 0.86, 86%, 6:7
16. 0.3, $\frac{3}{10}$, 30%
17. 0.02, 2%, 1:50
18. $\frac{3}{5}$, 60%, 3:5
19. $\frac{1}{25}$, 4%, 1:25
20. 0.1, $\frac{1}{10}$, 1:10

Review Set 8 from page 29.

1. 0.25
2. 0.9
3. 0.56
4. 1000
5. 0.7
6. 514.29
7. 2142.86
8. 500
9. 200
10. 50
11. 3
12. 0.63
13. 10
14. 0.67
15. 1.25
16. 31.25
17. 16.67
18. 240
19. 0.75
20. 2.27
21. 1
22. 6

Solutions—Review Set 8

1.
$$\frac{1000}{2} = \frac{125}{X}$$
$$\frac{1000}{2} \diagup\!\!\!\diagdown \frac{125}{X}$$
$$1000X = 2 \times 125$$
$$1000X = 250$$
$$\frac{1000X}{1000} = \frac{250}{1000}$$
$$X = 0.25$$

2.
$$\frac{500}{1.8} = \frac{250}{X}$$
$$\frac{500}{1.8} \diagup\!\!\!\diagdown \frac{250}{X}$$
$$500X = 1.8 \times 250$$
$$500X = 450$$
$$\frac{500X}{500} = \frac{450}{500}$$
$$X = 0.9$$

6.
$$\frac{X}{12} = \frac{1200}{28}$$
$$\frac{X}{12} \diagup\!\!\!\diagdown \frac{1200}{28}$$
$$28X = 12 \times 1200$$
$$28X = 14,400$$
$$\frac{28X}{28} = \frac{14,400}{28}$$
$$X = 514.285$$
$$X = 514.29$$

8.
$$\frac{2000}{X} = \frac{2}{0.5}$$
$$\frac{2000}{X} \diagup\!\!\!\diagdown \frac{2}{0.5}$$
$$2X = 2000 \times 0.5$$
$$2X = 1000$$
$$\frac{2X}{2} = \frac{1000}{2}$$
$$X = 500$$

9.
$$\frac{500}{X} = \frac{15}{6}$$
$$\frac{500}{X} \diagup\!\!\!\diagdown \frac{15}{6}$$
$$15X = 5000 \times 6$$
$$15X = 3000$$
$$\frac{15X}{15} = \frac{3000}{15}$$
$$X = 200$$

10.
$$\frac{\frac{1}{4}}{500} = \frac{\frac{2.5}{100}}{X}$$
$$\frac{\frac{1}{4}}{500} \diagup\!\!\!\diagdown \frac{\frac{2.5}{100}}{X}$$
$$\frac{1X}{4} = \frac{\overset{5}{\cancel{500}}}{1} \times \frac{2.5}{\underset{1}{\cancel{100}}}$$
$$\frac{1X}{4} = \frac{5}{1} \times \frac{2.5}{1}$$
$$\frac{1X}{4} \times \frac{4}{1} = 12.5 \times \frac{4}{1}$$
$$X = 12.5 \times \frac{4}{1}$$
$$X = \frac{12.5}{1} \times \frac{4}{1}$$
$$X = 50$$

14.
$$\frac{\frac{1}{100}}{1} \times \frac{\frac{1}{150}}{X}$$

$$\frac{1}{100}X = \frac{1}{150}$$

$$X = \frac{\frac{1}{150}}{\frac{1}{100}}$$

$$X = \frac{1}{150} \times \frac{100}{1} = \frac{100}{150}$$

$$X = \frac{2}{3} = 0.666 = 0.67$$

19.
$$\frac{6}{X} \times 0.5 = 4$$

$$\frac{6}{X} \times \frac{0.5}{1} = 4$$

$$\frac{3}{X} = \frac{4}{1}$$

$$\frac{3}{X} \times \frac{4}{1}$$

$$4X = 3$$

$$\frac{4X}{4} = \frac{3}{4}$$

$$X = 0.75$$

22.
$$\frac{5}{25\%} \times 30\% = X$$

$$\frac{5}{25\%} \times \frac{30\%}{1} = X$$

$$\frac{5 \times 0.3}{0.25 \times 1} = X$$

$$\frac{1.5}{0.25} = X$$

$$X = 6$$

Review Set 9 from pages 33 and 34.

1. metric
2. volume
3. weight
4. length
5. 0.001
6. 1000
7. 10
8. kilogram
9. milligram
10. 1000
11. 1
12. 2.2
13. 10
14. 0.3 g
15. 1.33 mL
16. 5 kg
17. 1.5 mm
18. 10 mg
19. microgram
20. milliliter
21. cubic centimeter
22. gram
23. millimeter
24. kilogram
25. centimeter

Review Set 10 from page 36.

1. dram
2. ounce
3. minim
4. one-half
5. grain
6. ℥ ss
7. gr $\frac{1}{6}$
8. ℥ iv
9. pt ii
10. qt i $\frac{1}{4}$
11. gr x
12. ℥ viiiss
13. gr ii
14. pt 16
15. gr iii
16. ℥ 32
17. gr viiss
18. 32
19. i
20. ii

Review Set 11 from page 37.

1. twenty drops
2. one thousand units
3. ten milliequivalents
4. four teaspoons
5. ten tablespoons
6. 4 gtt
7. 30 mEq
8. 5 T
9. 1500 U
10. 10 t
11. False
12. units, U
13. 3
14. 9
15. 1000

Review Set 12 from page 46.

1. 0.5
2. 15
3. 0.008
4. 0.01
5. 0.06
6. 0.3
7. 0.0002
8. 1200
9. 2.5
10. 65
11. 5
12. 1500
13. 2
14. 0.25
15. 2000
16. 56.08
17. 79.2
18. 1000
19. 1000
20. 0.001
21. 0.00023
22. 0.00105
23. 0.00001
24. 400
25. 0.025
26. 0.5
27. 10,000
28. 0.45
29. 0.005
30. 30,000

Solutions—Review Set 12

2.
$$\frac{1\,g}{1000\,mg} \times \frac{0.015\,g}{X\,mg}$$

$$1X = 0.015 \times 1000 = 0.015.$$

$$X = 15\,mg$$

3.
$$\frac{1\,g}{1000\,mg} \times \frac{X\,g}{8\,mg}$$

$$1000X = 8$$

$$\frac{1000X}{1000} = \frac{8}{1000} = .008.$$

$$X = 0.008\,g$$

7.
$$\frac{1\,g}{1000\,mg} \times \frac{X\,g}{0.2\,mg}$$

$$1000X = 0.2$$

$$\frac{1000X}{1000} = \frac{0.2}{1000} = .000.2$$

$$X = 0.0002\,g$$

9.
$$\frac{1\,kg}{1000\,g} \times \frac{0.0025\,kg}{X\,g}$$

$$1X = 0.0025 \times 1000 = 0.002.5$$

$$X = 2.5\,g$$

17.
$$\frac{1\,L}{1000\,mL} \times \frac{X\,L}{79,200\,mL}$$

$$1000X = 79,200$$

$$\frac{1000X}{1000} = \frac{79,200}{1000} = 79.200.$$

$$X = 79.2\,L$$

20.
$$\frac{1\,L}{1000\,mL} \times \frac{X\,L}{1\,mL}$$

$$1000X = 1$$

$$\frac{1000X}{1000} = \frac{1}{1000} = .001.$$

$$X = 0.001\,L$$

23.
$$\frac{1\,mg}{1000\,mcg} \times \frac{X\,mg}{0.01\,mcg}$$

$$1000X = 0.01$$

$$\frac{1000X}{1000} = \frac{0.01}{1000} = .000.01$$

$$X = 0.00001\,mg$$

Review Set 13 from pages 49 and 50.

1. 30, gr i = 60 mg
2. 45, gr i = 60 mg
3. $\frac{9}{20}$, 1 g = gr 15
4. 0.4, gr i = 60 mg
5. 0.5, 1 g = gr 15
6. $\frac{1}{4}$, gr i = 60 mg
7. 25, 1 t = 5 cc
8. ss, ℥ i = 30 cc
9. 75, ℥ i = 30 mL
10. iss, pt i = 500 mL
11. 12, 1 t = 5 mL
12. 60, 1 T = 15 cc
13. 19.8, 1 kg = 2.2 lb

14. 50, 1 kg = 2.2 lb
15. 96, 1 L = ℥ 32
16. 7.7, 1 kg = 2.2 lb
17. 30, 1 in = 2.5 cm
18. 2, qt i = 1 L
19. 15, 1 t = 5 mL
20. 45, 1 kg = 2.2 lb
21. $\frac{1}{150}$, gr i = 60 mg
22. $\frac{1}{100}$, gr i = 60 mg
23. 500, pt i = 500 mL (see No. 10)
24. 600, gr i = 60 mg
25. v, gr i = 60 mg

26. 12, 1 in = 2.5 cm
27. iss, gr i = 60 mg
28. ii, ℥ i = 30 mL
29. 10, gr i = 60 mg
30. ss, gr i = 60 mg
31. 2430
32. 1.25 mg
33. Dissolve 4 tablespoons or 2 ounces of Epsom Salts in 1 quart of water.
34. 2 t
35. 3 quarts of formula

Solutions—Review Set 13

2. $\dfrac{gr\ i}{60\ mg} \diagtimes \dfrac{gr\ \frac{3}{4}}{X\ mg}$

$1X = \frac{3}{4} \times \frac{60}{1}$

$X = 45\ mg$

3. $\dfrac{1\ g}{gr\ 15} \diagtimes \dfrac{0.03\ g}{gr\ X}$

$1X = \frac{3}{100} \times \frac{15}{1}$

$X = \frac{45}{100} = gr\ \frac{9}{20}$

4. $\dfrac{gr\ i}{60\ mg} \diagtimes \dfrac{gr\ \frac{1}{150}}{X\ mg}$

$1X = \frac{1}{150} \times \frac{60}{1} = \frac{60}{150}$

$150\overline{)60.0} = 0.4\ mg$ (quotient 0.4)

5. $\dfrac{1\ g}{gr\ 15} \diagtimes \dfrac{X\ g}{gr\ 7\frac{1}{2}}$

$15X = 7.5$

$\frac{15X}{15} = \frac{7.5}{15}$

$X = 0.5\ g$

6. $\dfrac{gr\ i}{60\ mg} \diagtimes \dfrac{gr\ X}{15\ mg}$

$60X = 15$

$\frac{60X}{60} = \frac{15}{60}$

$X = gr\ \frac{1}{4}$

9. $\dfrac{℥\ 1}{30\ mL} \diagtimes \dfrac{℥\ 2\frac{1}{2}}{X\ mL}$

$1X = 30 \times 2.5$

$X = 75\ mL$

11. $\dfrac{1\ t}{5\ mL} \diagtimes \dfrac{X\ t}{60\ mL}$

$5X = 60$

$\frac{5X}{5} = \frac{60}{5}$

$X = 12\ t$

16. $\dfrac{1\ kg}{2.2\ lb} \diagtimes \dfrac{3.5\ kg}{X\ lb}$

$1X = 3.5 \times 2.2$

$X = 7.7\ lb$

20. $\dfrac{1\ kg}{2.2\ lb} \diagtimes \dfrac{X\ kg}{99\ lb}$

$2.2X = 99$

$\frac{2.2X}{2.2} = \frac{99}{2.2}$

$2.2\overline{)99.0}$ = 45 kg

88
110
110

24. $\dfrac{gr\ 1}{60\ mg} \diagtimes \dfrac{gr\ 10}{X\ mg}$

$1X = 60 \times 10 = 60.0$

$X = 600\ mg$

28. $\dfrac{℥\ 1}{30\ mL} \diagtimes \dfrac{℥\ X}{60\ mL}$

$30X = 60$

$\frac{30X}{30} = \frac{60}{30} = 2$

$X = ℥\ ii$

31.
8 ounces
6 ounces
4 ounces
8 ounces
10 ounces
4 ounces
8 ounces
6 ounces
6 ounces
5 ounces
12 ounces
+ 4 ounces
81 ounces × 30 mL/oz = 2430 mL

32.

$$\frac{1 \text{ kg}}{2.2 \text{ lb}} \times \frac{X \text{ kg}}{55 \text{ lb}}$$

$$2.2X = 55$$

$$\frac{2.2X}{2.2} = \frac{55}{2.2}$$

$$X = 25 \text{ kg}$$

$$\frac{0.05 \text{ mg}}{1 \text{ kg}} \times \frac{X \text{ mg}}{25 \text{ kg}}$$

$$X = 0.05 \times 25$$

$$X = 1.25 \text{ mg}$$

33.

$$\frac{1 \text{ T}}{15 \text{ mL}} \times \frac{X \text{ T}}{60 \text{ mL}}$$

$$15X = 60$$

$$\frac{15X}{15} = \frac{60}{15}$$

$$X = 4 \text{ T Epsom Salts}$$

1 L (1000 mL) = qt i = 1 quart water

OR

$$\frac{ʒ i}{30 \text{ mL}} \times \frac{ʒ X}{60 \text{ mL}}$$

$$30X = 60$$

$$\frac{30X}{30} = \frac{60}{30}$$

$$X = ʒ 2 = 2 \text{ ounces Epsom Salts}$$
and 1 quart of water

Review Set 14 from pages 52 and 53.

1. 0.0005, 1 L = 1000 mL
2. 45, 1 g = gr 15
3. 38.18, 1 kg = 2.2 lb
4. 1.33, 1 g = gr 15
5. 7.5, gr i = 60 mg
6. iiss, ʒ i = 30 mL
7. iss, pt i = 500 mL
8. 45, ʒ i = 30 mL
9. $\frac{1}{4}$, gr i = 60 mg

10. 0.000625, 1 mg = 1000 mcg
11. $\frac{1}{2}$, 1 t = 5 mL
12. 30, gr i = 60 mg
13. $\frac{1}{8}$, gr i = 60 mg
14. $\frac{1}{100}$, gr i = 60 mg
15. 3, 1 in = 2.5 cm
16. 16,000, 1 g = 1000 mg
17. ss, ʒ i = 30 mL

18. ss, qt i = ʒ 32
19. 2, qt i = 1 L
20. ss, qt i = pt ii
21. ʒ v, ʒ i = 30 mL
22. 1, 1t = 5 mL
23. 8, ʒ viii = 250 mL
24. 22.73, 1 kg = 2.2 lb
25. 15, gr i = 60 mg

Solutions—Review Set 14

3. lb → kg or smaller → larger unit; therefore divide by conversion factor.

84 ÷ 2.2 = 38.18 kg

5. gr → mg or larger → smaller unit; therefore multiply by conversion factor.

$\frac{1}{8} \times 60 = \frac{60}{8} = 7.5$ mg

7. mL → pt or smaller → larger

$750 \div 500 = \text{pt } 1\frac{1}{2} = \text{pt iss}$

14. mg → gr or smaller → larger

$0.6 \div 60 = \frac{0.6}{60} = 0.01 = \text{gr} \frac{1}{100}$

(Remember that correct apothecary notation for amounts less than 1 is written in fractional form with $\frac{1}{2}$ written as ss.)

23. You know 8 ounces = 250 mL. Determine how many 8-ounce (250 mL) glasses of water are in 2000 mL.

mL → glasses or smaller → larger

$2000 \div 250 = \frac{2000}{250} = 8$ of the 8-ounce glasses of water

Review Set 15 from page 55.

1. 12:32 AM	6. 12:15 PM	11. 1330	16. 0345
2. 7:30 AM	7. 2:20 AM	12. 0004	17. 2400
3. 4:40 PM	8. 10:10 AM	13. 2145	18. 1530
4. 9:21 PM	9. 1:15 PM	14. 1200	19. 0620
5. 11:59 PM	10. 6:25 PM	15. 2315	20. 1745

Review Set 16 from page 57.

1. −17.8°	5. 22.2°	9. 176°	13. 39.2°
2. 185°	6. 37.2°	10. 97.5°	14. 34.6°
3. 212°	7. 39.8°	11. 37.8°	15. 39.3°
4. 89.6°	8. 104°	12. 66.2°	

Solutions—Review Set 16

1. $°C = \frac{F°-32}{1.8}$

   $°C = \frac{0-32}{1.8}$

   $°C = \frac{-32}{1.8}$

   $°C = -17.8°$

2. $°F = 1.8°C + 32$

   $°F = (1.8 \times 85) + 32$

   $°F = 153 + 32$

   $°F = 185°$

Review Set 17 from pages 69–71.

1. tuberculin
2. a. Yes
   b. Round 1.25 to 1.3 and measure on the cc scale as 1.3 cc.
3. No
4. 0.5

5. a. False
   b. The size of the drop varies according to the diameter of the hole at the end of the dropper.
6. No
7. Measure the oral liquid in an oral 3 cc syringe.
8. 5
9. Discard the excess prior to injecting the patient.
10. To prevent needlestick injury.

11.

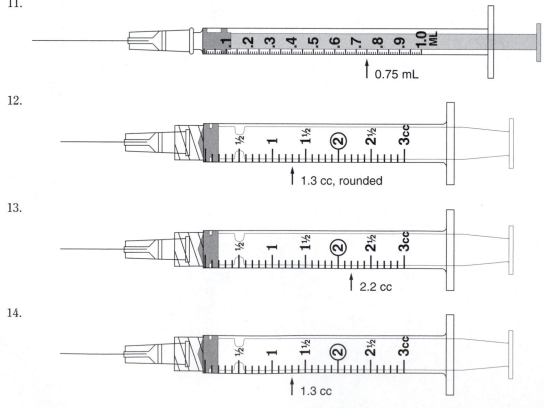

↑ 0.75 mL

12.

↑ 1.3 cc, rounded

13.

↑ 2.2 cc

14.

↑ 1.3 cc

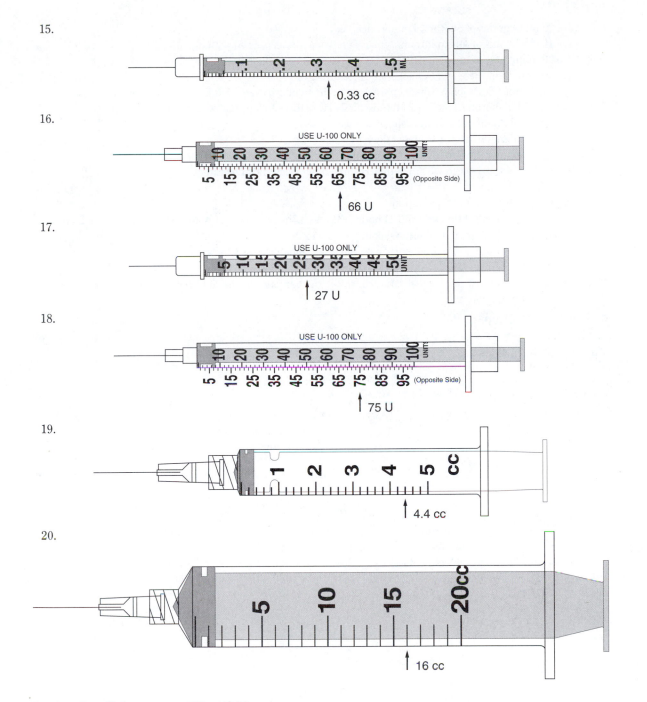

15.

0.33 cc

16.

USE U-100 ONLY

66 U

17.

USE U-100 ONLY

27 U

18.

USE U-100 ONLY

(Opposite Side)

75 U

19.

4.4 cc

20.

16 cc

Review Set 18 from pages 79 and 80.

1. 6 AM, 12 noon, 6 PM, 12 midnight
2. 9 AM
3. 7:30 AM, 11:30 AM, 4:30 PM, 9 PM
4. 9 AM, 5 PM
5. every 4 hours, as needed
6. 9/7/xx at 0900 (9 AM)
7. sublingual, under the tongue
8. once a day
9. 125 mcg
10. nitroglycerin, Darvocet-N 100, meperidine (Demerol), promethazine (Phenergan)
11. subcutaneous injection
12. once (at 9 AM)
13. Keflex
14. before breakfast (at 7:30 AM)
15. milliequivalent
16. Keflex and Slow K
17. Tylenol
18. twice (at 9 AM and 9 PM)
19. 0900 and 2100
20. 2400, 0600, 1200, and 1800
21. In the "One-Time Medication Dosage" section, lower left corner

Review Set 19 from pages 82 and 83.

1. Give 250 milligrams of naproxen orally two times a day.
2. Give 30 units of Humulin N U-100 insulin subcutaneously every day 30 minutes before breakfast.
3. Give 500 milligrams of Ceclor orally immediately and then give 250 milligrams every eight hours.

4. Give 25 micrograms of Synthroid orally once a day
5. Give 10 milligrams of Ativan intramuscularly every 4 hours as necessary for agitation.
6. Give 20 milligrams of furosemide intravenously (slowly) immediately.
7. Give 10 cubic centimeters of Gelusil orally at bedtime.
8. Give 2 drops of 1% atropine sulfate ophthalmic in the right eye every 15 minutes for four applications.
9. Give $\frac{1}{4}$ grain of morphine sulfate intramuscularly every three to four hours as needed for pain.
10. Give 0.25 milligrams of Lanoxin orally once a day.
11. Give 250 milligrams of tetracycline orally four times a day.
12. Give $\frac{1}{400}$ grain of nitroglycerin sublingually immediately.
13. Give 2 drops of Cortisporin Otic in both ears three times a day and at bedtime.
14. 1, 2, 6, 8, 9, 11, 12.
15. Contact the physician for clarification.
16. No; q.i.d. is given only 4 times during 24 hours, whereas q.4h means every 4 hours, which is 6 times in 24 hours.
17. Determined by drug order and hospital policy.
18. Patient, drug, dosage, route, frequency, date and time, signature of doctor/writer.
19. Parts 1–5
20. The right patient must receive the right drug in the right amount by the right route at the right time.

Review Set 20 from page 94.

1. B   2. D   3. C   4. A   5. E   6. F   7. G   8. 1 capsule
9. For IM or IV injection use.

Review Set 21 from pages 109–114.

1. 1 tablet   6. 2 tablets   10. 8 tablets   12. $\frac{1}{2}$ tablet
Note: The dose is correct;
but with such a large number   13. 2 capsules
2. 1 tablet   7. 2 tablets   of tablets, you would think
carefully and double-check   14. 1 tablet
3. $1\frac{1}{2}$ tablets   8. 2 tablets   your calculations.
4. $\frac{1}{2}$ tablet   9. $1\frac{1}{2}$ tablets   15. 2 capsules
5. $\frac{1}{2}$ tablet   11. 3.95 g or 4 g; 1 g; 2 tablets   16. $1\frac{1}{2}$ tablet

17. Select 10-mg tablets and give 1 tablet.   24. Select I and give 2 tablets.
18. Select 20-mg tablets and give $1\frac{1}{2}$ tablets (or give   25. Select C and give 1 tablet.
    1 10-mg and 1 20-mg tablets), 4 doses.   26. Select E and give 2 capsules.
19. Select 15-mg tablets and give 1 tablet.   27. Select D and give 2 capsules.
20. Select 60-mg tablets and give 1, q.4h *as needed*.   28. Select H and give 2 tablets
21. Select B and give 2 capsules.   29. Select A and give 1 capsule.
22. Select K and give 1 tablet.   30. Select C and give 1 tablet each dose.
23. Select F and give 1 tablet.

Solutions—Review Set 21

1. Convert: $\dfrac{1\,g}{1000\,mg} \diagdown\kern-1.2em\diagup \dfrac{0.1\,g}{X\,mg}$

   $X = 0.1 \times 1000 = 0.100. = 100\ mg$

   Order: $0.1\,g \nearrow \quad 100\ mg$

   Supply: 100 mg/tab

   Think: It is obvious you want to give 1 tablet.

   Calculate: $\dfrac{\text{Dosage on hand}}{\text{Amount on hand}} = \dfrac{\text{Dosage desired}}{\text{X Amount desired}}$

   $\dfrac{100\,mg}{1\,tab} \diagdown\kern-1.2em\diagup \dfrac{100\,mg}{X\,tab}$

   $100X = 100$

   $\dfrac{100X}{100} = \dfrac{100}{100}$

   $X = 1\ tab$

5. Order: 0.125 mg

   Supply: $\begin{array}{c}0.250\ mg\\0.25\ mg/tab\end{array}$ (Add 0 to compare 0.25 to 0.125)

   Calculate: $\dfrac{\text{Dosage on hand}}{\text{Amount on hand}} = \dfrac{\text{Dosage desired}}{\text{X Amount desired}}$

   $\dfrac{0.250\,mg}{1\,tab} \diagdown\kern-1.2em\diagup \dfrac{0.125\,mg}{X\,tab}$

   $0.250X = 0.125$

   $\dfrac{0.250X}{0.250} = \dfrac{0.125}{0.250}$

   $X = \dfrac{1}{2}\ tab$

10. Convert: $\dfrac{1\,g}{1000\,mg} \diagdown \dfrac{4\,g}{X\,mg}$

$X = 4 \times 1000 = 4.000. = 4000\,mg$

4000 mg

Order: 4 g

Supply: 500 mg/tab

Calculate: $\dfrac{\text{Dosage on hand}}{\text{Amount on hand}} = \dfrac{\text{Dosage desired}}{\text{X Amount desired}}$

$\dfrac{500\,mg}{1\,tab} \diagdown \dfrac{4000\,mg}{X\,tab}$

$500X = 4000$

$\dfrac{500X}{500} = \dfrac{4000}{500}$

$X = 8\ tabs$

11. Order: 0.06 g/kg/day

Weight: 145 lb

$\dfrac{1\,kg}{2.2\,lb} \diagdown \dfrac{X\,kg}{145\,lb}$

$2.2X = 145$

$\dfrac{2.2X}{2.2} = \dfrac{145}{2.2}$

$X = 65.9\ kg$

Now determine how many grams are needed for a person who weighs 65.9 kg.

$\dfrac{0.06\,g}{1\,kg} \diagdown \dfrac{X\,g}{65.9\,kg}$

$X = 0.06 \times 65.9 = 3.95\ g$ rounded to 4 g/day

Calculate: $\dfrac{\text{Dosage on hand}}{\text{Amount on hand}} = \dfrac{\text{Dosage desired}}{\text{X Amount desired}}$

Order: 4 g/day q.i.d. means 1 g/dose

Supply: 0.5 g/tab

$\dfrac{0.5\,g}{1\,tab} \diagdown \dfrac{1\,g}{X\,tab}$

$0.5X = 1$

$\dfrac{0.5X}{0.5} = \dfrac{1}{0.5}$

$X = 2\ tabs/dose$

14. Convert: $\dfrac{1\,mg}{1000\,mcg} \diagdown \dfrac{0.05\,mg}{X\,mcg}$

$X = 0.05 \times 1000 = 0.050. = 50\,mcg$

50 mcg

Order: 0.05 mg

Supply: 50 mcg/cap

Think: This answer is obvious. You want to give one capsule.

Calculate: $\dfrac{\text{Dosage on hand}}{\text{Amount on hand}} = \dfrac{\text{Dosage desired}}{\text{X Amount desired}}$

$\dfrac{50\,mcg}{1\,cap} \diagdown \dfrac{50\,mcg}{X\,cap}$

$50X = 50$

$\dfrac{50X}{50} = \dfrac{50}{50}$

$X = 1\ cap$

17. Convert: $\dfrac{gr\ 1}{60\,mg} \diagdown \dfrac{gr\ \frac{1}{6}}{X\,mg}$

$X = \dfrac{1}{6} \times 60 = \dfrac{60}{6} = 10\,mg$

10 mg

Order: gr $\frac{1}{6}$

Supply: 10 mg/tab and 2.5 mg/tab

Select: 10 mg and it is obvious you want to give 1 tablet.

Calculate: $\dfrac{\text{Dosage on hand}}{\text{Amount on hand}} = \dfrac{\text{Dosage desired}}{\text{X Amount desired}}$

$\dfrac{10\,mg}{1\,tab} \diagdown \dfrac{10\,mg}{X\,tab}$

$10X = 10$

$\dfrac{10X}{10} = \dfrac{10}{10}$

$X = 1\ tab$

28. Order: 0.5 mg

Convert: $\dfrac{1\,mg}{1000\,mcg} \diagdown \dfrac{X\,mg}{250\,mcg}$

$1000X = 250$

$\dfrac{1000X}{1000} = \dfrac{250}{1000}$

$X = 250 \div 1000 = .250. = 0.25\,mg$

0.25 mg

Supply: 250 mcg

Calculate: $\dfrac{\text{Dosage on hand}}{\text{Amount on hand}} = \dfrac{\text{Dosage desired}}{\text{X Amount desired}}$

$\dfrac{0.25\,mg}{1\,tab} \diagdown \dfrac{0.5\,mg}{X\,tab}$

$0.25X = 0.50$ (Add 0 to compare 0.5 and 0.25)

$\dfrac{0.25X}{0.25} = \dfrac{0.50}{0.25}$

$X = 2\ tab$

30. Weight: 176 lb

$\dfrac{1\,kg}{2.2\,lb} \diagdown \dfrac{X\,kg}{176\,lb}$

$2.2X = 176$

$\dfrac{2.2X}{2.2} = \dfrac{176}{2.2}$

$X = 80\ kg$

q.6h doses: 4 doses/day

Order: 50 mg/kg/day

$\dfrac{1\,kg}{50\,mg} \diagdown \dfrac{80\,kg}{X\,mg}$

$X = 50 \times 80 = 4000\,mg/day$

4000 mg/day, q.6h means

$\dfrac{4000\,mg}{4\,doses}$ or 1000 mg/dose

Supply: 1000 mg/tab

Think: It is obvious you want to give 1 tablet.

Calculate: $\dfrac{\text{Dosage on hand}}{\text{Amount on hand}} = \dfrac{\text{Dosage desired}}{\text{X Amount desired}}$

$\dfrac{1000\,mg}{1\,tab} \diagdown \dfrac{1000\,mg}{X\,tab}$

$1000X = 1000$

$\dfrac{1000X}{1000} = \dfrac{1000}{1000}$

$X = 1\ tab$

Review Set 22 from pages 117–120.

1. 7.5	5. 1	9. C; 2 mL	13. 47 doses
2. 5	6. 20	10. A; 2 mL	14. 5 mL
3. 20	7. 2t	11. 5 mL	15. 4 containers; 0900,
4. 4	8. B; 2.5 mL ($\frac{1}{2}$ t)	12. 30 mL	1300, 1900

Solutions—Review Set 22

2. Convert: $\dfrac{gr\ i}{60\ mg} \diagdown \dfrac{gr\ \frac{1}{6}}{X\ mg}$

$X = \frac{1}{6} \times 60 = 10\ mg$

Order: $gr\ \frac{1}{6} \overset{10\ mg}{\nearrow}$

Supply: 10 mg/5 mL

Calculate: $\dfrac{\text{Dosage on hand}}{\text{Amount on hand}} = \dfrac{\text{Dosage desired}}{\text{X Amount desired}}$

$\dfrac{10\ mg}{5\ mL} \diagdown \dfrac{10\ mg}{X\ mL}$

$10X = 50$

$\dfrac{10X}{10} = \dfrac{50}{10}$

$X = 5\ mL$

4. Order: 100 mg

Supply: 125 mg/5 mL

Calculate: $\dfrac{\text{Dosage on hand}}{\text{Amount on hand}} = \dfrac{\text{Dosage desired}}{\text{X Amount desired}}$

$\dfrac{125\ mg}{5\ mL} \diagdown \dfrac{100\ mg}{X\ mL}$

$125X = 500$

$\dfrac{125X}{125} = \dfrac{500}{125}$

$X = 4\ mL$

6. Order: 25 mg

Convert: 1 t = 5 mL

Supply: 6.25 mg/t $\overset{6.25\ mg/5\ mL}{\searrow}$

Calculate: $\dfrac{\text{Dosage on hand}}{\text{Amount on hand}} = \dfrac{\text{Dosage desired}}{\text{X Amount desired}}$

$\dfrac{6.25\ mg}{5\ mL} \diagdown \dfrac{25\ mg}{X\ mL}$

$6.25X = 125$

$\dfrac{6.25X}{6.25} = \dfrac{125}{6.25}$

$X = 20\ mL$

7. Order: 125 mg

Supply: 62.5 mg/5 mL

Calculate: $\dfrac{\text{Dosage on hand}}{\text{Amount on hand}} = \dfrac{\text{Dosage desired}}{\text{X Amount desired}}$

$\dfrac{62.5\ mg}{5\ mL} \diagdown \dfrac{125\ mg}{X\ mL}$

$62.5X = 625$

$\dfrac{62.5X}{62.5} = \dfrac{625}{62.5}$

$X = 10\ mL$

Convert: $\dfrac{1\ t}{5\ mL} \diagdown \dfrac{X\ t}{10\ mL}$

$5X = 10$

$\dfrac{5X}{5} = \dfrac{10}{5}$

$X = 2\ t$

Give 10 mL or 2 t.

Review Set 23 from pages 139–143.

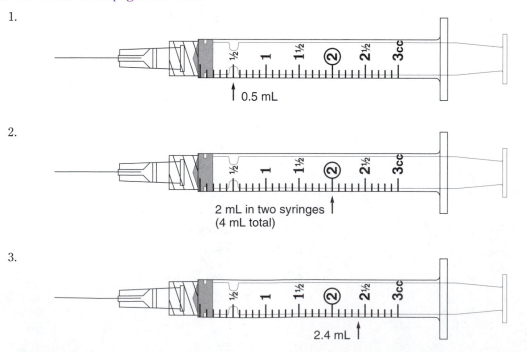

1.

↑ 0.5 mL

2.

2 mL in two syringes ↑
(4 mL total)

3.

2.4 mL ↑

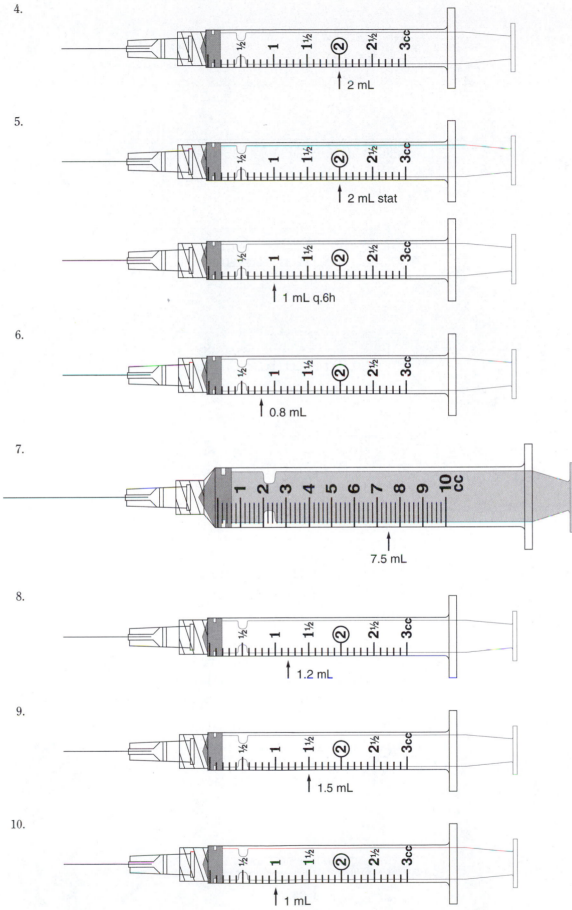

4.

½ 1 1½ ② 2½ 3cc
↑ 2 mL

5.

½ 1 1½ ② 2½ 3cc
↑ 2 mL stat

½ 1 1½ ② 2½ 3cc
↑ 1 mL q.6h

6.

½ 1 1½ ② 2½ 3cc
↑ 0.8 mL

7.

1 2 3 4 5 6 7 8 9 10 cc
↑ 7.5 mL

8.

½ 1 1½ ② 2½ 3cc
↑ 1.2 mL

9.

½ 1 1½ ② 2½ 3cc
↑ 1.5 mL

10.

½ 1 1½ ② 2½ 3cc
↑ 1 mL

11.

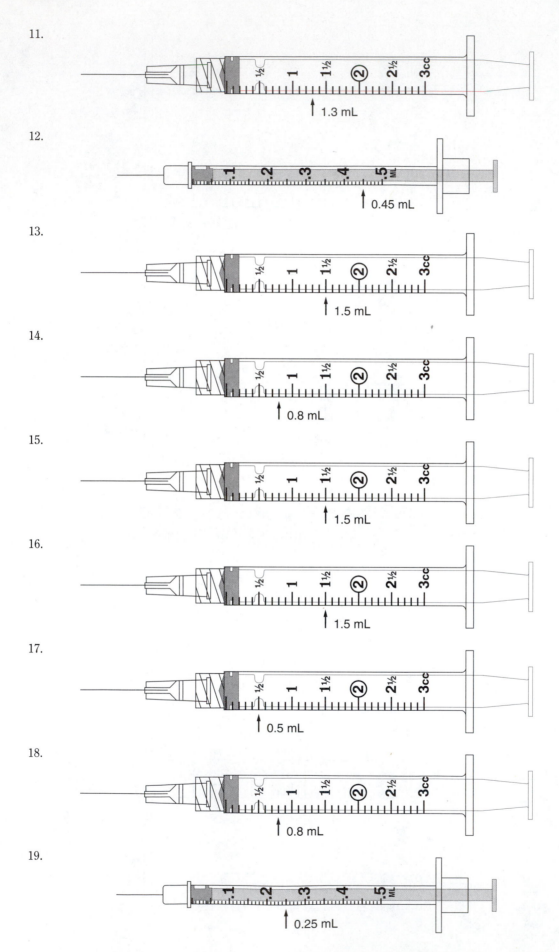

1.3 mL

12.

0.45 mL

13.

1.5 mL

14.

0.8 mL

15.

1.5 mL

16.

1.5 mL

17.

0.5 mL

18.

0.8 mL

19.

0.25 mL

20.

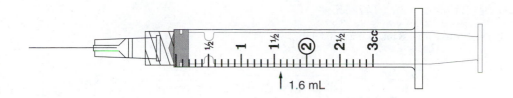

$\uparrow$ 1.6 mL

Solutions—Review Set 23

1. Convert:

$$\frac{gr\ 1}{60\ mg} \times \frac{gr\ \frac{1}{4}}{X\ mg}$$

$$X = 60 \times \frac{1}{4} = 15\ mg$$

Order: gr $\frac{1}{4}$ → 15 mg

Supply: 30 mg/mL

Calculate: $\dfrac{\text{Dosage on hand}}{\text{Amount on hand}} = \dfrac{\text{Dosage desired}}{\text{X Amount desired}}$

$$\frac{30\ mg}{1\ mL} \times \frac{15\ mg}{X\ mL}$$

$$30X = 15$$

$$\frac{30X}{30} = \frac{15}{30}$$

$$X = \frac{1}{2} = 0.5\ mL$$

3. Order: 600 mcg

Supply: 500 mcg/2 mL

Calculate: $\dfrac{\text{Dosage on hand}}{\text{Amount on hand}} = \dfrac{\text{Dosage desired}}{\text{X Amount desired}}$

$$\frac{500\ mcg}{2\ mL} \times \frac{600\ mcg}{X\ mL}$$

$$500X = 1200$$

$$\frac{500X}{500} = \frac{1200}{500}$$

$$X = 2.4\ mL$$

6. Order: 8,000 U

Supply: 10,000 U/mL

Calculate: $\dfrac{\text{Dosage on hand}}{\text{Amount on hand}} = \dfrac{\text{Dosage desired}}{\text{X Amount desired}}$

$$\frac{10,000\ U}{1\ mL} \times \frac{8000\ U}{X\ mL}$$

$$10,000X = 8000$$

$$\frac{10,000X}{10,000} = \frac{8000}{10,000}$$

$$X = 0.8\ mL$$

8. Order: 60 mg

Supply: 75 mg/1.5 mL

Calculate: $\dfrac{\text{Dosage on hand}}{\text{Amount on hand}} = \dfrac{\text{Dosage desired}}{\text{X Amount desired}}$

$$\frac{75\ mg}{1.5\ mL} \times \frac{60\ mg}{X\ mL}$$

$$75X = 90$$

$$\frac{75X}{75} = \frac{90}{75}$$

$$X = 1.2\ mL$$

9. Convert:

$$\frac{gr\ 1}{60\ mg} \times \frac{gr\ \frac{1}{100}}{X\ mg}$$

$$X = 60 \times \frac{1}{100} = \frac{60}{100} = .60. = 0.6\ mg$$

Order: gr $\frac{1}{100}$ → 0.6 mg

Supply: 0.4 mg/mL

Calculate: $\dfrac{\text{Dosage on hand}}{\text{Amount on hand}} = \dfrac{\text{Dosage desired}}{\text{X Amount desired}}$

$$\frac{0.4\ mg}{1\ mL} \times \frac{0.6\ mg}{X\ mL}$$

$$0.4X = 0.6$$

$$\frac{0.4X}{0.4} = \frac{0.6}{0.4}$$

$$X = 1.5\ mL$$

11. Order: 400,000 U

Supply: 300,000 U/mL

Calculate: $\dfrac{\text{Dosage on hand}}{\text{Amount on hand}} = \dfrac{\text{Dosage desired}}{\text{X Amount desired}}$

$$\frac{300,000\ U}{1\ mL} \times \frac{400,000\ U}{X\ mL}$$

$$300,000X = 400,000$$

$$\frac{300,000X}{300,000} = \frac{400,000}{300,000}$$

$$X = 1.33 = 1.3\ mL$$

19. Order: 12.5 mg

Supply: 50 mg/mL

Calculate: $\dfrac{\text{Dosage on hand}}{\text{Amount on hand}} = \dfrac{\text{Dosage desired}}{\text{X Amount desired}}$

$$\frac{50\ mg}{1\ mL} \times \frac{12.5\ mg}{X\ mL}$$

$$50X = 12.5$$

$$\frac{50X}{50} = \frac{12.5}{50}$$

$$X = 0.25\ mL$$

Review Set 24 from pages 147–152.

1. Reconstitute with 1.5 mL and give 0.89 mL.

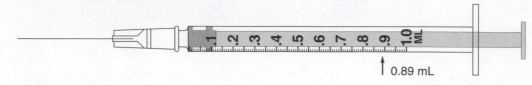

0.89 mL

2. Reconstitute with 5 mL and give 1.5 mL.

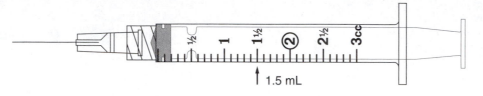

1.5 mL

3. Reconstitute with 2 mL and give 0.5 mL.

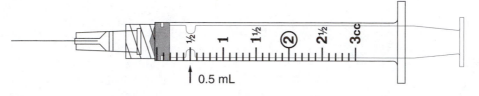

0.5 mL

4. Reconstitute with 50 mL and give 12.5 mL.

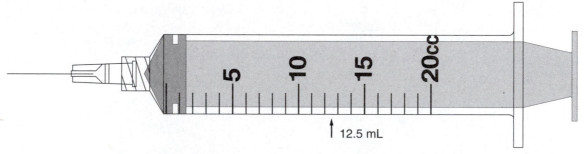

12.5 mL

5. Reconstitute with 50 mL and give 15 mL.

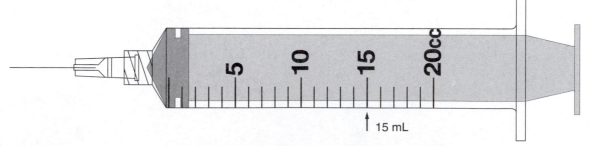

15 mL

6. Reconstitute with 3.5 mL diluent and give 2 mL.

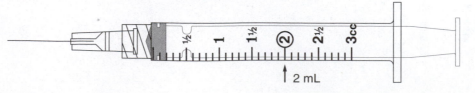

2 mL

7. Reconstitute with 8 mL diluent and give 2.8 mL.

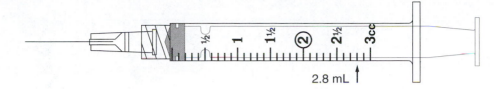

2.8 mL

8. Reconstitute with 4 mL diluent and give 0.5 mL.

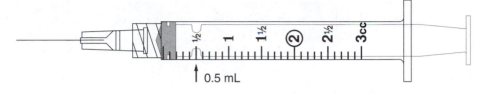

0.5 mL

9. Reconstitute with 1.6 mL diluent and give 1 mL.

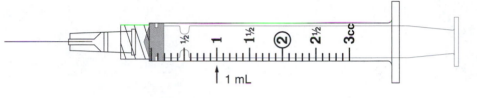

1 mL

10. Reconstitute with 1 mL diluent and give 1.2 mL.

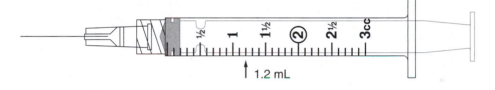

1.2 mL

11. Reconstitute with 1.6 mL diluent and give 0.8 mL.

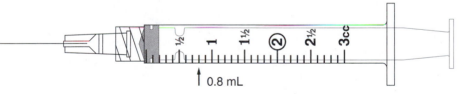

0.8 mL

12. Reconstitute with 2.5 mL diluent and give 1.5 mL.

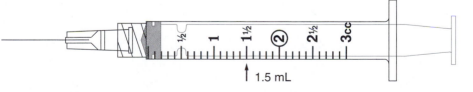

1.5 mL

13. Reconstitute with 6.6 mL diluent and give 2 mL.

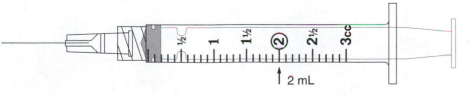

2 mL

14. Reconstitute with 10 mL diluent and give 0.5 mL.

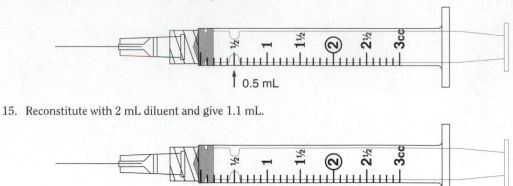

↑ 0.5 mL

15. Reconstitute with 2 mL diluent and give 1.1 mL.

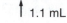

↑ 1.1 mL

Solutions—Review Set 24

1. Order : 250 mg

   Supply : 280 mg/mL

   Calculate : $\dfrac{\text{Dosage on hand}}{\text{Amount on hand}} = \dfrac{\text{Dosage desired}}{\text{X Amount desired}}$

   $\dfrac{280 \text{ mg}}{1 \text{ mL}} \diagdown\!\!\!\!\diagup \dfrac{250 \text{ mg}}{\text{X mL}}$

   $280X = 250$

   $\dfrac{280X}{280} = \dfrac{250}{280}$

   $X = 0.89 \text{ mL}$

2. Select 5 mL diluent to be added in order to give patient smallest dosage you can measure exactly in a 3-cc syringe. If you select 4 mL, then 1 g = 2.5 mL and you would need to give 1.25 mL for 500 mg dose; a 3-cc syringe does not have 1.25 mL calibration. Therefore, select 5 mL diluent and 1 g = 3 mL; give 1.5 mL:

   Order: 500 mg

   Convert: 1 g = 1000 mg

   Supply: 1000 mg/3 mL ⤸
   1 g/3 mL ⤶

   Calculate : $\dfrac{\text{Dosage on hand}}{\text{Amount on hand}} = \dfrac{\text{Dosage desired}}{\text{X Amount desired}}$

   $\dfrac{1000 \text{ mg}}{3 \text{ mL}} \diagdown\!\!\!\!\diagup \dfrac{500 \text{ mg}}{\text{X mL}}$

   $1000X = 1500$

   $\dfrac{1000X}{1000} = \dfrac{1500}{1000}$

   $X = 1.5 \text{ mL}$

8. Order: 200 mg

   Convert: 1 g = 1000 mg

   Supply: ⤹1000 mg/2.5 mL
   ⤷1 g/2.5 mL

   Calculate: $\dfrac{\text{Dosage on hand}}{\text{Amount on hand}} = \dfrac{\text{Dosage desired}}{\text{X Amount desired}}$

   $\dfrac{1000 \text{ mg}}{2.5 \text{ mL}} \diagdown\!\!\!\!\diagup \dfrac{200 \text{ mg}}{\text{X mL}}$

   $1000X = 500$

   $\dfrac{1000X}{1000} = \dfrac{500}{1000}$

   $X = 0.5 \text{ mL}$

15. Order : 250 mg

    Supply : 225 mg/1 mL

    Calculate : $\dfrac{\text{Dosage on hand}}{\text{Amount on hand}} = \dfrac{\text{Dosage desired}}{\text{X Amount desired}}$

    $\dfrac{225 \text{ mg}}{1 \text{ mL}} \diagdown\!\!\!\!\diagup \dfrac{250 \text{ mg}}{\text{X mL}}$

    $225X = 250$

    $\dfrac{225X}{225} = \dfrac{250}{225}$

    $X = 1.1 \text{ mL}$

Review Set 25 from pages 157–159.

1. In a U-100 insulin syringe
2. Lo-Dose U-100 insulin syringe
3. 0.2 mL
4. 0.6 mL

5. 0.25 mL
6. insulin
7. False
8. 68 U

9. 15 U
10. 23 U
11. 57 U

12.

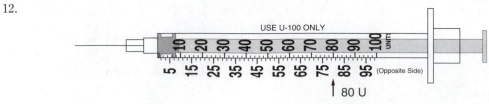

↑ 80 U

13.

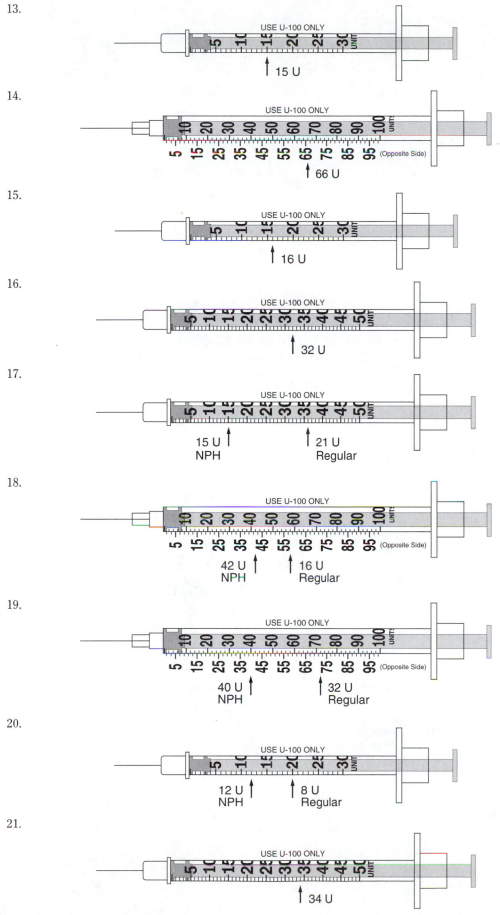

14.

15.

16.

17.

18.

19.

20.

21.

22.

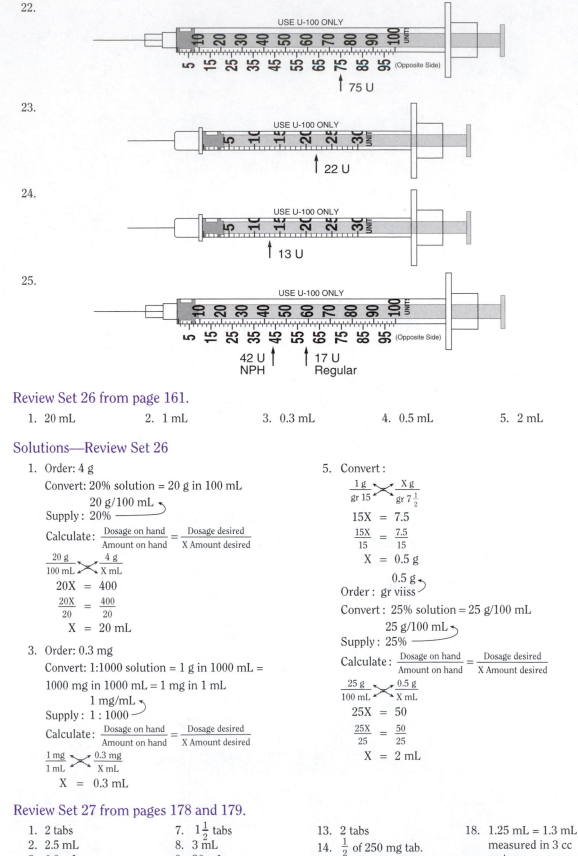

↑ 75 U

23.

↑ 22 U

24.

↑ 13 U

25.

42 U ↑   ↑ 17 U
NPH   Regular

Review Set 26 from page 161.

1. 20 mL   2. 1 mL   3. 0.3 mL   4. 0.5 mL   5. 2 mL

Solutions—Review Set 26

1. Order: 4 g
    Convert: 20% solution = 20 g in 100 mL
    $\qquad\qquad$ 20 g/100 mL
    Supply: 20%
    Calculate: $\dfrac{\text{Dosage on hand}}{\text{Amount on hand}} = \dfrac{\text{Dosage desired}}{\text{X Amount desired}}$

    $\dfrac{20\ g}{100\ mL} \times \dfrac{4\ g}{X\ mL}$

    $20X = 400$

    $\dfrac{20X}{20} = \dfrac{400}{20}$

    $X = 20\ mL$

3. Order: 0.3 mg
    Convert: 1:1000 solution = 1 g in 1000 mL =
    1000 mg in 1000 mL = 1 mg in 1 mL
    $\qquad\qquad$ 1 mg/mL
    Supply: 1 : 1000
    Calculate: $\dfrac{\text{Dosage on hand}}{\text{Amount on hand}} = \dfrac{\text{Dosage desired}}{\text{X Amount desired}}$

    $\dfrac{1\ mg}{1\ mL} \times \dfrac{0.3\ mg}{X\ mL}$

    $X = 0.3\ mL$

5. Convert:

    $\dfrac{1\ g}{gr\ 15} \times \dfrac{X\ g}{gr\ 7\frac{1}{2}}$

    $15X = 7.5$

    $\dfrac{15X}{15} = \dfrac{7.5}{15}$

    $X = 0.5\ g$

    $\qquad\qquad$ 0.5 g
    Order: gr viiss
    Convert: 25% solution = 25 g/100 mL
    $\qquad\qquad$ 25 g/100 mL
    Supply: 25%
    Calculate: $\dfrac{\text{Dosage on hand}}{\text{Amount on hand}} = \dfrac{\text{Dosage desired}}{\text{X Amount desired}}$

    $\dfrac{25\ g}{100\ mL} \times \dfrac{0.5\ g}{X\ mL}$

    $25X = 50$

    $\dfrac{25X}{25} = \dfrac{50}{25}$

    $X = 2\ mL$

Review Set 27 from pages 178 and 179.

1. 2 tabs
2. 2.5 mL
3. 0.8 mL
4. 0.7 mL
5. 7.5 mL
6. 0.6 mL

7. $1\frac{1}{2}$ tabs
8. 3 mL
9. 30 mL
10. 1.6 mL
11. 3 mL
12. 0.5 mL

13. 2 tabs
14. $\frac{1}{2}$ of 250 mg tab.
15. 2.4 mL
16. 2 tabs
17. 8 mL

18. 1.25 mL = 1.3 mL
    measured in 3 cc
    syringe.
19. 16 mL
20. 7 mL

Solutions—Review Set 27

2.
$$\frac{D}{H} \times Q = X$$
$$\frac{\overset{1}{\cancel{150}\text{ mg}}}{\underset{2}{\cancel{300}\text{ mg}}} \times 5\text{ mL} = X$$
$$\frac{5}{2}\text{ mL} = X$$
$$X = 2.5\text{ mL}$$

5.
$$\frac{D}{H} \times Q = X$$
$$\frac{\overset{3}{\cancel{12}\text{ mEq}}}{\underset{2}{\cancel{8}\text{ mEq}}} \times 5\text{ mL} = X$$
$$\frac{15}{2}\text{ mL} = X$$
$$X = 7.5\text{ mL}$$

6.
$$\frac{D}{H} \times Q = X$$
$$\frac{2.4\text{ mg}}{4\text{ mg}} \times 1\text{ mL} = X$$
$$X = 0.6\text{ mL}$$

9.
$$\frac{D}{H} \times Q = X$$
$$\frac{\overset{2}{\cancel{160}\text{ mg}}}{\underset{1}{\cancel{80}\text{ mg}}} \times 15\text{ mL} = X$$
$$\frac{30}{1}\text{ mL} = X$$
$$X = 30\text{ mL}$$

13. 1) Convert: gr to mg. Equivalent: gr i = 60 mg
gr → mg = larger → smaller: multiply
60 is the conversion factor
$$\text{gr ss} = \text{gr } \frac{1}{2}$$
$$\frac{1}{2} \times 60\text{ mg} = 30\text{ mg}$$

2)
$$\frac{D}{H} \times Q = X$$
$$\frac{\overset{2}{\cancel{30}\text{ mg}}}{\underset{1}{\cancel{15}\text{ mg}}} \times 1\text{ tab} = X$$
$$\frac{2}{1}\text{ tab} = X$$
$$X = 2\text{ tablets}$$

16. 1) Convert: mg to mcg. Equivalent: 1 mg = 1000 mcg
mg → mcg = larger to smaller: multiply
1000 is the conversion factor
$$0.15 \times 1000 = 0.150. = 150\text{ mcg}$$

2)
$$\frac{D}{H} \times Q = X$$
$$\frac{\overset{2}{\cancel{150}\text{ mcg}}}{\underset{1}{\cancel{75}\text{ mcg}}} \times 1\text{ tablet} = X$$
$$X = \frac{2}{1}\text{ tab}$$
$$X = 2\text{ tablets}$$

19.
$$\frac{D}{H} \times Q = X$$
$$\frac{8\text{ mg}}{2.5\text{ mg}} \times 5\text{ mL} = X$$
$$\frac{40}{2.5}\text{ mL} = X$$
$$X = 16\text{ mL}$$

Review Set 28 from pages 191 and 192.

1. 156 mg
2. 12.5 mL
3. 25 mg
4. 0.25 mL
5. 375 mg
6. 1.5 mL
7. 2 mL
8. 8 mg
9. 0.2 mL
10. 125 mg; 2.5 mL
11. 20 to 40 mg / kg / day
12. 3 (q.8h = 3 doses in 24 hours)
13. Yes. Correct single dose dosage range = 45.33 mg to 90.66 mg.
14. 1.5 mL
15. No. There are only 10 single doses of 1.5 mL each available in the 15 mL bottle. Three bottles would be needed.
16. 15 kg/mg/day or 60 mg/day
17. Yes
18. 0.8 mL
19. 800 mg/day
20. 1600 mg/day
21. 200–400 mg/dose
22. Yes, the dosage is safe.
23. 90–180 mg/day
24. Yes, the dosage is safe.

Solutions—Review Set 28

1. 1) Calculate: Child's weight in kg.
Equivalent: 1 kg = 2.2 lb
$$\frac{1\text{ kg}}{2.2\text{ lb}} \times \frac{X\text{ kg}}{55\text{ lb}}$$
$$2.2X = 55$$
$$\frac{2.2X}{2.2} = \frac{55}{2.2}$$
$$X = 25\text{ kg}$$

2) Calculate: The equivalent desired dosage based on the recommended dosage of 25 mg/kg/day, divided into 4 q.6h doses.
$$\frac{25\text{ mg}}{1\text{ kg}} \times \frac{X\text{ mg}}{25\text{ kg}}$$
$$X = 25 \times 25 = 625\text{ mg}$$

3) Calculate: One dose.
$$\frac{625}{4} = 156.25 = 156\text{ mg}$$

2.
$$\frac{62.5\text{ mg}}{5\text{ mL}} \times \frac{156\text{ mg}}{X\text{ mL}}$$
$$62.5X = 780$$
$$\frac{62.5X}{62.5} = \frac{780}{62.5}$$
$$X = 12.48 = 12.5\text{ mL}$$

16. 1) Calculate: Child's weight in kg.
$$\frac{1\text{ kg}}{2.2\text{ lb}} \times \frac{X\text{ kg}}{9\text{ lb}}$$
$$2.2X = 9$$
$$\frac{2.2X}{2.2} = \frac{9}{2.2}$$
$$X = 4.09 = 4\text{ kg}$$

2) Calculate: Daily dosage for 4 kg child.
$$\frac{15\text{ mg}}{1\text{ kg}} \times \frac{X\text{ mg}}{4\text{ kg}}$$
$$X = 60\text{ mg/day}$$

17. 60 mg/day divided into two doses =

$\frac{60}{2} = 30$ mg/dose. Yes, the 30 mg order is safe.

18.
$$\frac{75 \text{ mg}}{2 \text{ mL}} \times \frac{30 \text{ mg}}{\text{X mL}}$$
$$75X = 60$$
$$\frac{75X}{75} = \frac{60}{75}$$
$$X = 0.8 \text{ mL}$$

Or, $\frac{D}{H} \times Q = X$

$$\frac{30 \text{ mg}}{75 \text{ mg}} \times 2 \text{ mL} = 0.8 \text{ mL}$$

19.
$$\frac{100 \text{ mg}}{1 \text{ kg}} \times \frac{\text{X mg}}{8 \text{ kg}}$$
$$X = 800 \text{ mg/day}$$

20.
$$\frac{200 \text{ mg}}{1 \text{ kg}} \times \frac{\text{X mg}}{8 \text{ kg}}$$
$$X = 1600 \text{ mg/day}$$

21.
$$\frac{800 \text{ mg}}{4} = 200 \text{ mg minimum}$$
$$\frac{1600 \text{ mg}}{4} = 400 \text{ mg maximum}$$

23.
$$\frac{6 \text{ mg}}{1 \text{ kg}} \times \frac{\text{X mg}}{15 \text{ kg}}$$
$$X = 90 \text{ mg minimum}$$
$$\frac{12 \text{ mg}}{1 \text{ kg}} \times \frac{\text{X mg}}{15 \text{ kg}}$$
$$X = 180 \text{ mg maximum}$$

24.
$$\frac{16 \text{ mg}}{1 \text{ mL}} \times \frac{90 \text{ mg}}{\text{X mL}}$$
$$16X = 90$$
$$\frac{16X}{16} = \frac{90}{16}$$
$$X = 5.6 \text{ mL minimum dosage; therefore,}$$
the dosage ordered is safe.

Review Set 29 from page 195.

1. 0.56 m^2
2. 330 mg
3. 40 mg
4. 1 m^2
5. 250 mg
6. 2.5 mL
7. 1.2 mL
8. 235 mg

Solutions—Review Set 29

2. $\frac{\text{Child BSA}}{1.7 \text{m}^2} \times \text{Adult dose} =$

$$\frac{0.56 \text{m}^2}{1.7 \text{m}^2} \times 1000 \text{ mg} = 330 \text{ mg}$$

3. BSA = 0.27 m^2

$$\frac{0.27 \text{m}^2}{1.7 \text{m}^2} \times 250 \text{ mg} = 39.7 = 40 \text{ mg}$$

6. 30 inches, 25 pounds = 0.5 m^2 BSA
250 mg × 0.5 m^2 = 125 mg

$$\frac{50 \text{ mg}}{1 \text{ mL}} \times \frac{125 \text{ mg}}{\text{X mL}}$$
$$50X = 125$$
$$\frac{50X}{50} = \frac{125}{50}$$
$$X = \frac{\overset{5}{\cancel{125}}}{\underset{2}{\cancel{50}}}$$
$$X = 2.5 \text{ mL}$$

Or, $\frac{D}{H} \times Q = \frac{125 \text{ mg}}{50 \text{ mg}} \times 1 \text{ mL} = 2.5 \text{ mL}$

7. 45 inches, 55 pounds = 0.9 m^2 BSA
3.3 mg × 0.9 m^2 = 2.97 mg (round to 3 mg)

$$\frac{5 \text{ mg}}{2 \text{ mL}} \times \frac{3 \text{ mg}}{\text{X mL}}$$
$$5X = 6$$
$$\frac{5X}{5} = \frac{6}{5}$$
$$X = \frac{6}{5}$$
$$X = 1.2 \text{ mL}$$

Or, $\frac{D}{H} \times Q = \frac{3 \text{ mg}}{5 \text{ mg}} \times 2 \text{ mL} = \frac{6}{5} = 1.2 \text{ mL}$

Review Set 30 from pages 205–207.

1. normal saline; C
2. dextrose 5%, water; E
3. dextrose 5%, normal saline (0.9% sodium chloride); G
4. dextrose 5%, 0.45% sodium chloride; D
5. dextrose 5%, 0.225% sodium chloride; A
6. dextrose 5%, Ringer's Lactate; H
7. dextrose 5%, 0.45% sodium chloride, potassium chloride 20 mEq per liter; B
8. dextrose 5%, normal saline (0.9% sodium chloride), potassium chloride 20 mEq per liter; F

Review Set 31 from page 209.

1. 50 g dextrose; 9 g NaCl
2. 25 g dextrose; 2.25 g NaCl
3. 25 g dextrose
4. 6.75 g NaCl

Solutions—Review Set 31

2. $\dfrac{5\,g}{100\,mL} \diagdown\!\!\!\!\diagup \dfrac{X\,g}{500\,mL}$

$100X = 2500$

$\dfrac{100X}{100} = \dfrac{2500}{100}$

$X = 25\,g\ dextrose$

$\dfrac{0.45\,g}{100\,mL} \diagdown\!\!\!\!\diagup \dfrac{X\,g}{500\,mL}$

$100X = 225$

$\dfrac{100X}{100} = \dfrac{225}{100}$

$X = 2.25\,g\ NaCl$

4. $\dfrac{0.9\,g}{100\,mL} \diagdown\!\!\!\!\diagup \dfrac{X\,g}{750\,mL}$

$100X = 675$

$\dfrac{100X}{100} = \dfrac{675}{100}$

$X = 6.75\,g\ NaCl$

Review Set 32 from page 215.

1. 100 mL/h   2. 120 mL/h   3. 83 mL/h   4. 200 mL/h   5. 120 mL/h   6. 125 mL/h

Solutions—Review Set 32

1. $1\,L = 1000\,mL$

$\dfrac{mL}{h} = \dfrac{1000\,mL}{10\,h} = 100\ mL/h$

2. $\dfrac{mL}{h} = \dfrac{1800\,mL}{15\,h} = 120\ mL/h$

3. $\dfrac{mL}{h} = \dfrac{2000\,mL}{24\,h} = 83.33 = 83\ mL/h$

4. $\dfrac{100\,mL}{30\,min} \diagdown\!\!\!\!\diagup \dfrac{X\,mL}{60\,min}$

$30X = 6000$

$\dfrac{30X}{30} = \dfrac{6000}{30}$

$X = 200\ mL/60\ min\ or\ 200\ mL/h$

5. $\dfrac{30\,mL}{15\,min} \diagdown\!\!\!\!\diagup \dfrac{X\,mL}{60\,min}$

$15X = 1800$

$\dfrac{15X}{15} = \dfrac{1800}{15}$

$X = 120\ mL/60\ min\ or\ 120\ mL/h$

6. $2.5\,L = 2500\,mL$

$\dfrac{mL}{h} = \dfrac{2500\,mL}{20\,h} = 125\ mL/h$

Review Set 33 from page 216.

1. 15 gtt/mL   2. 20 gtt/mL   3. 60 gtt/mL   4. 60 gtt/mL   5. 10 gtt/mL

Review Set 34 from page 218.

1. $\dfrac{V}{T} \times C = R$ 3. 50 gtt/min   5. 25 gtt/min   6. 83 gtt/min   7. 34 gtt/min

2. 21 gtt/min   4. 50 gtt/min

Solutions—Review Set 34

1. $\dfrac{Total\ Volume}{Total\ Time\ in\ Min} \times Drop\ Factor\ Calibration = Rate$

   Total *volume* divided by *total time* in minutes, multiplied by the *drop factor calibration* in drops per milliliter, equals the flow *rate* in drops per minute.

2. $24\,h = 24 \times 60 = 1440\,min$

   $\dfrac{V}{T} \times C = R$

   $\dfrac{3000\,mL}{1440\,min} \times 10\ gtt/mL = 20.8 = 21\,gtt/min$

3. $5\,h = 5 \times 60 = 300\,min$

   $\dfrac{250\,mL}{300\,min} \times 60\ gtt/mL = 50\,gtt/min$

4. $\dfrac{100\,mL}{40\,min} \times 20\ gtt/mL = 50\,gtt/min$

5. $1hr = 60\,min$

   $\dfrac{25\,mL}{60\,min} \times 60\ gtt/mL = 25\,gtt/min$

6. $4\,h = 4 \times 60 = 240\,min$
   Two 500 mL units of blood = 1000 mL total volume

   $\dfrac{1000\,mL}{240\,min} \times 20\ gtt/mL = 83.3 = 83\,gtt/min$

7. $12\,hr = 12 \times 60 = 720\,min$

   $\dfrac{1240\,mL}{720\,min} \times 20\ gtt/mL = 34.4 = 34\,gtt/min$

Review Set 35 from page 220.

1. 60   3. 3   5. 6   7. 63 gtt/min   9. 28 gtt/min
2. 1   4. 4   6. $\dfrac{mL/h}{\text{Drop factor constant}}$ 8. 42 gtt/min   10. 60 gtt/min

Solutions—Review Set 35

2. $\dfrac{60}{60} = 1$

3. $\dfrac{60}{20} = 3$

4. $\dfrac{60}{15} = 4$

5. $\dfrac{60}{10} = 6$

6. mL per hour divided by drop factor constant = gtt/min

7. $mL/h = \dfrac{1000\ mL}{4\ h} = 250\ mL/h$

   $\dfrac{mL/h}{\text{Drop factor constant}} = \dfrac{250}{4} = 62.5 = 63\ gtt/min$

8. $mL/h = \dfrac{750\ mL}{6\ h} = 125\ mL/h$

   $\dfrac{mL/h}{\text{Drop factor constant}} = \dfrac{125}{3} = 41.66 = 42\ gtt/min$

9. $mL/h = \dfrac{500\ mL}{3\ h} = 167\ mL/h$

   $\dfrac{167\ mL}{6\ h} = 27.83 = 28\ gtt/min$

10. $\dfrac{60}{1} = 60\ gtt/min$

Review Set 36 from pages 221 and 222.

1. 31 gtt/min   3. 33 gtt/min   5. 31 gtt/min   7. 35 gtt/min   9. 25 gtt/min   11. 83 mL/h
2. 100 gtt/min   4. 42 gtt/min   6. 125 mL/h   8. 28 gtt/min   10. 125 mL/h   12. 125 mL/h

Solutions—Review Set 36

1. $\dfrac{V}{T} \times C = R$

   $\dfrac{3000\ mL}{1440\ min} \times 15\ gtt/mL = 31.25 = 31\ gtt/min$

2. $\dfrac{V}{T} \times C = R$

   $\dfrac{200\ mL}{120\ min} \times 60\ gtt/mL = 100\ gtt/min$

3. $\dfrac{V}{T} \times C = R$

   $\dfrac{800\ mL}{480\ min} \times 20\ gtt/mL = 33.33 = 33\ gtt/min$

4. $\dfrac{V}{T} \times C = R$

   $\dfrac{1000\ mL}{1440\ min} \times 60\ gtt/mL = 41.66 = 42\ gtt/min$

5. $\dfrac{V}{T} \times C = R$

   $\dfrac{1500\ mL}{720\ min} \times 15\ gtt/mL = 31.25 = 31\ gtt/min$

6. $\dfrac{V}{T} \times C = R$

   $\dfrac{250\ mL}{120\ min} \times 60\ gtt/mL = 125\ mL/h$

7. $mL/h = \dfrac{2500\ mL}{24\ h} = 104.16 = 104\ mL/h$

   $\dfrac{mL/h}{\text{Drop factor constant}} =$

   $\dfrac{104}{3} = 34.66 = 35\ gtt/min$

8. $mL/h = \dfrac{500\ mL}{3\ h} = 166.67 = 167\ mL/h$

   $\dfrac{mL/h}{\text{Drop factor constant}} =$

   $\dfrac{167}{6} = 27.77 = 28\ gtt/min$

9. $mL/h = \dfrac{1200\ mL}{8\ h} = 150\ mL/h$

   $\dfrac{mL/h}{\text{Drop factor constant}} =$

   $\dfrac{150}{6} = 25\ gtt/min$

10. $mL/h = \dfrac{1000\ mL}{8\ h} = 125\ mL/h$

11. $mL/h = \dfrac{2000\ mL}{24\ h} = 83.33 = 83\ mL/h$

12. $mL/h = \dfrac{500\ mL}{4\ h} = 125\ mL/h$

Review Set 37 from pages 223 and 224.

1. 42 gtt/min; reset to 47 gtt/min after you assess patient and determine condition is stable.
2. 42 gtt/min; reset to 45 gtt/min after you assess patient and determine condition is stable.
3. 42 gtt/min. Ask my supervisor or the physician for a revised order, since the new rate would be 67 gtt/min (an increase of 60%).
4. 28 gtt/min; reset to 31 gtt/min after you assess patient and determine condition is stable.
5. 25 gtt/min. Ask my supervisor or the physician for a revised order, since the new rate would be 36 gtt/min (an increase of 44%).

Solutions—Review Set 37

1. $\frac{V}{T} \times C = R$

    $\frac{1500 \text{ mL}}{720 \text{ min}} \times 20 \text{ gtt/mL} = 41.66 = 42 \text{ gtt/min}$

    After the sixth hour, 6 hours remaining.

    $\frac{850 \text{ mL}}{360 \text{ min}} \times 20 \text{ gtt/mL} = 47.22 = 47 \text{ gtt/min}$

    Reset to 47 gtt/min ($\frac{47-42}{42} = 12\%$ faster than original rate).

2. $\frac{V}{T} \times C = R$

    $\frac{1000 \text{ mL}}{360 \text{ min}} \times 15 \text{ gtt/mL} = 41.66 = 42 \text{ gtt/min}$

    After 4 hours, 2 hours remain.

    $\frac{360 \text{ mL}}{120 \text{ min}} \times 15 \text{ gtt/mL} = 45 \text{ gtt/min}$

    Reset to 45 gtt/min ($\frac{45-42}{42} = 7\%$ faster than original rate).

3. $\frac{V}{T} \times C = R$

    $\frac{1000 \text{ mL}}{480 \text{ min}} \times 20 \text{ gtt/mL} = 41.66 = 42 \text{ gtt/min}$

    After 4 hours, 4 hours remain.

    $\frac{800 \text{ mL}}{240 \text{ min}} \times 20 \text{ gtt/mL} = 66.66 = 67 \text{ gtt/min}$

    ($\frac{67-42}{42} = 60\%$ faster)

    Call supervisor or physician for a revised order.

4. $\frac{V}{T} \times C = R$

    $\frac{2000 \text{ mL}}{720 \text{ min}} \times 10 \text{ gtt/mL} = 27.77 = 28 \text{ gtt/min}$

    After 8 hours, 4 hours remain.

    $\frac{750 \text{ mL}}{240 \text{ min}} \times 10 \text{ gtt/mL} = 31.25 = 31 \text{ gtt/min}$

    ($\frac{31-28}{28} = 11\%$ faster)

    Reset to 31 gtt/min

5. $\frac{V}{T} \times C = R$

    $\frac{100 \text{ mL}}{240 \text{ min}} \times 60 \text{ gtt/mL} = 25 \text{ gtt/min}$

    After 90 min, 150 min remain.

    $\frac{90 \text{ mL}}{150 \text{ min}} \times 60 \text{ gtt/mL} = 36 \text{ gtt/min}$

    ($\frac{36-25}{25} = 44\%$ faster)

    Call supervisor or physician for a revised order.

Review Set 38 from page 225.

1. 133 gtt/min
2. 133 mL/h
3. 50 gtt/min
4. 200 mL/h
5. 100 gtt/min

Solutions—Review Set 38

1. $\frac{V}{T} \times C = R$

    $\frac{100}{45} \times 60 = 133.33 = 133 \text{ gtt/min}$

2. mL/h

    $\frac{100 \text{ mL}}{45 \text{ min}} \times \frac{X}{60 \text{ min}}$

    $45X = 6000$

    $X = 133.33 = 133 \text{ mL/h}$

3. $\frac{V}{T} \times C = R$

    $\frac{50}{15} \times 15 = 50 \text{ gtt/min}$

4. mL/h

    $\frac{50 \text{ mL}}{15 \text{ min}} \times \frac{X}{60 \text{ min}}$

    $15X = 3000$

    $\frac{15X}{15} = \frac{3000}{15}$

    $X = 200 \text{ mL/h}$

5. $\frac{V}{T} \times C = R$

    $\frac{50}{30} \times 60 = 100 \text{ gtt/min}$

Review Set 39 from pages 235 and 236.

1. 5 h and 33 min or about $5\frac{1}{2}$ h
2. $6\frac{2}{3}$ h or 6 h and 40 min
3. 8 h
4. 6 h; 20 gtt/min
5. 4 h; 20 gtt/min
6. 11 hours later or 0300 approximately, the next day
7. 21 gtt/min; 16 hours later or 0730
8. 1008 mL
9. 1152 mL
10. 3024 mL

Solutions—Review Set 39

1. $\frac{V}{T} \times C = R$

$\frac{500 \text{ mL}}{T \text{ min}} \times 20 \text{ gtt/mL} = 30 \text{ gtt/min}$

$\frac{500}{T} \times \frac{20}{1} = 30$

$\frac{10000}{T} \diagdown \frac{30}{1}$

$30T = 10000$

$\frac{30T}{30} = \frac{10000}{30}$

$T = 333 \text{ min}$

Convert: min → h

$\frac{60 \text{ min}}{1 \text{ h}} \diagdown \frac{333 \text{ min}}{X \text{ h}}$

$60X = 333$

$X = 5.55 \text{ h} = 5 \text{ h and } 33 \text{ min or about } 5\frac{1}{2} \text{ h}$

2. $\frac{V}{T} \times C = R$

$\frac{1000 \text{ mL}}{T \text{ min}} \times \frac{10 \text{ gtt/mL}}{1} = 25 \text{ gtt/min}$

$\frac{10000}{T} \diagdown \frac{25}{1}$

$25 T = 10000$

$\frac{25 T}{25} = \frac{10000}{25}$

$T = 400 \text{ min}$

Convert: min → h

$\frac{60 \text{ min}}{1 \text{ h}} \diagdown \frac{400 \text{ min}}{X \text{ h}}$

$60X = 400$

$\frac{60 X}{60} = \frac{400}{60}$

$X = 6.67 = 6\frac{2}{3} \text{ h or } 6 \text{ h} + 40 \text{ min}$

3. $\frac{V}{T} \times C = R$

$\frac{800 \text{ mL}}{T \text{ min}} \times 15 \text{ gtt/mL} = 25$

$\frac{12000}{T} \diagdown \frac{25}{1}$

$25 T = 12000$

$\frac{25 T}{25} = \frac{12000}{25}$

$T = 480 \text{ min}$

Convert: min → h

$\frac{60 \text{ min}}{1 \text{ h}} \diagdown \frac{480 \text{ min}}{X \text{ h}}$

$60X = 480$

$\frac{60 X}{60} = \frac{480}{60}$

$X = 8 \text{ h}$

4. Time: 120 mL @ 20 mL/h

$\frac{120 \text{ mL}}{20 \text{ mL/h}} = 6 \text{ h}$

Rate: $\frac{V}{T} \times C = R$

$\frac{120 \text{ mL}}{\cancel{360} \text{ min}} \times \overset{1}{\cancel{60}} \text{ gtt/mL} = 20 \text{ gtt/min}$

5. $\frac{80 \text{ mL}}{20 \text{ mL/h}} = 4 \text{ h}$

$\frac{80}{\underset{4}{\cancel{240}}} \times \overset{1}{\cancel{60}} = 20 \text{ gtt/min}$

6. $\frac{V}{T} \times C = R$

$\frac{1200 \text{ mL}}{T \text{ min}} \times 15 \text{ gtt/mL} = 27 \text{ gtt/min}$

$\frac{18000}{T} \diagdown \frac{27}{1}$

$27T = 18000$

$\frac{27T}{27} = \frac{18000}{27}$

$T = 667 \text{ min}$

$T = \frac{667}{60} = 11.1$

$= 11 \text{ h}$

$1600 + 1100 (11 \text{ h}) = 2700;$

$2700 - 2400 = 0300 \text{ next day}$

7. Time: 2000 mL @125 mL/h $= \frac{2000 \text{ mL}}{125 \text{ mL/h}} = 16 \text{ h}$

$1530 + 1600 = 3130; 3130 - 2400 = 0730 \text{ next day}$

Rate: $\frac{2000 \text{ mL}}{960 \text{ min}} \times 10 \text{ gtt/mL} = 20.83 = 21 \text{ gtt/min}$

8. $\frac{V}{T} \times C = R$

$\frac{V \text{ mL}}{1440 \text{ min}} \times 60 \text{ gtt/mL} = 42 \text{ gtt/min}$

$\frac{60 V}{1440} \diagdown \frac{42}{1}$

$60 V = 60480$

$\frac{60V}{60} = \frac{60480}{60}$

$V = 1008 \text{ mL}$

9. $\frac{V}{T} \times C = R$

$\frac{V \text{ mL}}{1440 \text{ min}} \times 15 \text{ gtt/mL} = 12 \text{ gtt/min}$

$\frac{15 V}{1440} \diagdown \frac{12}{1}$

$15 V = 17280$

$\frac{15V}{15} = \frac{17280}{15}$

$V = 1152 \text{ mL}$

10. $\frac{V}{T} \times C = R$

$\frac{V \text{ mL}}{1440 \text{ min}} \times 10 \text{ gtt/mL} = 21 \text{ gtt/min}$

$\frac{10 V}{1440} \diagdown \frac{21}{1}$

$10 V = 30240$

$\frac{10V}{10} = \frac{30240}{10}$

$V = 3024 \text{ mL}$

Review Set 40 from pages 238 and 239.

1. 87 gtt/min; 48 mL
2. 75 gtt/min; 57 mL
3. 120 gtt/min; 22 mL
4. 23 mL
5. 8 mL

Solutions—Review Set 40

1. Total volume = 50 + 15 = 65 mL

   $\frac{V}{T} \times C = \frac{65 \text{ mL}}{45 \text{ min}} \times 60 \text{ gtt/mL} = 86.66 = 87 \text{ gtt/min}$

   Volume IV fluid to add to chamber = 50 − 2 = 48 mL

2. Total volume = 60 + 15 = 75 mL

   $\frac{V}{T} \times C = \frac{75 \text{ mL}}{60 \text{ min}} \times 60 \text{ gtt/mL} = 75 \text{ gtt/min}$

   Volume IV fluid to add to chamber = 60 − 3 = 57 mL

3. Total volume = 25 + 15 = 40 mL

   $\frac{V}{T} \times C = \frac{40 \text{ mL}}{20 \text{ min}} \times 60 \text{ gtt/mL} = 120 \text{ gtt/min}$

   Volume IV fluid to add to chamber = 25 − 3 = 22 mL

4. $\frac{50 \text{ mL}}{60 \text{ min}} \times \frac{X \text{ mL}}{30 \text{ min}}$

   $60X = 1500$

   $\frac{60X}{60} = \frac{1500}{60}$

   X = 25 mL total dilution volume

Calculate: Amount of drug to administer

$\frac{125 \text{ mg}}{1 \text{ mL}} \times \frac{250 \text{ mg}}{X \text{ mL}}$

$125X = 250$

$\frac{125X}{125} = \frac{250}{125}$

$X = 2 \text{ mL}$

Add 23 mL 0.9% NaCl and 2 mL Ancef

5. $\frac{30 \text{ mL}}{60 \text{ min}} \times \frac{X \text{ mL}}{20 \text{ min}}$

   $60X = 600$

   $\frac{60X}{60} = \frac{600}{60}$

   X = 10 mL total dilution volume

   Add 8 mL D$_5$W and 2 mL Medication X.

Review Set 41 from pages 240 and 241.

1. 5 mEq
2. 2.5 mL
3. 0.3 mEq/h
4. 250 mg
5. 10 mL
6. 20 mg/h
7. 20 mg/h
8. Yes

Solutions—Review Set 41

1. $\frac{20 \text{ mEq}}{1000 \text{ mL}} \times \frac{X \text{ mEq}}{250 \text{ mL}}$

   $1000X = 5000$

   $\frac{1000X}{1000} = \frac{5000}{1000}$

   $X = 5 \text{ mEq per 250 mL}$

2. $\frac{2 \text{ mEq}}{1 \text{ mL}} \times \frac{5 \text{ mEq}}{X \text{ mL}}$

   $2X = 5$

   $\frac{2X}{2} = \frac{5}{2}$

   $X = 2.5 \text{ mL}$

3. The total volume is now 252.5 mL (250 mL D$_5$W + 2.5 mL KCl).

   $\frac{5 \text{ mEq}}{252.5 \text{ mL}} \times \frac{X \text{ mEq}}{15 \text{ mL}}$

   $252.5 X = 75$

   $\frac{252.5X}{252.5} = \frac{75}{252.5}$

   $X = 0.297 \text{ mEq} = 0.3 \text{ mEq}$

   The child receives 0.3 mEq per hour.

4. $\frac{1000 \text{ mg}}{1000 \text{ mL}} \times \frac{X \text{ mg}}{250 \text{ mL}}$

   $1000X = 250000$

   $\frac{1000X}{1000} = \frac{250,000}{1000}$

   $X = 250 \text{ mg}$

5. $\frac{500 \text{ mg}}{20 \text{ mL}} \times \frac{250 \text{ mg}}{X \text{ mL}}$

   $500X = 5000$

   $\frac{500X}{500} = \frac{5000}{500}$

   $X = 10 \text{ mL}$

6. The total volume is now 260 mL (250 mL D$_5$NS + 10 mL aminophylline).

   $\frac{250 \text{ mg}}{260 \text{ mL}} \times \frac{X \text{ mg}}{20 \text{ mL}}$

   $260X = 5000$

   $X = 19 \text{ mg}$

   The child receives 19 mg per hour.

7. $1 \text{ kg} = 2.2 \text{ lb}$

   $\frac{44}{2.2} = 20 \text{ kg}$

   $1 \text{ mg/kg/h} = 20 \text{ mg/h}$

8. Yes, the dosage is exactly right.

Review Set 42 from page 243.

1. 4 mL   2. 6.3 mL   3. 67 mL/h   4. 48 mL/h

Solutions—Review Set 42

1. $\dfrac{100\ mg}{1\ mL} \diagdown \diagup \dfrac{400\ mg}{X\ mL}$

$100X = 400$

$\dfrac{100X}{100} = \dfrac{400}{100}$

$X = 4\ mL$

2. $\dfrac{4\ mg}{1\ mL} \diagdown \diagup \dfrac{25\ mg}{X\ mL}$

$4X = 25$

$\dfrac{4X}{4} = \dfrac{25}{4}$

$X = 6.25\ mL = 6.3\ mL$

3. For the first 10 kg at 100 mL/kg/day

$\dfrac{100\ mL}{1\ kg} \diagdown \diagup \dfrac{X\ mL}{10\ kg}$

$X = 10 \times 100 = 10.00. = 1000\ mL$ for first 10 kg

For the next 10 kg at 50 mL/kg/day

$\dfrac{50\ mL}{1\ kg} \diagdown \diagup \dfrac{X\ mL}{10\ kg}$

$X = 50 \times 10 = 50.0. = 500\ mL$ for next 10 kg

25 kg – 20 kg = 5 kg remaining. For the remaining 5 kg at 20 mL/kg/day

$\dfrac{20\ mL}{1\ kg} \diagdown \diagup \dfrac{X\ mL}{5\ kg}$

$X = 20 \times 5 = 100\ mL$ for each kg above 20 kg

$\begin{array}{r} 1000 \\ 500 \\ +\ 100 \\ \hline 1600\ mL/24h \end{array}$

$\dfrac{1600\ mL}{24\ h} = 66.6 = 67\ mL/h$ for the 25 kg patient

4. For the first 10 kg at 100 mL/kg/day

$\dfrac{100\ mL}{1\ kg} \diagdown \diagup \dfrac{X\ mL}{10\ kg}$

$X = 100 \times 10 = 100.0. = 1000\ mL$

For the remaining 3 kg at 50 mL/kg/day

$\dfrac{50\ mL}{1\ kg} \diagdown \diagup \dfrac{X\ mL}{3\ kg}$

$X = 50 \times 3 = 150\ mL$

$\begin{array}{r} 1000 \\ +\ 150 \\ \hline 1150\ \ mL/24\ h \end{array}$

$\dfrac{1150\ mL}{24\ h} = 47.9 = 48\ mL/h$

Review Set 43 from pages 246 and 247.

1. 40 mL/h, Yes
2. 14 mL/h, Yes
3. 10 mL/h, No

4. Yes, setting is accurately set for order. No, hourly dosage is not safe. Contact the physician to review the order.

5. No
6. Yes
7. No
8. Yes

9. No
10. No
11. 10 mL/h
12. 50 mL/h

Solutions—Review Set 43

1. $\dfrac{25,000\ U}{1000\ mL} \diagdown \diagup \dfrac{1000\ U}{X\ mL}$

$25,000X = 1,000,000$

$\dfrac{25,000X}{25,000} = \dfrac{1,000,000}{25,000}$

$X = 40\ mL/h$

$\dfrac{1000\ U}{1\ h} \diagdown \diagup \dfrac{X\ U}{24\ h}$

$X = 1000 \times 24 = 24.000. = 24,000\ U/24\ h$

Normal adult dosage = 20,000 – 40,000 U/day.

2. $\dfrac{40,000\ U}{500\ mL} \diagdown \diagup \dfrac{1100\ U}{X\ mL}$

$40,000X = 550,000$

$\dfrac{40,000X}{40,000} = \dfrac{550,000}{40,000}$

$X = 14\ mL/h$

$\dfrac{1100\ U}{1\ h} \diagdown \diagup \dfrac{X\ U}{24\ h}$

$X = 1100 \times 24 = 26,400\ U/24\ h$

3. $\dfrac{25,000\ U}{500\ mL} \diagdown \diagup \dfrac{500\ U}{X\ mL}$

$25,000X = 250,000$

$\dfrac{25,000X}{25,000} = \dfrac{250,000}{25,000}$

$X = 10\ mL/h$

$\dfrac{500\ U}{1\ h} \diagdown \diagup \dfrac{X\ U}{24\ h}$

$X = 500 \times 24 = 12,000\ U/24\ h$

4. $\dfrac{40,000\ U}{500\ mL} \diagdown \diagup \dfrac{2500\ U}{X\ mL}$

$40,000X = 1,250,000$

$\dfrac{40,000X}{40,000} = \dfrac{1,250,000}{40,000}$

$X = 31\ mL/h$

$\dfrac{2500\ U}{1\ h} \diagdown \diagup \dfrac{X\ U}{24\ h}$

$X = 2500 \times 24 = 60,000\ U/24\ h$

5.

$$\dfrac{25{,}000\ U}{1000\ mL} \bowtie \dfrac{X\ U}{120\ mL}$$

$$1000X = 3{,}000{,}000\ U$$

$$\dfrac{1000X}{1000} = \dfrac{3{,}000{,}000}{1000}$$

$$X = 3000\ U/h$$

$$\dfrac{3000\ U}{1\ h} \bowtie \dfrac{X\ U}{24\ h}$$

$$X = 3000 \times 24 = 72{,}000\ U/24\ h$$

6.

$$\dfrac{30{,}000\ U}{500\ mL} \bowtie \dfrac{X\ U}{25\ mL}$$

$$500X = 750{,}000$$

$$\dfrac{500X}{500} = \dfrac{750{,}000}{500}$$

$$X = 1500\ U/h$$

$$\dfrac{1500\ U}{1\ h} \bowtie \dfrac{X\ U}{24\ h}$$

$$X = 1500 \times 24 = 36{,}000\ U/24\ h$$

7.

$$\dfrac{40{,}000\ U}{1000\ mL} \bowtie \dfrac{X\ U}{80\ mL}$$

$$1000X = 3{,}200{,}000$$

$$\dfrac{1000X}{1000} = \dfrac{3{,}200{,}000}{1000}$$

$$X = 3200\ U/h$$

$$\dfrac{3200\ U}{1\ h} \bowtie \dfrac{X\ U}{24\ h}$$

$$X = 3200 \times 24 = 76{,}800\ U/24\ h$$

8.

$$\dfrac{20{,}000\ U}{1000\ mL} \bowtie \dfrac{X\ U}{60\ mL}$$

$$1000X = 1{,}200{,}000\ U$$

$$\dfrac{1000X}{1000} = \dfrac{1{,}200{,}000}{1000}$$

$$X = 1200\ U/h$$

$$\dfrac{1200\ U}{1\ h} \bowtie \dfrac{X\ U}{24\ h}$$

$$X = 1200 \times 24 = 28{,}800\ U/24\ h$$

9.

$$\dfrac{30{,}000\ U}{500\ mL} \bowtie \dfrac{X\ U}{96\ mL/h}$$

$$500X = 2{,}880{,}000\ U$$

$$\dfrac{500X}{500} = \dfrac{2{,}880{,}000}{500}$$

$$X = 5760\ U/h$$

$$\dfrac{5760\ U}{1\ h} \bowtie \dfrac{X\ U}{24\ h}$$

$$X = 5760 \times 24 = 138{,}240\ U/24\ h$$

10.

$$\dfrac{10{,}000\ U}{1000\ mL} \bowtie \dfrac{X\ U}{80\ mL}$$

$$1000X = 800{,}000$$

$$\dfrac{1000X}{1000} = \dfrac{800{,}000}{1000}$$

$$X = 800\ mL/h$$

$$\dfrac{800\ mL}{1\ h} \bowtie \dfrac{X\ mL}{24\ h}$$

$$X = 800 \times 24 = 19{,}200\ U/24\ h$$

11.

$$\dfrac{500\ U}{500\ mL} \bowtie \dfrac{10\ U}{X\ mL}$$

$$500X = 5000$$

$$\dfrac{500X}{500} = \dfrac{5000}{500}$$

$$X = 10\ mL/h$$

12.

$$\dfrac{40\ mEq}{1000\ mL} \bowtie \dfrac{2\ mEq}{X\ mL}$$

$$40X = 2000\ mEq$$

$$\dfrac{40X}{40} = \dfrac{2000}{40}$$

$$X = 50\ mL/h$$

Review Set 44 from page 252.

1. 120 mL/h
2. 60 mL/h
3. 75 mL/h
4. 24 mL/h
5. 40 mL/h
6. 142.5 – 570 mcg/min
7. 0.14 – 0.57 mg/min
8. Yes
9. 4 mg/min
10. Yes
11. 100 mL/h; 25 mL/h
12. 1 mL/h

Solutions—Review Set 44

1. 1) Convert: $g \to mg$

$$\dfrac{1\ g}{1000\ mg} \bowtie \dfrac{2\ g}{X\ mg}$$

$$X = 2 \times 1000 = 2.000. = 2000\ mg$$

2) Calculate: mL/min

$$\dfrac{2000\ mg}{1000\ mL} \bowtie \dfrac{4\ mg}{X\ mL}$$

$$2000X = 4000$$

$$\dfrac{2000X}{2000} = \dfrac{4000}{2000}$$

$$X = 2\ mL$$

2 mL of IV fluid delivers 4 mg of medication.
4 mg/min are delivered by 2 mL/min.

3) Calculate: mL/h

$$\dfrac{2\ mL}{1\ min} \bowtie \dfrac{X\ mL}{60\ min}$$

$$X = 120\ mL/60\ min \text{ or } 120\ mL/h$$

2. 1) Convert: $g \to mg$

$$\dfrac{1\ g}{1000\ mg} \bowtie \dfrac{0.5\ g}{X\ mg}$$

$$X = 0.5 \times 1000 = 0.500. = 500\ mg$$

2) Calculate: mL/min

$$\dfrac{500\ mg}{250\ mL} \bowtie \dfrac{2\ mg}{X\ mL}$$

$$500X = 500$$

$$\dfrac{500X}{500} = \dfrac{500}{500}$$

$$X = 1\ mL$$

1 mL of IV fluid contains 2 mg of medication.
4 mg/min are delivered by 1 mL/min.

3) Calculate: mL/h

$$\dfrac{1\ mL}{1\ min} \bowtie \dfrac{X\ mL}{60\ min}$$

$$X = 60\ mL/60\ min \text{ or } 60\ mL/h$$

3. 1) Convert: mg → mcg

$$\frac{1\ mg}{1000\ mcg} \diagdown \frac{2\ mg}{X\ mcg}$$

$$X = 2 \times 1000 = 2.000. = 2000\ mcg$$

2) Calculate: mL/min

$$\frac{2000\ mcg}{500\ mL} \diagdown \frac{5\ mcg}{X\ mL}$$

$$2000X = 2500$$

$$\frac{2000X}{2000} = \frac{2500}{2000}$$

$$X = 1.25\ mL$$

1.25 mL of IV fluid contains 5 mcg of medication.
5 mcg/min are delivered by 1.25 mL/min.

3) Calculate: mL/h

$$\frac{1.25\ mL}{1\ min} \diagdown \frac{X\ mL}{60\ min}$$

$$X = 75\ mL/60\ min\ or\ 75\ mL/h$$

4. 1) Convert: lb → mg

$$\frac{1\ kg}{2.2\ lb} \diagdown \frac{X\ kg}{198\ lb}$$

$$2.2X = 198$$

$$\frac{2.2X}{2.2} = \frac{198}{2.2}$$

$$X = 90\ kg$$

2) Convert: mg → mcg

$$\frac{1\ mg}{1000\ mcg} \diagdown \frac{450\ mg}{X\ mcg}$$

$$X = 450 \times 1000 = 450.000.$$

$$= 450,000\ mcg$$

3) Calculate: mcg/min

$$\frac{4\ mcg}{1\ kg} \diagdown \frac{X\ mcg}{90\ kg}$$

$$X = 360\ mcg\ per\ 90\ kg\ patient$$

4 mcg/kg/min = 360 mcg/min for this patient.

4) Calculate: mL/min

$$\frac{450,000\ mcg}{500\ mL} \diagdown \frac{360\ mcg}{X\ mL}$$

$$450,000X = 180,000$$

$$\frac{450,000X}{450,000} = \frac{180,000}{450,000}$$

$$X = 0.4\ mL$$

0.4 mL contains 360 mcg. 0.4 mL must be administered per min to provide the 360 mcg/min; therefore, 0.4 mL/min.

5) Calculate: mL/h

$$\frac{0.4\ mL}{1\ min} \diagdown \frac{X\ mL}{60\ min}$$

$$X = 24\ mL/h$$

5. 1) Convert: mg → mcg

$$\frac{1\ mg}{1000\ mcg} \diagdown \frac{800\ mg}{X\ mcg}$$

$$X = 800 \times 1000 = 800.000.$$

$$= 800,000\ mcg$$

2) Calculate: mcg/min

$$\frac{15\ mcg}{1\ kg} \diagdown \frac{X\ mcg}{70\ kg}$$

$$X = 1050\ mcg\ per\ 70\ kg\ patient;$$
to be administered per min;
1050 mcg/min

3) Calculate: mL/min

$$\frac{800,000\ mcg}{500\ mL} \diagdown \frac{1050\ mcg}{X\ mL}$$

$$800,000X = 525,000$$

$$\frac{800,000X}{800,000} = \frac{525,000}{800,000}$$

$$X = 0.656 = 0.66\ mL$$

0.66 mL contains 1050 mcg; 0.66 mL/min delivers 1050 mcg/min

4) Calculate: mL/h

$$\frac{0.66\ mL}{1\ min} \diagdown \frac{X\ mL}{60\ min}$$

$$X = 39.6 = 40\ mL/60\ min\ or\ 40\ mL/h$$

6. 1) Convert: lb → kg

$$\frac{1\ kg}{2.2\ lb} \diagdown \frac{X\ kg}{125\ lb}$$

$$2.2X = 125$$

$$\frac{2.2X}{2.2} = \frac{125}{2.2}$$

$$X = 56.8 = 57\ kg$$

2) Calculate: Minimum mcg/min

$$\frac{2.5\ mcg}{1\ kg} \diagdown \frac{X\ mcg}{57\ kg}$$

$$X = 142.5\ mcg\ per\ 57\ kg;$$
to be administered per min;
142.5 mcg/min

3) Calculate: Maximum mcg/min

$$\frac{10\ mcg}{1\ kg} \diagdown \frac{X\ mcg}{57\ kg}$$

$$X = 570\ mcg\ per\ 57\ kg;$$
to be administered per min;
570 mcg/min

7. 1) Calculate: Minimum mg/min

$$\frac{1\ mg}{1000\ mcg} \diagdown \frac{X\ mg}{142.5\ mcg}$$

$$1000X = 142.5$$

$$\frac{1000X}{1000} = \frac{142.5}{1000}$$

$$X = \frac{142.5}{1000} = .142.5 = 0.14\ mg/min$$

2) Calculate: Maximum mg/min

$$\frac{1\ mg}{1000\ mcg} \diagdown \frac{X\ mg}{570\ mcg}$$

$$1000X = 570$$

$$\frac{1000X}{1000} = \frac{570}{1000}$$

$$X = \frac{570}{1000} = .570. = 0.57\ mg/min$$

8. 1) Calculate: mg/h

$$\frac{500 \text{ mg}}{500 \text{ mL}} \diagup\hspace{-0.9em}\diagdown \frac{X \text{ mg}}{15 \text{ mL}}$$

$$500X = 7500$$

$$\frac{500X}{500} = \frac{7500}{500}$$

$$X = 15 \text{ mg, which when dispersed at}$$
15 mL per hour, is 15 mg/h
or 15 mg/60 min

2) Calculate: mg/min

$$\frac{15 \text{ mg}}{60 \text{ min}} \diagup\hspace{-0.9em}\diagdown \frac{X \text{ mg}}{1 \text{ min}}$$

$$60X = 15$$

$$\frac{60X}{60} = \frac{15}{60}$$

$$X = 0.25 \text{ mg/min} = 250 \text{ mcg/min}$$

Yes, the order is within the safe range (142.5–570 mcg/min) for this patient.

9. 1) Convert: g → mg

$$\frac{1 \text{ g}}{1000 \text{ mg}} \diagup\hspace{-0.9em}\diagdown \frac{2 \text{ g}}{X \text{ mg}}$$

$$X = 2 \times 1000 = 2.000. = 2000 \text{ mg}$$

2) Calculate: mg/h

$$\frac{2000 \text{ mg}}{500 \text{ mL}} \diagup\hspace{-0.9em}\diagdown \frac{X \text{ mg}}{60 \text{ mL}}$$

$$500X = 120,000$$

$$\frac{500X}{500} = \frac{120,000}{500}$$

$$X = 240 \text{ mg}$$

At 60 mL/h 240 mg are administered per hour or 240 mg/60 min

3) Calculate: mg/min

$$\frac{240 \text{ mg}}{60 \text{ min}} \diagup\hspace{-0.9em}\diagdown \frac{X \text{ mg}}{1 \text{ min}}$$

$$60X = 240$$

$$\frac{60X}{60} = \frac{240}{60}$$

$$X = 4 \text{ mg/min}$$

10. Yes, 4 mg/min is within the normal range of 2–6 mg/min.

11. 1) Calculate: g/mL for bolus

$$\frac{20 \text{ g}}{500 \text{ mL}} \diagup\hspace{-0.9em}\diagdown \frac{2 \text{ g}}{X \text{ mL}}$$

$$20X = 1000$$

$$\frac{20X}{20} = \frac{1000}{20}$$

$$X = 50 \text{ mL delivers the 2 g of medication.}$$
2 g/30 min are 50 mL/30 min.

2) Calculate: mL/h for bolus

$$\frac{50 \text{ mL}}{30 \text{ min}} \diagup\hspace{-0.9em}\diagdown \frac{X \text{ mL}}{60 \text{ min}}$$

$$30X = 3000$$

$$\frac{30X}{30} = \frac{3000}{30}$$

$$X = 100 \text{ mL/60 min or 100 mL/h}$$

3) Calculate: g/mL for continuous infusion

$$\frac{20 \text{ g}}{500 \text{ mL}} \diagup\hspace{-0.9em}\diagdown \frac{1 \text{ g}}{X \text{ mL}}$$

$$20X = 500$$

$$\frac{20X}{20} = \frac{500}{20}$$

$$X = 25 \text{ mL}$$

1 g of medication is in 25 mL. 1 g/h is delivered by 25 mL/h.

12. 1) Convert: U → mU

$$\frac{1 \text{ U}}{1000 \text{ mU}} \diagup\hspace{-0.9em}\diagdown \frac{15 \text{ U}}{X \text{ mU}}$$

$$X = 15 \times 1000 = 15.000. = 15,000 \text{ mU}$$

2) Calculate: mL/min

$$\frac{15,000 \text{ mU}}{250 \text{ mL}} \diagup\hspace{-0.9em}\diagdown \frac{1 \text{ mU}}{X \text{ mL}}$$

$$15,000X = 250$$

$$\frac{15,000X}{15,000} = \frac{250}{15,000}$$

$$X = 0.017 \text{ mL}$$

1 mU is in 0.017 mL. Infuse 1 mU/min and 0.017 mL/min is delivered.

3) Calculate: mL/h

$$\frac{0.017 \text{ mL}}{1 \text{ min}} \diagup\hspace{-0.9em}\diagdown \frac{X \text{ mL}}{60 \text{ min}}$$

$$X = 1.02 = 1 \text{ mL/60 min or 1 mL/h}$$

Review Set 45 from pages 254 and 255.

1. IV PB @ 33 gtt/min; IV @ 19 gtt/min
2. IV PB @ 40 gtt/min; IV @ 42 gtt/min
3. IV PB @ 25 gtt/min; IV @ 32 gtt/min
4. IV PB @ 50 gtt/min; IV @ 90 gtt/min
5. IV PB @ 50 gtt/min; IV @ 40 gtt/min
6. IV PB @ 100 mL/h; IV @ 100 mL/h
7. IV PB @ 200 mL/h; IV @ 76 mL/h
8. IV PB @ 200 mL/h; IV @ 122 mL/h

Solutions—Review Set 45

1. Step 1.   IV PB rate: $\frac{V}{T} \times C = R$

$$\frac{100 \text{ mL}}{30 \text{ min}} \times 10 \text{ gtt/mL} = 33 \text{ gtt/min}$$

Step 2.   IV PB time: q.4h × 30 min =
$$6 \times 30 = 180 \text{ min} = 3 \text{ h}$$

Step 3.   IV PB volume: 6 × 100 = 600 mL

Step 4.   Regular IV volume: 3000 − 600 = 2400 mL

Step 5.   Regular IV time: 24 − 3 = 21 h

Step 6.   Regular IV rate: $\dfrac{\text{mL/h}}{\text{drop factor constant}}$

$$\frac{2400 \text{ mL}}{21 \text{ h}} = 114 \text{ mL/h}$$

$$\frac{114}{6} = 19 \text{ gtt/min}$$

2. Step 1.   IV PB rate: $\frac{V}{T} \times C = R$

$\frac{40 \text{ mL}}{60 \text{ min}} \times 60 \text{ gtt/mL} = 40 \text{ gtt/min}$

Step 2.   IV PB time: q.i.d. = 4 times/day = 4 h

Step 3.   IV PB volume: $4 \times 40 \text{ mL} = 160 \text{ mL}$

Step 4.   Regular IV volume: $1000 - 160 = 840 \text{ mL}$

Step 5.   Regular IV time: $24 - 4 = 20 \text{ h} = 1200 \text{ min}$

Step 6.   Regular IV rate: $\frac{V}{T} \times C = R$

$\frac{840 \text{ mL}}{1200 \text{ min}} \times 60 \text{ gtt/mL} = \frac{840}{20} = 42 \text{ gtt/min}$

3. Step 1.   IV PB rate:

$\frac{50 \text{ mL}}{30 \text{ min}} \times 15 \text{ gtt/mL} = 25 \text{ gtt/min}$

Step 2.   IV PB time: q.6h $\times 30 \text{ min} = 4 \times 30 = 120 \text{ min} = 2 \text{ h}$

Step 3.   IV PB volume: $4 \times 50 = 200 \text{ mL}$

Step 4.   Reg. IV volume: $3000 - 200 = 2800 \text{ mL}$

Step 5.   Reg. IV time: $24 - 2 = 22 \text{ h}$

Step 6.   Reg. IV rate: $\frac{\text{mL/h}}{\text{dropfactor constant}}$

$\frac{2800 \text{ mL}}{22 \text{ h}} = 127 \text{ mL/h}$

$\frac{127}{4} = 31.75 = 32 \text{ gtt/min}$

4. Step 1.   IV PB rate: 50 mL/h = 50 gtt/min

Step 2.   IV PB time: q.6h = 4x/day = 4 h

Step 3.   IV PB volume: $50 \times 4 = 200 \text{ mL}$

Step 4.   Reg. IV volume: $2000 - 200 = 1800 \text{ mL}$

Step 5.   Reg. IV time: $24 - 4 = 20 \text{ h}$

Step 6.   Reg. IV rate: $\frac{1800 \text{ mL}}{20 \text{ h}} = 90 \text{ mL/h} = 90 \text{ gtt/min}$

5. Step 1.   IV PB rate: 50 mL/h = 50 gtt/min

Step 2.   IV PB time: q.8 h = 3x/day = 3 h

Step 3.   IV PB volume: $50 \times 3 = 150 \text{ mL}$

Step 4.   Reg. IV volume: $1000 - 150 = 850 \text{ mL}$

Step 5.   Reg. IV time: $24 - 3 = 21 \text{ h}$

Step 6.   Reg. IV rate: $\frac{850 \text{ mL}}{21 \text{ h}} = 40.48 \text{ mL/h}$
$= 40 \text{ gtt/min}$

6. Step 1.   IV PB rate:

$\frac{50 \text{ mL}}{30 \text{ min}} \diagdown \diagup \frac{X \text{ mL}}{60 \text{ min}}$

$30X = 3000$

$\frac{30X}{30} = \frac{3000}{30}$

$X = 100 \text{ mL/60 min or } 100 \text{ mL/h}$

Step 2.   IV PB time: q.6 h = 4x/day = $4 \times 30 = 120 \text{ min} = 2 \text{ h}$

Step 3.   IV PB volume: $50 \times 4 = 200 \text{ mL}$

Step 4.   Reg. IV volume: $2400 - 200 = 2200 \text{ mL}$

Step 5.   Reg. IV time: $24 - 2 = 22 \text{ h}$

Step 6.   Reg IV rate: $\frac{2200 \text{ mL}}{22 \text{ h}} = 100 \text{ mL/h}$

7. Step 1.   IV PB rate:

$\frac{100 \text{ mL}}{30 \text{ min}} \diagdown \diagup \frac{X \text{ mL}}{60 \text{ min}}$

$30X = 6000$

$\frac{30X}{30} = \frac{6000}{30}$

$X = 200 \text{ mL/60 min or } 200 \text{ mL/h}$

Step 2.   IV PB time: q.8 h = 3x/day = $3 \times 30 = 90 \text{ min} = 1\frac{1}{2} \text{ h}$

Step 3.   IV PB volume: $100 \times 3 = 300 \text{ mL}$

Step 4.   Reg. IV volume: $2000 - 300 = 1700 \text{ mL}$

Step 5.   Reg. IV time: $24 - 1\frac{1}{2} = 22\frac{1}{2}$

Step 6.   Reg IV rate: $\frac{1700 \text{ mL}}{22.5 \text{ h}} = 75.56 = 76 \text{ mL/h}$

8. Step 1.   IV PB rate

$\frac{50 \text{ mL}}{15 \text{ min}} \diagdown \diagup \frac{X \text{ mL}}{60 \text{ min}}$

$15X = 3000$

$\frac{15X}{15} = \frac{3000}{15}$

$X = 200 \text{ mL/60 min or } 200 \text{ mL/h}$

Step 2.   IV PB time: q.6 h = 4x/day = $4 \times 15 \text{ min} = 60 \text{ min} = 1 \text{ h}$

Step 3.   IV PB volume: $50 \times 4 = 200 \text{ mL}$

Step 4.   Reg. IV volume: $3000 - 200 = 2800 \text{ mL}$

Step 5.   Reg. IV time: $24 - 1 = 23 \text{ h}$

Step 6.   Reg. IV rate: $\frac{2800 \text{ mL}}{23 \text{ h}} = 121.74 = 122 \text{ mL/h}$

Practice Problems

Practice Problems—Chapter 1 from pages 29 and 30.

1. XIV
2. XXV
3. VIII
4. XX
5. 7
6. 24
7. 19
8. 30
9. $\frac{11}{12}$
10. $\frac{47}{63}$
11. 1
12. $\frac{1}{2}$
13. 45.78
14. 59.24
15. 0.09
16. 12
17. $\frac{2}{3}$
18. $\frac{1}{2}$
19. 0.02
20. 0.64
21. $\frac{1}{10}, \frac{1}{6}, \frac{1}{5}, \frac{1}{3}, \frac{1}{2}$
22. $\frac{2}{3}, \frac{3}{4}, \frac{5}{6}, \frac{7}{8}, \frac{9}{10}$
23. 0.009, 0.125, 0.1909, 0.25, 0.3
24. $\frac{1}{2}$%, 0.9%, 50%, 100%, 500%
25. 0.01
26. 0.04
27. 0.9%
28. $\frac{1}{3}$
29. 5:9
30. $\frac{1}{20}$
31. 1:200
32. $\frac{2}{3}$
33. 75%
34. 40%
35. 0.17
36. 1.21
37. 1.3
38. 2.5
39. 0.67
40. 100
41. 4
42. 20,000
43. 3.3
44. 300
45. 8.33
46. 5
47. 11
48. $2.42
49. 12
50. 8

Solutions—Chapter 1

17. $\frac{1}{150} \div \frac{1}{100} = \frac{1}{150} \times \frac{100}{1} = \frac{100}{150} = \frac{2}{3}$

20. $\frac{16\%}{\frac{1}{4}} = 16\% \times \frac{4}{1} = 0.16 \times 4 = 0.64$

33. $3:4 = \frac{3}{4} = 4\overline{)3.00} = 75\%$

$$\begin{array}{r} 0.75 \\ 4\overline{)3.00} \\ \underline{2\ 8} \\ 20 \\ \underline{20} \end{array}$$

37. $\frac{0.3}{2.6} \times \frac{0.15}{X}$

$0.3X = 2.6 \times 0.15$
$0.3X = 0.39$
$\frac{0.3X}{0.3} = \frac{0.39}{0.3}$
$X = 1.3$

42. $\frac{\frac{1}{2}\%}{1000} = \frac{10\%}{X}$

$\frac{0.005}{1000} = \frac{0.1}{X}$

$\frac{0.005}{1000} \times \frac{0.1}{X}$

$0.005X = 1000 \times 0.1$
$0.005X = 100$
$\frac{0.005X}{0.005} = \frac{100}{0.005}$
$X = 20,000$

46. proportion:

$\frac{1\ \text{nurse}}{6\ \text{patients}} = \frac{X\ \text{nurses}}{30\ \text{patients}}$

$\frac{1}{6} = \frac{X}{30}$

Practice Problems—Chapter 2 from pages 39 and 40.

1. milli
2. micro
3. centi
4. kilo
5. meter
6. gram
7. liter
8. drop
9. ounce
10. minim
11. grain
12. milligram
13. microgram
14. unit
15. milliequivalent
16. teaspoon
17. dram
18. milliliter
19. cubic centimeter
20. pint
21. tablespoon
22. millimeter
23. gram
24. centimeter
25. liter
26. meter
27. kilogram
28. gr ss
29. 2 t
30. $3\frac{1}{3}$
31. 500 mU
32. 0.5 L
33. gr $\frac{1}{4}$
34. gr $\frac{1}{200}$
35. 0.05 mg

Practice Problems—Chapter 3 from pages 58 and 59.

1. 500
2. 10
3. 7.5
4. 3
5. 0.004
6. 0.5
7. ss
8. 0.3
9. 70
10. 149.6
11. 180
12. 105
13. 0.3
14. 15
15. 6
16. 90
17. 32.05
18. 7.99 or 8
19. 0.008
20. 2
21. 95
22. viiss
23. $\frac{1}{100}$
24. 0.67
25. 68.18
26. i
27. 1
28. 500
29. 2
30. iii
31. 30
32. 30
33. 1
34. 1
35. 1
36. 1500
37. 45
38. iss
39. $\frac{1}{6}$
40. 0.025
41. 4300
42. 0.06
43. 15
44. 45
45. 0.8
46. 3600
47. 0.0036
48. 0.01
49. 10
50. 0.17
51. 5:30 PM
52. 2030
53. 9:15 AM
54. 36.7°
55. 230°
56. 86°
57. −16.7°
58. 8:01 PM
59. 1930
60. 0645
61. 2400
62. 9 full doses
63. 8 full doses
64. 840 mL
65. 100%; all of it

Solutions—Chapter 3

62. $ʒ$ iv = 4 × 30 = 120 mL/bottle ($ʒ$ i = 30 mL)
each dose = $2\frac{1}{2}$ t = $2\frac{1}{2} \times 5 = 12.5$ mL
(1 t = 5 mL)
proportion:

$\frac{1\ \text{dose}}{12.5\ \text{mL}} = \frac{X\ \text{doses}}{120\ \text{mL}}$

Bottle holds 120 mL; each dose is 12.5 mL.

$12.5X = 120$

$\frac{12.5X}{12.5} = \frac{120}{12.5}$

$X = 9.6$ or 9 *full* doses.

65. gr$\frac{1}{6} = \frac{1}{6} \times \frac{60}{1} = \frac{60}{6} = 10$ mg ordered (gr i = 60 mg)
The ampule contains 10 mg, and the doctor orders gr$\frac{1}{6}$ or 10 mg; therefore, the patient should receive all of the solution in the ampule.

Practice Problems—Chapter 4 from pages 72–74.

1. 1 cc
2. hundredths or 0.01
3. No. The tuberculin syringe has a maximum capacity of 1 mL.
4. Round to 1.3 mL and measure at 1.3 mL.
5. 30 mL or 1 oz
6. 1 mL tuberculin
7. 0.75 cc
8. False
9. False
10. True

11.

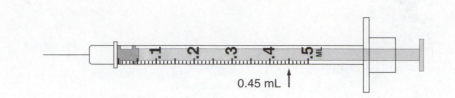

0.45 mL

12.

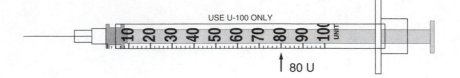

USE U-100 ONLY

80 U

13.

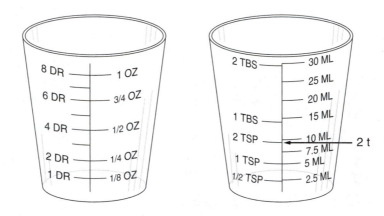

14.

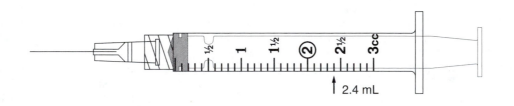

2.4 mL

15.

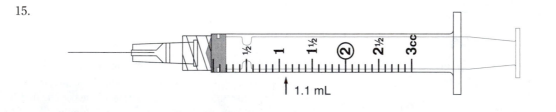

1.1 mL

16.

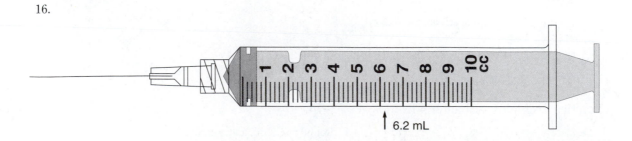

6.2 mL

Practice Problems—Chapter 5 from pages 85–88.

1. ounce
2. per rectum
3. before meals
4. after
5. three times a day
6. every four hours
7. when necessary
8. by mouth, orally
9. once a day, every day
10. right eye
11. immediately
12. freely, as desired
13. hour of sleep, bedtime
14. intramuscular
15. without
16. ss
17. gtt
18. mL
19. gr
20. g
21. $\bar{c}$
22. q.i.d.
23. O.U.
24. SC
25. tsp (t)
26. b.i.d.
27. q.3h
28. p.c.
29. $\bar{a}$
30. kg

31. Give 60 milligrams of Toradol intramuscularly immediately and every 6 hours.
32. Give 300,000 units of procaine penicillin G intramuscularly four times a day.
33. Give 5 milliliters of Mylanta orally 1 hour before and 1 hour after meals, at bedtime, and every 2 hours as needed at night.
34. Give 25 milligrams of Librium orally every 6 hours when necessary for agitation.
35. Give 5,000 units of heparin subcutaneously immediately.
36. Give 50 milligrams of Demerol intramuscularly every 3–4 hours when necessary for pain.
37. Give 0.25 milligram of digoxin orally every day.
38. Give 2 drops of 10% Neosynephrine to the left eye every 30 minutes for 2 applications.
39. Give 40 milligrams of Lasix intramuscularly immediately.
40. Give 4 milligrams of Decadron intravenously twice a day.
41. 12:00 midnight, 8:00 AM, 4:00 PM
42. 20 units
43. SC–subcutaneous
44. Give 500 milligrams of Cipro orally every 12 hours.
45. 8:00 AM, 12:00 noon, 6:00 PM
46. Digoxin 0.125 mg p.o. q.d.
47. with, $\bar{c}$
48. Give 150 milligrams of ranitidine tablets orally twice daily with breakfast and supper.
49. Vancomycin
50. 12 hours

Practice Problems—Chapter 6 from pages 97–99.

1. 8 mEq per tab
2. Summit Pharmaceuticals of Ciba-Geigy Corporation
3. ampicillin sodium/sulbactam sodium
4. Reconstitute with up to 100 mL of an appropriate diluent cited in the package insert.
5. 10 mL
6. 25 mg/mL
7. Keflin
8. cephalothin sodium
9. fluid intramuscular solution
10. 10 mL
11. Roche Laboratories
12. capsule
13. April, 2000
14. 80 mg
15. J
16. H
17. H
18. oral
19. 0666060
20. 80 mg/tablet

Practice Problems—Chapter 7 from pages 123–132.

1. $\frac{1}{2}$ tablet
2. 2 tablets
3. $\frac{1}{2}$ tablet
4. 2.5 mL
5. 10 mL
6. 2 tablets
7. 10 mL
8. $1\frac{1}{2}$ tablets
9. $1\frac{1}{2}$ tablets
10. $\frac{1}{2}$ tablet
11. $1\frac{1}{2}$ tablets
12. 1 tablet
13. $1\frac{1}{2}$ tablets
14. 1 tablet
15. 1 tablet
16. Select 5 mg and give $1\frac{1}{2}$ tablets
17. 7.5 mL or $1\frac{1}{2}$ t
18. $1\frac{1}{2}$ tablets
19. 2 tablets
20. 2 capsules
21. Select 0.75 mg tablets and give 1 tablet
22. $\frac{1}{2}$ tablet
23. 2 tablets
24. 2 tablets
25. 2 tablets
26. D; 1 tablet
27. A; 1 tablet
28. C; 1 tablet
29. B; 2 tablets
30. J; 2 tablets
31. G; 2 tablets
32. F; 5 mL
33. H; 2 tablets
34. E; 30 mL
35. M; 2 capsules
36. N; 1 tablet
37. L; 2 capsules
38. K; 1 tablet
39. O; 1 tablet
40. P; 1 tablet
41. B; 1 tablet
42. 1 tablet
43. A; 1 tablet
44. 1 tablet
45. B; 1 mL

Solutions—Chapter 7

2. Convert :

$$\frac{gr\ 1}{60\ mg} \times \frac{gr\ \frac{1}{2}}{X\ mg}$$

$$X = 60 \times \frac{1}{2} = 30\ mg$$

Order : $gr\ ss = gr\ \frac{1}{2}$ 30 mg

Supply : 15 mg/tab

Calculate : $\dfrac{\text{Dosage on hand}}{\text{Amount on hand}} = \dfrac{\text{Dosage desired}}{\text{X Amount desired}}$

$$\frac{15\ mg}{1\ tab} \times \frac{30\ mg}{X\ tab}$$

$$15X = 30$$

$$\frac{15X}{15} = \frac{30}{15}$$

$$X = 2\ tabs$$

3. Convert :

$$\frac{1\ mg}{1000\ mcg} \times \frac{0.075\ mg}{X\ mcg}$$

$$X = 0.075 \times 1000 = 0.075. = 75\ mcg$$

Order : 0.075 mg   75 mcg

Supply : 150 mcg/tab

Calculate : $\dfrac{\text{Dosage on hand}}{\text{Amount on hand}} = \dfrac{\text{Dosage desired}}{\text{X Amount desired}}$

$$\frac{150\ mcg}{1\ tab} \times \frac{75\ mcg}{X\ tab}$$

$$150X = 75$$

$$\frac{150X}{150} = \frac{75}{150}$$

$$X = \frac{1}{2}\ tab$$

8. Order :   150 mg

Convert :

$$\frac{1\ g}{1000\ mg} \times \frac{0.1\ g}{X\ mg}$$

$$X = 0.1 \times 1000 = 0.100. = 100\ mg$$

100 mg/tab

Supply : 0.1 g/tab

Calculate : $\dfrac{\text{Dosage on hand}}{\text{Amount on hand}} = \dfrac{\text{Dosage desired}}{\text{X Amount desired}}$

$$\frac{100\ mg}{1\ tab} \times \frac{150\ mg}{X\ tab}$$

$$100X = 150$$

$$\frac{100X}{100} = \frac{150}{100}$$

$$X = 1\frac{1}{2}\ tab$$

9. Convert :

$$\frac{gr\ 1}{60\ mg} \times \frac{gr\ \frac{3}{4}}{X\ mg}$$

$$X = 60 \times \frac{3}{4} = 45\ mg$$

45 mg

Order : $gr\ \frac{3}{4}$

Supply : 30 mg/tab

Calculate : $\dfrac{\text{Dosage on hand}}{\text{Amount on hand}} = \dfrac{\text{Dosage desired}}{\text{X Amount desired}}$

$$\frac{30\ mg}{1\ tab} \times \frac{45\ mg}{X\ tab}$$

$$30X = 45$$

$$\frac{30X}{30} = \frac{45}{30}$$

$$X = 1\frac{1}{2}\ tab$$

14. Convert :

$$\frac{gr\ 1}{60\ mg} \times \frac{gr\ \frac{1}{8}}{X\ mg}$$

$$X = 60 \times \frac{1}{8} = 7.5\ mg$$

7.5 mg

Order : $gr\ \frac{1}{8}$

Supply : 7.5 mg tab

Think : It is obvious you want to give 1 tablet.

Calculate : $\dfrac{\text{Dosage on hand}}{\text{Amount on hand}} = \dfrac{\text{Dosage desired}}{\text{X Amount desired}}$

$$\frac{7.5\ mg}{1\ tab} \times \frac{7.5\ mg}{X\ tab}$$

$$7.5X = 7.5$$

$$\frac{7.5X}{7.5} = \frac{7.5}{7.5}$$

$$X = 1\ tab$$

17. Order : 300,00 U

Supply : 200,000 U/5 mL

Calculate : $\dfrac{\text{Dosage on hand}}{\text{Amount on hand}} = \dfrac{\text{Dosage desired}}{\text{X Amount desired}}$

$$\frac{200,000\ U}{5\ mL} \times \frac{300,000\ U}{X\ mL}$$

$$200,000X = 1,500,000$$

$$\frac{200,000X}{200,000} = \frac{1,500,000}{200,000}$$

$$X = 7.5\ mL$$

Convert : $\dfrac{1\ t}{5\ mL} = \dfrac{X\ t}{7.5\ mL}$

$$5X = 7.5$$

$$\frac{5X}{5} = \frac{7.5}{5}$$

$$X = 1\frac{1}{2}\ t$$

34. Order : 40 mEq

Supply : 20 mEq/15 mL

Calculate : $\dfrac{\text{Dosage on hand}}{\text{Amount on hand}} = \dfrac{\text{Dosage desired}}{\text{X Amount desired}}$

$$\frac{20\ mEq}{15\ mL} \times \frac{40\ mEq}{X\ mL}$$

$$20X = 600$$

$$\frac{20X}{20} = \frac{600}{20}$$

$$X = 30\ mL\ or\ ʒ\ i$$

Practice Problems—Chapter 8 from pages 165–174.

1. 0.4 mL; 0.5 mL TB syringe
2. 1 mL; 3 cc syringe
3. 2.4 mL; 3 cc syringe
4. 0.6 mL; 1 mL TB or 3 cc syringe
5. 2 mL; 3 cc syringe
6. 2 mL; 3 cc syringe
7. 15 mL; 20 cc syringe
8. 2 mL; 3 cc syringe
9. 15 mL; 20 cc syringe
10. 0.8 mL; 1 mL TB or 3 cc syringe
11. 1 mL; 3 cc syringe
12. 1 mL; 3 cc syringe
13. 0.5 mL; 1 mL TB or 3 cc syringe
14. 1.5 mL; 3 cc syringe
15. 0.6 mL; 1 mL TB or 3 cc syringe
16. 0.6 mL; 1 mL TB or 3 cc syringe
17. 1.9 mL; 3 cc syringe
18. 0.6 mL; 1 mL TB or 3 cc syringe
19. 1 mL; 3 cc syringe
20. 1.2 mL; 3 cc syringe
21. 1.5 mL; 3 cc syringe
22. 1 mL; 3 cc syringe
23. 1.2 mL; 3 cc syringe
24. 0.7 mL; 1 mL TB or 3 cc syringe
25. 0.75 mL; 1 mL TB or 3 cc syringe
26. 1.5 mL; 3 cc syringe
27. 0.7 mL; 1 mL TB or 3 cc syringe
28. 0.8 mL; 1 mL TB or 3 cc syringe
29. 1 mL; 3 cc syringe
30. 3.8 mL; 5 cc syringe
31. 0.8 mL; 1 mL TB or 3 cc syringe
32. 1.6 mL; 3 cc syringe
33. 6 mL; 10 cc syringe
34. 0.8 mL; 1 mL TB or 3 cc syringe
35. 1.5 mL; 3 cc syringe
36. 5 mL; 5 cc syringe
37. 1.3 mL; 3 cc syringe
38. 1 mL; 3 cc syringe
39. 0.7 mL; 1 mL TB or 3 cc syringe
40. 1 mL; 3 cc syringe
41. 30 mL; 20 cc syringe (2 syringes)
42. 16 U; Lo-Dose 30 U U-100 insulin syringe
43. 70 units; standard U-100 insulin syringe
44. 25 units; Lo-Dose 50 U U-100 insulin syringe

45.

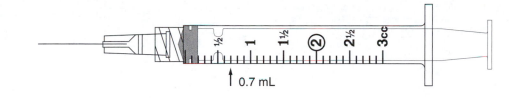

↑ 0.7 mL

46.

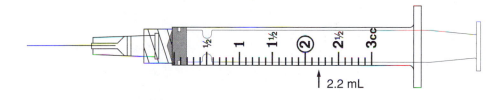

↑ 2.2 mL

47.

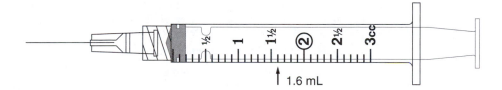

↑ 1.6 mL

48.

2.5 mL in two syringes ↑
(5 mL total)

49.

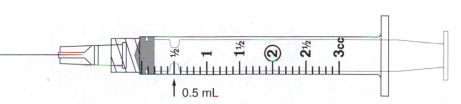

↑ 0.5 mL

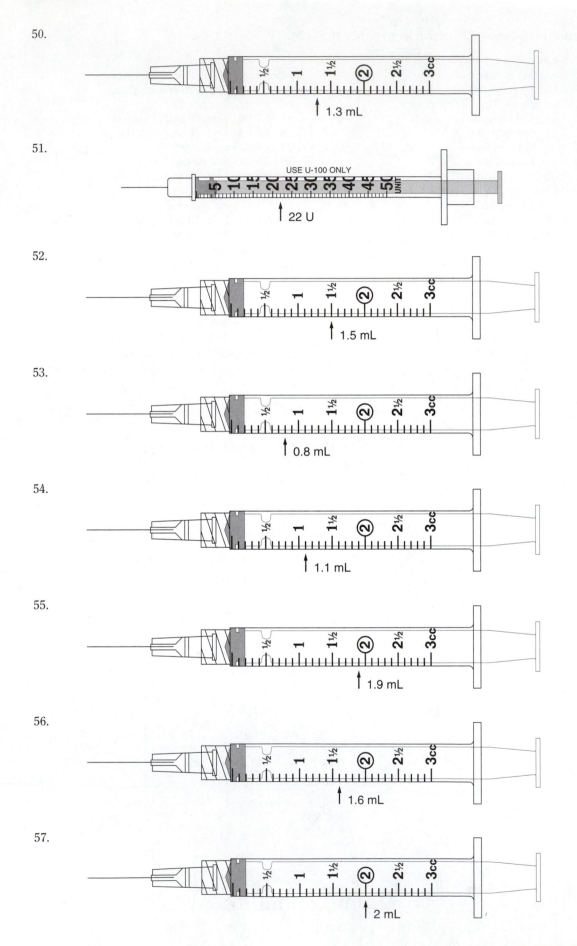

50.

↑ 1.3 mL

51.

USE U-100 ONLY

↑ 22 U

52.

↑ 1.5 mL

53.

↑ 0.8 mL

54.

↑ 1.1 mL

55.

↑ 1.9 mL

56.

↑ 1.6 mL

57.

↑ 2 mL

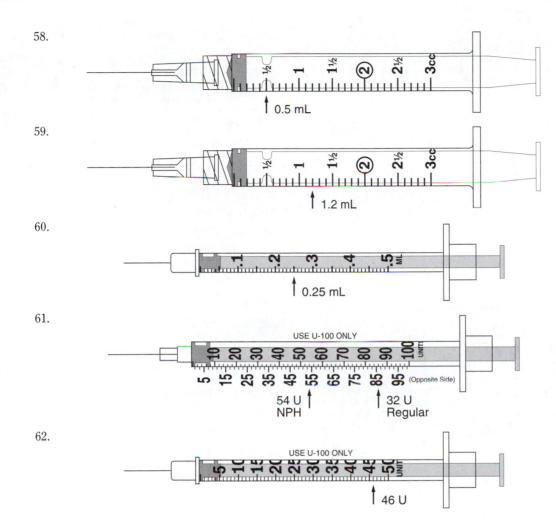

58.

↑ 0.5 mL

59.

↑ 1.2 mL

60.

↑ 0.25 mL

61.

USE U-100 ONLY

(Opposite Side)

54 U ↑
NPH

↑ 32 U
Regular

62.

USE U-100 ONLY

↑ 46 U

Solutions—Chapter 8

3. Convert: $\dfrac{1 \text{ mg}}{1000 \text{ mcg}} \diagdown\diagup \dfrac{0.6 \text{ mg}}{X \text{ mcg}}$

$X = 0.6 \times 1000 = 0.600. = 600 \text{ mcg}$

Order: 0.6 mg ⟶ 600 mcg

Supply: 500 mcg/2 mL

Calculate: $\dfrac{\text{Dosage on hand}}{\text{Amount on hand}} = \dfrac{\text{Dosage desired}}{\text{X Amount desired}}$

$\dfrac{500 \text{ mcg}}{2 \text{ mL}} \diagdown\diagup \dfrac{600 \text{ mcg}}{X \text{ mL}}$

$500X = 1200$

$\dfrac{500X}{500} = \dfrac{1200}{500}$

$X = 2.4 \text{ mL}$

7. Order: 3 mg

Supply: 1 mg/5 mL

Calculate: $\dfrac{\text{Dosage on hand}}{\text{Amount on hand}} = \dfrac{\text{Dosage desired}}{\text{X Amount desired}}$

$\dfrac{1 \text{ mg}}{5 \text{ mL}} \diagdown\diagup \dfrac{3 \text{ mg}}{X \text{ mL}}$

$X = 15 \text{ mL}$

14. Convert: $\dfrac{\text{gr } 1}{60 \text{ mg}} \diagdown\diagup \dfrac{\text{gr } \frac{1}{100}}{X \text{ mg}}$

$X = 60 \times \dfrac{1}{100} = 0.6 \text{ mg}$

Order: gr $\frac{1}{100}$ ⟶ 0.6 mg

Supply: 0.4 mg/mL

Calculate: $\dfrac{\text{Dosage on hand}}{\text{Amount on hand}} = \dfrac{\text{Dosage desired}}{\text{X Amount desired}}$

$\dfrac{0.4 \text{ mg}}{1 \text{ mL}} \diagdown\diagup \dfrac{0.6 \text{ mg}}{X \text{ mL}}$

$0.4X = 0.6$

$\dfrac{0.4X}{0.4} = \dfrac{0.6}{0.4}$

$X = 1.5 \text{ mL}$

17. Order: 75 mg

Supply: 80 mg/2 mL

Calculate: $\dfrac{\text{Dosage on hand}}{\text{Amount on hand}} = \dfrac{\text{Dosage desired}}{\text{X Amount desired}}$

$\dfrac{80 \text{ mg}}{2 \text{ mL}} \diagdown\diagup \dfrac{75 \text{ mg}}{X \text{ mL}}$

$80X = 150 \text{ mL}$

$\dfrac{80X}{80} = \dfrac{150}{80}$

$X = 1.88 = 1.9 \text{ mL}$

18. Convert: $\dfrac{\text{gr } 1}{60 \text{ mg}} \diagdown \dfrac{\text{gr }\frac{1}{10}}{\text{X mg}}$

$\quad\quad X = 60 \times \dfrac{1}{10} = 6 \text{ mg}$

Order: gr $\frac{1}{10}$ → 6 mg

Supply: 10 mg/mL

Calculate: $\dfrac{\text{Dosage on hand}}{\text{Amount on hand}} = \dfrac{\text{Dosage desired}}{\text{X Amount desired}}$

$\dfrac{10 \text{ mg}}{1 \text{ mL}} \diagdown \dfrac{6 \text{ mg}}{\text{X mL}}$

$\quad 10X = 6$

$\quad \dfrac{10X}{10} = \dfrac{6}{10}$

$\quad\quad X = 0.6 \text{ mL}$

23. Order: 60 mg

Supply: 75 mg/1.5 mL

Calculate: $\dfrac{\text{Dosage on hand}}{\text{Amount on hand}} = \dfrac{\text{Dosage desired}}{\text{X Amount desired}}$

$\dfrac{75 \text{ mg}}{1.5 \text{ mL}} \diagdown \dfrac{60 \text{ mg}}{\text{X mL}}$

$\quad 75X = 90 \text{ mg}$

$\quad \dfrac{75X}{75} = \dfrac{90}{75}$

$\quad\quad X = 1.2 \text{ mL}$

30. Order: 750 mg

Supply: 1 g → 1000 mg

Calculate: $\dfrac{\text{Dosage on hand}}{\text{Amount on hand}} = \dfrac{\text{Dosage desired}}{\text{X Amount desired}}$

$\dfrac{1000 \text{ mg}}{5 \text{ mL}} \diagdown \dfrac{750 \text{ mg}}{\text{X mL}}$

$\quad 1000X = 3750$

$\quad \dfrac{1000X}{1000} = \dfrac{3750}{1000}$

$\quad\quad X = 3.75 = 3.8 \text{ mL}$

32. Convert: $\dfrac{1 \text{ mg}}{1000 \text{ mcg}} \diagdown \dfrac{0.4 \text{ mg}}{\text{X mcg}}$

$\quad\quad X = 0.4 \times 1000 = 0.400. = 400 \text{ mcg}$

Order: 0.4 mg → 400 mcg

Supply: 500 mcg/2 mL

Calculate: $\dfrac{\text{Dosage on hand}}{\text{Amount on hand}} = \dfrac{\text{Dosage desired}}{\text{X Amount desired}}$

$\dfrac{500 \text{ mcg}}{2 \text{ mL}} \diagdown \dfrac{400 \text{ mcg}}{\text{X mL}}$

$\quad 500X = 800$

$\quad \dfrac{500X}{500} = \dfrac{800}{500}$

$\quad\quad X = 1.6 \text{ mL}$

36. Convert: 10% = 10 g/100 mL

Order: 0.5 g

Supply: 10 g/100 mL

Calculate: $\dfrac{\text{Dosage on hand}}{\text{Amount on hand}} = \dfrac{\text{Dosage desired}}{\text{X Amount desired}}$

$\dfrac{10 \text{ g}}{100 \text{ mL}} \diagdown \dfrac{0.5 \text{ g}}{\text{X mL}}$

$\quad 10X = 50$

$\quad \dfrac{10X}{10} = \dfrac{50}{10}$

$\quad\quad X = 5 \text{ mL}$

37. Order: 400,000 U

Supply: 300,000 U/mL

Calculate: $\dfrac{\text{Dosage on hand}}{\text{Amount on hand}} = \dfrac{\text{Dosage desired}}{\text{X Amount desired}}$

$\dfrac{300,000 \text{ U}}{1 \text{ mL}} \diagdown \dfrac{400,000 \text{ U}}{\text{X mL}}$

$\quad 300,00X = 400,000$

$\quad \dfrac{300,000X}{300,000} = \dfrac{400,000}{300,000}$

$\quad\quad X = 1.33 = 1.3 \text{ mL}$

40. Order: 0.5 mg

Convert: 1 : 2000 = 1 g/2000 mL

Convert: 1 g = 1000 mg

Supply: 1000 mg/2000 mL

Calculate: $\dfrac{\text{Dosage on hand}}{\text{Amount on hand}} = \dfrac{\text{Dosage desired}}{\text{X Amount desired}}$

$\dfrac{1000 \text{ mg}}{2000 \text{ mL}} \diagdown \dfrac{0.5 \text{ mg}}{\text{X mL}}$

$\quad 1000X = 1000$

$\quad \dfrac{1000X}{1000} = \dfrac{1000}{1000}$

$\quad\quad X = 1 \text{ mL}$

47. Order: 65 mg

Supply: 80 mg/2 mL

Calculate: $\dfrac{\text{Dosage on hand}}{\text{Amount on hand}} = \dfrac{\text{Dosage desired}}{\text{X Amount desired}}$

$\dfrac{80 \text{ mg}}{2 \text{ mL}} \diagdown \dfrac{65 \text{ mg}}{\text{X mL}}$

$\quad 80X = 130$

$\quad \dfrac{80X}{80} = \dfrac{130}{80}$

$\quad\quad X = 1.63 = 1.6 \text{ mL}$

Practice Problems—Chapter 9 from pages 180–182.

1. 45 mL
2. 2 mL
3. 1.6 mL
4. $\frac{1}{2}$ t
5. 2.5 mL
6. 16 mL
7. 1.4 mL
8. 0.7 mL
9. 2.3 mL
10. 0.13 mL, measured in a tuberculin syringe
11. 1.6 mL
12. 1.5 mL
13. 1.3 mL
14. 2.5 mL
15. 1.6 mL
16. 7.5 mL
17. 1.6 mL
18. 2 tabs
19. 8 mL
20. 4.5 mL
21. 30 mL
22. 1.4 mL
23. 15 mL
24. 20 mL
25. 12 mL

Solutions—Chapter 9

1. $\dfrac{D}{H} \times Q = X$

    $\dfrac{30\ g}{3.33\ g} \times 5\ mL = X$

    $\dfrac{150}{3.33}\ mL = X$

    $X = 45\ mL$

2. $\dfrac{D}{H} \times Q = X$

    $\dfrac{\overset{1}{\cancel{500,000}}\ U}{\underset{10}{\cancel{5,000,000}}\ U} \times 20\ mL = X$

    $\dfrac{20}{10}\ mL = X$

    $X = 2\ mL$

6. $\dfrac{D}{H} \times Q = X$

    $\dfrac{40\ mg}{12.5\ mg} \times 5\ mL = X$

    $\dfrac{200}{12.5}\ mL = X$

    $X = 16\ mL$

7. $\dfrac{D}{H} \times Q = X$

    $\dfrac{\overset{7}{\cancel{350,000}}\ U}{\underset{10}{\cancel{500,000}}\ U} \times 2\ mL = X$

    $\dfrac{14}{10}\ mL = X$

    $X = 1.4\ mL$

8. $\dfrac{D}{H} \times Q = X$

    $\dfrac{3.5\ mg}{10\ mg} \times 2\ mL = X$

    $\dfrac{7}{10}\ mL = X$

    $X = 0.7\ mL$

9. $\dfrac{D}{H} \times Q = X$

    $\dfrac{90\ mg}{\underset{40}{\cancel{80}}\ mg} \times \overset{1}{\cancel{2}}\ mL = X$

    $\dfrac{90}{40}\ mL = X$

    $X = 2.25\ mL$

    $= 2.3\ mL$ measured in a 3 cc syringe

13. 1) Convert: g → mg. Equivalent: 1 g = 1000 mg

    2) $\dfrac{D}{H} \times Q = X$

    $\dfrac{\overset{1}{\cancel{500}}\ mg}{\underset{2}{\cancel{1000}}\ mg} \times 2.5\ mL = X$

    $\dfrac{2.5}{2}\ mL = X$

    $X = 1.25\ mL = 1.3\ mL$

16. $\dfrac{D}{H} \times Q = X$

    $\dfrac{\overset{1}{\cancel{10}}\ mEq}{\underset{2}{\cancel{20}}\ mEq} \times 15\ mL = X$

    $\dfrac{15}{2}\ mL = X$

    $X = 7.5\ mL$

18. 1) Convert: mg → mcg. Equivalent: 1 mg = 1000 mcg

    $0.075 \times 1000 = 0.075. = 75\ mcg$

    2) $\dfrac{D}{H} \times Q = X$

    $\dfrac{150\ mcg}{75\ mcg} \times 1\ tablet = X$

    $\dfrac{150}{75}\ tablets = X$

    $X = 2\ tablets$

Practice Problems—Chapter 10 from pages 198–201.

1. 1.8 mL
2. No; none, consult with the physician or your supervisor before administering any of this drug.
3. 0.62 mL
4. 125 mg
5. 0.5 mL
6. 175 mg
7. 0.7mL
8. 235 mg
9. 0.94 mL
10. 83 mL
11. 6 mL
12. 13 mL
13. 1.8 mL
14. 5 kg
15. 75 mg
16. 37.5 mg
17. yes
18. 1 mL
19. Yes
20. No, contact the physician.
21. 120 mg
22. 3.75 mL
23. Yes, the dosage is safe.
24. Yes, the dosage is safe.
25. 0.04 mg/dose
26. 0.8 mL
27. 112.5 mg/day
28. 37.5 mg/dose
29. 22–44 mg/day up to 22–44 mg/dose
30. 0.33 m²
31. 59.4 mg q.6h
32. 150–300 mg/day
33. 75–150 mg q.12h
34. Yes, the dosage is safe.

Solutions—Chapter 10

2. 1) Calculate: Child's weight in kg

    $\dfrac{1\ kg}{2.2\ lb} \diagdown\diagup \dfrac{X\ kg}{66\ lb}$

    $2.2X = 66$

    $\dfrac{2.2X}{2.2} = \dfrac{66}{2.2}$

    $X = 30\ kg$

    2) Calculate: Dosage

    $\dfrac{3\ mg}{1\ kg} \diagdown\diagup \dfrac{X\ mg}{30\ kg}$

    $X = 90\ mg$

    $105 - 90 = 15;\ \dfrac{15}{90} = 17\%$ more than recommended.

3. Child's BSA: 0.52 m²

$$\frac{0.52\ m^2}{1.7\ m^2}\times 100\ mg\ =\ 31\ mg$$

$$\frac{50\ mg}{1\ mL}\diagdown\diagup\frac{31\ mg}{X\ mL}$$

$$50X\ =\ 31$$

$$\frac{50X}{50}\ =\ \frac{31}{50}$$

$$X\ =\ 0.62\ mL$$

4. Child's BSA = 0.42 m²

$$\frac{0.42\ m^2}{1.7\ m^2}\times 500\ mg = 125\ mg$$

5. $$\frac{250\ mg}{1\ mL}\diagdown\diagup\frac{125\ mg}{X\ mL}$$

$$250X\ =\ 125$$

$$\frac{250X}{250}\ =\ \frac{125}{250}$$

$$X\ =\ 0.5\ mL$$

6. Child's BSA: 0.6 m²

Equivalent: 1 g = 1000 mg

$$0.5\ g = 0.5\times 1000 = 0.500. = 500\ mg$$

$$\frac{0.6\ m^2}{1.7\ m^2}\times 500\ mg = 175\ mg$$

7. $$\frac{250\ mg}{1\ mL}\diagdown\diagup\frac{175\ mg}{X\ mL}$$

$$250X\ =\ 175$$

$$\frac{250X}{250}\ =\ \frac{175}{250}$$

$$X\ =\ 0.7\ mL$$

10. 1) Calculate: Child's weight in kg

$$\frac{1\ kg}{2.2\ lb}\diagdown\diagup\frac{X\ kg}{55\ lb}$$

$$2.2X\ =\ 55$$

$$\frac{2.2X}{2.2}\ =\ \frac{55}{2.2}$$

$$X\ =\ 25\ kg$$

2) Calculate: Dosage

$$\frac{0.2\ g}{1\ kg}\diagdown\diagup\frac{X\ g}{25\ kg}$$

$$X\ =\ 5\ g$$

3) Calculate: Amount to give

$$\frac{6\ g}{100\ mL}\diagdown\diagup\frac{5\ g}{X\ mL}$$

$$6X\ =\ 500$$

$$\frac{6X}{6}\ =\ \frac{500}{6}$$

$$X\ =\ 83\ mL$$

Or, $$\frac{D}{H}\times Q = X$$

$$\frac{5\ g}{6\ g}\times 100\ mL = \frac{500}{6} = 83\ mL$$

11. 1) Calculate: Child's weight in kg.

$$\frac{1\ kg}{2.2\ lb}\diagdown\diagup\frac{X\ kg}{26\ lb}$$

$$2.2X\ =\ 26$$

$$\frac{2.2X}{2.2}\ =\ \frac{26}{2.2}$$

$$X\ =\ 11.8 = 12\ kg$$

2) Calculate: Dosage.

$$\frac{50\ mg}{1\ kg}\diagdown\diagup\frac{X\ mg}{12\ kg}$$

$$X\ =\ 600\ mg\ \text{divided into 4 q.6h doses}$$

$$\frac{600}{4}\ =\ 150\ mg/dose$$

3) Calculate: Amount to give.

$$\frac{125\ mg}{5\ mL}\diagdown\diagup\frac{150\ mg}{X\ mL}$$

$$125X\ =\ 750$$

$$\frac{125X}{125}\ =\ \frac{750}{125}$$

$$X\ =\ 6\ mL$$

Or, $$\frac{D}{H}\times Q = X$$

$$\frac{150\ mg}{125\ mg}\times 5\ mL = \frac{750}{125} = 6\ mL$$

13. BSA = 0.9 m²

$$2\ mg/m^2\times 0.9\ m^2\ =\ 1.8\ mg$$

$$\frac{1\ mg}{1\ mL}\diagdown\diagup\frac{1.8\ mg}{X\ mL}$$

$$X\ =\ 1.8\ mL$$

Or, $$\frac{D}{H}\times Q = X$$

$$\frac{1.8\ mg}{1\ mg}\times 1\ mL = 1.8\ mL$$

21. $$\frac{10\ mg}{1\ kg}\diagdown\diagup\frac{X\ mg}{12\ kg}$$

$$X\ =\ 120\ mg$$

22. $$\frac{80\ mg}{2.5\ mL}\diagdown\diagup\frac{120\ mg}{X\ mL}$$

$$80X\ =\ 300$$

$$\frac{80X}{80}\ =\ \frac{300}{80}$$

$$X\ =\ 3.75\ mL$$

23. $$\frac{10\ mcg}{1\ kg}\diagdown\diagup\frac{X\ mcg}{4\ kg}$$

$$X\ =\ 40\ mcg\ \text{minimum dosage}$$

$$\frac{12\ mcg}{1\ kg}\diagdown\diagup\frac{X\ mcg}{4\ kg}$$

$$X\ =\ 48\ mcg\ \text{maximum dosage}$$

Convert: mg → mcg

Equivalent: 1 mg = 1000 mcg

$$\frac{1\ mg}{1000\ mcg}\diagdown\diagup\frac{0.048\ mg}{X\ mcg}$$

$$X\ =\ 0.048\times 1000 = 0.048. = 48\ mcg$$

Yes, the dosage is safe.

24. $$\frac{0.08\ mg}{1\ kg}\diagdown\diagup\frac{X\ mg}{14\ kg}$$

$$X\ =\ 1.12\ mg\ \text{minimum dosage}$$

$$\frac{0.2\ mg}{1\ kg}\diagdown\diagup\frac{X\ mg}{14\ kg}$$

$$X\ =\ 2.8\ mg\ \text{maximum dosage}$$

Yes, the dosage is safe.

25. $\dfrac{0.001 \text{ mg}}{1 \text{ kg}} \diagup\!\!\!\!\diagdown \dfrac{X \text{ mg}}{40 \text{ kg}}$

   X = 0.04 mg/dose

26. $\dfrac{0.05 \text{ mg}}{1 \text{ mL}} \diagup\!\!\!\!\diagdown \dfrac{0.04 \text{ mg}}{X \text{ mL}}$

   0.05X = 0.04

   $\dfrac{0.05X}{0.05} = \dfrac{0.04}{0.05}$

   X = 0.8 mL

27. $\dfrac{7.5 \text{ mg}}{1 \text{ kg}} \diagup\!\!\!\!\diagdown \dfrac{X \text{ mg}}{15 \text{ kg}}$

   X = 112.5 mg/day

28. q.8h = 3 doses/day

   $\dfrac{112.5}{3} = 37.5$ mg/dose

29. $\dfrac{1 \text{ mg}}{1 \text{ kg}} \diagup\!\!\!\!\diagdown \dfrac{X \text{ mg}}{22 \text{ kg}}$

   X = 22 mg minimum dosage

   $\dfrac{2 \text{ mg}}{1 \text{ kg}} \diagup\!\!\!\!\diagdown \dfrac{X \text{ mg}}{22 \text{ kg}}$

   X = 44 mg maximum dosage

30. 6 kg and 60 cm = 0.33 m²

31. 180 mg/m² × 0.33 m² = 59.4 mg

32. $\dfrac{6 \text{ mg}}{1 \text{ kg}} \diagup\!\!\!\!\diagdown \dfrac{X \text{ mg}}{25 \text{ kg}}$

   X = 150 mg/day minimum dosage

   $\dfrac{12 \text{ mg}}{1 \text{ kg}} \diagup\!\!\!\!\diagdown \dfrac{X \text{ mg}}{25 \text{ mg}}$

   X = 300 mg/day maximum dosage

33. q.12h = 2 doses/day

   $\dfrac{150}{2} = 75$ mg q.12h minimum

   $\dfrac{300}{2} = 150$ mg q.12h maximum

34. Yes, the dosage is safe.

   $\dfrac{16 \text{ mg TMP}}{1 \text{ mL}} \diagup\!\!\!\!\diagdown \dfrac{X \text{ mg TMP}}{9.3 \text{ mL}}$

   X = 16 × 9.3 = 148.9 mg TMP per dose, the upper limit of the safe range.

Practice Problems—Chapter 11 from pages 230–232.

1. 17 gtt/min
2. 42 gtt/min
3. 42 gtt/min
4. 8 gtt/min
5. 125 mL/h
6. Assess patient. If stable, recalculate and reset to 114 mL/h.
7. 31 gtt/min
8. 42 gtt/min
9. Assess patient. If stable, recalculate and reset to 50 gtt/min.
10. 3000 mL
11. Abbott
12. 15 gtt/mL
13. 4
14. $\dfrac{\text{mL/h}}{\text{drop factor constant}} : \dfrac{500 \text{ mL}}{4 \text{ h}} = 125 \text{ mL/h}; \dfrac{125 \text{ mL/h}}{4} = 31.25 = 31$ gtt/min
15. $\dfrac{V}{T} \times C = R : \dfrac{500}{240} \times 15 = 31.25 = 31$ gtt/min
16. 1930 or 7:30 P.M.
17. 250 mL
18. Recalculate 210 mL to infuse over remaining 2 hours. Reset IV to 26 gtt/min.
19. 125 mL/h
20. 100 mL/h
21. dextrose 2.5% in 0.45% sodium chloride
22. 25 g dextrose; 4.5 g NaCl
23. A central line is a special catheter inserted to access a large vein in the chest.
24. A primary line is the IV tubing used to set up a primary IV infusion. It is long enough to reach from the IV bag to the hub of the IV catheter.
25. The purpose of a saline/heparin lock is to administer IV medications when the patient does not require IV fluids.
26. milliequivalent (mEq)
27. The purpose of the PCA pump is to allow the patient to self-administer IV medication for pain without having to call the nurse for a p.r.n. medication.
28. Advantages of the syringe pump are that a small amount of medication can be delivered directly from the syringe, and a specified time can be programmed in the pump.
29. phlebitis and infiltration
30. hourly (q.1h)
31. Blood loss occurring due to surgery, trauma, or hemorrhage; bone marrow depression in cancer patients; plasma clotting factors in hemophilia.
32. A, B, O, AB
33. At the bedside two nurses verify the identification band, blood bank number, blood type of donor, blood type of patient, donor number, ordered component, and expiration date of the blood. Both nurses sign the blood tag.
34. The Y-set system has two ports that allow normal saline to be infused to prime the IV line and ensure all the blood is infused to the patient. The Y-set also contains a filter to remove debris or tiny clots.
35. Monitor for transfusion reactions.

Solutions—Chapter 11

1. $\frac{V}{T} \times C = R : \frac{200}{120} \times 10 = 16.66 = 17$ gtt/min

2. $\frac{V}{T} \times C = R : \frac{1000}{1440} \times 60 = 41.66 = 42$ gtt/min

3. $\frac{V}{T} \times C = R : \frac{1500}{720} \times 20 = 41.66 = 42$ gtt/min

4. $\frac{V}{T} \times C = R : \frac{200}{1440} \times 60 = 8.33 = 8$ gtt/min

5. $\frac{\text{Total mL}}{\text{Total hours}} = \frac{1000 \text{ mL}}{8 \text{ h}} = 125$ mL/h

6. $\frac{800 \text{ mL}}{7 \text{ h}} = 114.28 = 114$ mL/h

   $\frac{114-125}{125}$ gives 9% *decrease* in flow rate; within safe limits of 25% variance. Assess patient; if stable reset infusion rate to 114 mL/h.

7. $\frac{V}{T} \times C = R : 1000 + 2000 = 3000$ mL

   $\frac{3000 \text{ mL}}{1440 \text{ min}} \times 15 \text{ gtt/mL} = \frac{45,000}{1440} = 31.25 = 31$ gtt/min

8. $\frac{\text{mL/h}}{\text{Drop factor constant}} = \frac{125 \text{ mL/h}}{3} = 41.66 = 42$ gtt/min

9. $\frac{V}{T} \times C = R$

   $\frac{1000 \text{ mL}}{360 \text{ min}} \times 15 \text{ gtt/mL} = \frac{15,000}{360} = 41.67 = 42$ gtt/min

   $6 - 2 = 4$ hours remaining

   $\frac{800 \text{ mL}}{240 \text{ min}} \times 15 \text{ gtt/mL} = \frac{12,000}{240} = 50$ gtt/min

   $\frac{50-42}{42} = 19\%$ increase; within safe limits of 25% variance. Assess patient; if condition is stable reset infusion rate to 50 gtt/min.

10. q.4 h = 6 times/24 h = 6×500 mL = 3000 mL

13. $\frac{60}{15} = 4$

16. 1530 + 4 h = 1530 + 0400 = 1930 − 1200 = 7:30 P.M.

17. $\frac{500 \text{ mL}}{4 \text{ h}} \diagdown \diagup \frac{X \text{ mL}}{2 \text{ h}}$

    $4X = 1000$

    $\frac{4X}{4} = \frac{1000}{4}$

    $X = 250$ mL

    or, 500 mL/4 h = 125 mL/h

    125 mL/h × 2 h = 250 mL

18. $\frac{210 \text{ mL}}{120 \text{ min}} \times 15 \text{ gtt/mL} = \frac{3150}{120} = 26.25 = 26$ gtt/min

    $\frac{26-31}{31} = 16\%$ *decrease* in rate; within safe limits of 25% variance. Assess patient; if condition is stable, reset infusion rate to 26 gtt/min.

19. $\frac{500 \text{ mL}}{4 \text{ h}} = 125$ mL/h

20. $\frac{50 \text{ mL}}{30 \text{ min}} \diagdown \diagup \frac{X \text{ mL}}{60 \text{ min}}$

    $30X = 3000$

    $\frac{30X}{30} = \frac{3000}{30}$

    $X = 100$ mL/h

Practice Problems—Chapter 12 from pages 258–260.

1. 60 gtt/mL
2. 5 mL
3. 20 mL
4. 50 gtt/min
5. one
6. 12 mL/h; Yes
7. 15 mL/h
8. 2.5 mL
9. 4000 U/h, No
10. 6 h & 15 min
11. 60 mL/h
12. 45 mL/h
13. 60 mL/h
14. 24 mL/h
15. Yes
16. IV PB: 17 gtt/min; Regular IV: 22 gtt/min
17. IV PB: 100 gtt/min; Regular IV: 127 gtt/min
18. 102 mL/h
19. 8 mEq
20. 2 mL/min
21. 1 h and 40 min
22. 1932 hours
23. 1536 mL
24. 15 h
25. 50 mL/h; 50 gtt/min
26. 75 mL/h; No
27. 7.4 mL
28. 33 mL/h
29. 150 mL/h: 50 mL/h
30. 2 mL/h

Solutions—Chapter 12

1. Volume control sets are microdrip infusion sets.

2. $\frac{1 \text{ g}}{5 \text{ mL}} \diagdown \diagup \frac{1 \text{ g}}{X \text{ mL}}$

   It is obvious you would infuse 5 mL over 30 min.

3. $\frac{50 \text{ mL}}{60 \text{ min}} \diagdown \diagup \frac{X \text{ mL}}{30 \text{ min}}$

   $60X = 1500$

   $\frac{60X}{60} = \frac{1500}{60}$

   $X = 25$ mL total dilution volume

   $25 - 5 = 20$ mL

4. $\frac{\text{mL/h}}{\text{drop factor constant}} = \frac{50}{1} = 50$ gtt/min

5. once at 1200 hours

6. $\frac{25,000 \text{ U}}{250 \text{ mL}} \diagdown \diagup \frac{1200 \text{ U}}{X \text{ mL}}$

   $25,000X = 300,000$

   $\frac{25,000X}{25,000} = \frac{300,000}{25,000}$

   $X = 12$ mL/h

   $\frac{1200 \text{ U}}{1 \text{ h}} \diagdown \diagup \frac{X \text{ U}}{24 \text{ h}}$

   $X = 28,800$ U/24 h

   1200 U are in 12 mL; 1200 U/h are delivered by 12 mL/h. (normal range = 20,000–40,000 U)

7. $\frac{500 \text{ mg}}{250 \text{ mL}} \diagdown \diagup \frac{30 \text{ mg}}{X \text{ mL}}$

   $500X = 7500$

   $\frac{500X}{500} = \frac{7500}{500}$

   $X = 15$ mL

   30 mg are in 15 mL; 30 mg/h are delivered by 15 mL/h

8.
$$\frac{20\ mEq}{100\ mL} \diagdown\!\!\!\!\diagup \frac{X\ mEq}{250\ mL}$$

$$1000X\ =\ 5000$$

$$\frac{1000X}{1000}\ =\ \frac{5000}{1000}$$

$$X\ =\ 5\ mEq$$

$$\frac{2\ mEq}{1\ mL} \diagdown\!\!\!\!\diagup \frac{5\ mEq}{X\ mL}$$

$$2X\ =\ 5$$

$$\frac{2X}{2}\ =\ \frac{5}{2}$$

$$X\ =\ 2.5\ mL$$

9.
$$\frac{40,000\ U}{1000\ mL} \diagdown\!\!\!\!\diagup \frac{X\ U}{100\ mL}$$

$$1000X\ =\ 4,000,000$$

$$\frac{1000X}{1000}\ =\ \frac{4,000,000}{1000}$$

$$X\ =\ 4000\ U/h$$

$$\frac{4000\ U}{1\ h} \diagdown\!\!\!\!\diagup \frac{X\ U}{24\ h}$$

$$X\ =\ 96,000\ U/24\ h$$

4000 U are in 100 mL; 4000 U/h are delivered by 100 mL/h (normal range = 20,000–40,000 U)

10. 1) Convert: L → mL

$$\frac{1\ L}{1000\ mL} \diagdown\!\!\!\!\diagup \frac{1.5\ L}{X\ mL}$$

$$X\ =\ 1.5\times1000 = 1.500. = 1500\ mL$$

2) Calculate: time

$$\frac{4\ mL}{1\ min} \diagdown\!\!\!\!\diagup \frac{1500\ mL}{X\ min}$$

$$4X\ =\ 1500$$

$$\frac{4X}{4}\ =\ \frac{1500}{4}$$

$$X\ =\ 375\ min$$

3) Convert: min → h

$$\frac{60\ min}{1\ h} \diagdown\!\!\!\!\diagup \frac{375\ min}{X\ h}$$

$$60X\ =\ 375$$

$$\frac{60X}{60}\ =\ \frac{375}{60}$$

$$X\ =\ 6.25\ h\ or\ 6\ h\ and\ 15\ min$$

11. 1) Convert: g → mg

$$\frac{1\ g}{1000\ mg} \diagdown\!\!\!\!\diagup \frac{2\ g}{X\ mg}$$

$$X\ =\ 2\times1000 = 2.000. = 2000\ mg$$

2) Calculate: mL/min

$$\frac{2000\ mg}{500\ mL} \diagdown\!\!\!\!\diagup \frac{4\ mg}{X\ mL}$$

$$2000X\ =\ 2000$$

$$\frac{2000X}{2000}\ =\ \frac{2000}{2000}$$

$$X\ =\ 1\ mL$$

4 mg are in 1 mL; 4 mg/min are administered by 1 mL/min

3) Calculate: mL/h

$$\frac{1\ mL}{1\ min}\ =\ \frac{X\ mL}{60\ min}$$

It is obvious that it is 60 mL/60 min or 60 mL/h.

12. 1) Convert g → mg: 1 g = 1000 mg
2) Calculate: mL/min

$$\frac{1000\ mg}{250\ mL} \diagdown\!\!\!\!\diagup \frac{3\ mg}{X\ mL}$$

$$1000X\ =\ 750$$

$$\frac{1000X}{1000}\ =\ \frac{750}{1000}$$

$$X\ =\ 750 \div 1000 = .750. = 0.75\ mL$$

3 mg are in 0.75 mL; 3 mg/min are administered by 0.75 mL/min

3) Calculate: mL/h

$$\frac{0.75\ mL}{1\ min} \diagdown\!\!\!\!\diagup \frac{X\ mL}{60\ min}$$

$$X\ =\ 45\ mL/60\ min\ or\ 45\ mL/h$$

13. 1) Convert: g → mg: 1 g = 1000 mg
2) Calculate: mL/min

$$\frac{1000\ mg}{500\ mL} \diagdown\!\!\!\!\diagup \frac{2\ mg}{X\ mL}$$

$$1000X\ =\ 1000$$

$$\frac{1000X}{1000}\ =\ \frac{1000}{1000}$$

$$X\ =\ 1\ mL$$

2 mg are in 1 mL; 2 mg/min are administered by 1 mL/min.

3) Calculate: mL/h

$$\frac{1\ mL}{1\ min} \diagdown\!\!\!\!\diagup \frac{X\ mL}{60\ min}$$

$$X\ =\ 60\ mL/60\ min = 60\ mL/h$$

14. 1) Calculate: mcg/min

$$\frac{5\ mcg/min}{1\ kg} \diagdown\!\!\!\!\diagup \frac{X\ mcg/min}{80\ kg}$$

$$X\ =\ 400\ mcg/min$$

2) Convert: mg → mcg

$$\frac{1\ mg}{1000\ mcg} \diagdown\!\!\!\!\diagup \frac{250\ mg}{X\ mcg}$$

$$X\ =\ 250\times1000 = 250.000.$$
$$=\ 250,000\ mcg$$

3) Calculate: mL/min

$$\frac{250,000\ mcg}{250\ mL} \diagdown\!\!\!\!\diagup \frac{400\ mcg}{X\ mL}$$

$$250,000X\ =\ 100,000$$

$$\frac{250,000X}{250,000}\ =\ \frac{100,000}{250,000}$$

$$X\ =\ 0.4\ mL$$

400 mcg are in 0.4 mL.
400 mcg/min are administered by 0.4 mL/min.

4) Calculate: mL/h

$$\frac{0.4\ mL}{1\ min} \diagdown\!\!\!\!\diagup \frac{X\ mL}{60\ min}$$

$$X\ =\ 24\ mL/60\ min\ or\ 24\ mL/h$$

15.
$$\frac{2000\ mg}{1000\ mL} \diagdown\!\!\!\!\diagup \frac{X\ mg}{75\ mL}$$

$$1000X\ =\ 150,000$$

$$\frac{1000X}{1000}\ =\ \frac{150,000}{1000}$$

$$X\ =\ 150\ mg;\ 75\ mL\ contain\ 150\ mg,$$
$$75\ mL/h\ deliver\ 150\ mg/h\ or$$
$$150\ mg/60\ min$$

$$\frac{150 \text{ mg}}{60 \text{ min}} \times \frac{X \text{ mg}}{1 \text{ min}}$$

$$60X = 150$$

$$\frac{60X}{60} = \frac{150}{60}$$

$$X = 2.5 \text{ mg/min (within normal range of } 1\text{–}4 \text{ mg/min)}$$

16. IV PB flow rate:

$$\frac{\text{mL}/\text{h}}{\text{drop factor constant}} = \frac{100}{6} = 16.67 = 17 \text{ gtt/min}$$

IV PB time: q.6 h = 4x/day = 4 h

IV PB volume: 100 mL × 4 = 400 mL

Regular IV volume: 3000 − 400 = 2600 mL

Regular IV time: 24 − 4 = 20 h = 1200 min

Regular IV rate: $\frac{\text{mL}/\text{h}}{\text{drop factor constant}} : \frac{2600}{20} =$

130 mL/h; $\frac{130}{6} = 21.67 = 22$ gtt/min

17. IV PB rate: $\frac{V}{T} \times C = R: \frac{50}{\overset{1}{\underset{}{30}}} \times \overset{2}{60} = 100$ gtt/min

IV PB time: q.i.d. = 4x/day

4 × 30 min = 120 min = 2 h

IV PB volume: 50 mL × 4 = 200 mL

Regular IV volume: 3000 − 200 = 2800 mL

Regular IV time: 24 − 2 = 22 h × 60 min = 1320 min

Regular IV rate: $\frac{V}{T} \times C = R \; \frac{2800}{1320} \times 60 = 127$ gtt/min

18. 1) Convert: lb → kg

$$\frac{1 \text{ kg}}{2.2 \text{ lb}} \times \frac{X \text{ kg}}{125 \text{ lb}}$$

$$2.2X = 125$$

$$\frac{2.2X}{2.2} = \frac{125}{2.2}$$

$$X = 56.8 = 57 \text{ kg}$$

2) Calculate: mcg/min

$$\frac{3 \text{ mcg/min}}{1 \text{ kg}} \times \frac{X \text{ mcg/min}}{57 \text{ kg}}$$

$$X = 171 \text{ mcg/min}$$

3) Convert: mg → mcg

$$\frac{1 \text{ mg}}{1000 \text{ mcg}} \times \frac{50 \text{ mg}}{X \text{ mcg}}$$

$$X = 50 \times 1000 = 50.000.$$
$$= 50,000 \text{ mcg}$$

4) Calculate: mL/min

$$\frac{50,000 \text{ mcg}}{500 \text{ mL}} \times \frac{171 \text{ mcg}}{X \text{ mL}}$$

$$50,000X = 85,500$$

$$\frac{50,000X}{50,000} = \frac{85,500}{50,000}$$

$$X = 1.7 \text{ mL}$$

171 mcg/min are administered by 1.7 mL/min.

5) Calculate: mL/h

$$\frac{1.7 \text{ mL}}{1 \text{ min}} \times \frac{X \text{ mL}}{60 \text{ min}}$$

$$X = 102 \text{ mL/60 min or } 102 \text{ mL/h}$$

19. 1000 − 800 = 200 mL infused

$$\frac{40 \text{ mEq}}{1000 \text{ mL}} \times \frac{X \text{ mEq}}{200 \text{ mL}}$$

$$1000X = 8000$$

$$\frac{1000X}{1000} = \frac{8000}{1000}$$

$$X = 8 \text{ mEq}$$

20.
$$\frac{125 \text{ mL}}{60 \text{ min}} \times \frac{X \text{ mL}}{1 \text{ min}}$$

$$60X = 125$$

$$\frac{60X}{60} = \frac{125}{60}$$

$$X = 2.08 = 2 \text{ mL/min}$$

21. $\frac{V}{T} \times C = R$

$$\frac{250 \text{ mL}}{T \text{ min}} \times 10 \text{ gtt/mL} = 25 \text{ gtt/min}$$

$$\frac{2500}{T} \times \frac{25}{1}$$

$$25T = 2500$$

$$\frac{25T}{25} = \frac{2500}{25}$$

$$T = 100 \text{ min}$$

Convert: min → h

$$\frac{60 \text{ min}}{1 \text{ h}} \times \frac{100 \text{ min}}{X \text{ h}}$$

$$60 X = 100$$

$$\frac{60X}{60} = \frac{100}{60}$$

$$X = 1.67 \text{ h} = 1\frac{2}{3} \text{ h or}$$
$$1 \text{ h and 40 min remaining}$$

22.
$$\frac{100 \text{ mL}}{T \text{ min}} \times 60 \text{ gtt/mL} = 33 \text{ gtt/min}$$

$$\frac{6000}{T} \times \frac{33}{1}$$

$$33T = 6000$$

$$\frac{33T}{33} = \frac{6000}{33}$$

$$T = 181.82 = 182 \text{ min}$$

Convert: min → h

$$\frac{60 \text{ min}}{1 \text{ h}} \times \frac{182 \text{ min}}{X \text{ h}}$$

$$60 X = 182$$

$$\frac{60X}{60} = \frac{182}{60}$$

$$X = 3 \text{ h and 2 min or 0302 h}$$

1630 + 0302 = 1932 hours

23. $\frac{V}{T} \times C = R$

$$\frac{V \text{ mL}}{480 \text{ min}} \times 15 \text{ gtt/mL} = 48 \text{ gtt/min}$$

$$\frac{15V}{480} \times \frac{48}{1}$$

$$15V = 23040$$

$$\frac{15V}{15} = \frac{23,040}{15}$$

$$V = 1536 \text{ mL}$$

24.
$$\frac{100 \text{ mL}}{1 \text{ h}} \times \frac{1500 \text{ mL}}{X \text{ h}}$$

$$100X = 1500$$

$$\frac{100X}{100} = \frac{1500}{100}$$

$$X = 15 \text{ h}$$

25.
$$\frac{40 \text{ mEq}}{1000 \text{ mL}} \diagdown \frac{2 \text{ mEq}}{\text{X mL}}$$

$$40\text{X} = 2000$$

$$\frac{40\text{X}}{40} = \frac{2000}{40}$$

$$\text{X} = 50 \text{ mL}$$

20 mEq/h are delivered by 50 mL/h.
Drop factor constant is 1.
50 mL/h = 50 gtt/min

26.
$$\frac{50,000 \text{ U}}{1000 \text{ mL}} \diagdown \frac{3750 \text{ U}}{\text{X mL}}$$

$$50,000\text{X} = 3,750,000$$

$$\frac{50,000\text{X}}{50,000} = \frac{3,750,000}{50,000}$$

$$\text{X} = 75 \text{ mL}; 3750 \text{ U are in } 75 \text{ mL};$$
$$75 \text{ mL/h deliver } 3750 \text{ U/h}$$

$$\frac{3750 \text{ U}}{1 \text{ h}} \diagdown \frac{\text{X U}}{24}$$

$$\text{X} = 3750 \times 24 = 90,000 \text{ U/24 h}$$

No, dosage is too high.

27.
$$\frac{5 \text{ mg}}{1 \text{ mL}} \diagdown \frac{37 \text{ mg}}{\text{X mL}}$$

$$5\text{X} = 37$$

$$\frac{5\text{X}}{5} = \frac{37}{5}$$

$$\text{X} = 7.4 \text{ mL}$$

28.
$$\frac{100 \text{ mL/24 h}}{1 \text{ kg}} \diagdown \frac{\text{X mL/24 h}}{8 \text{ kg}}$$

$$\text{X} = 800 \text{ mL/24 h}$$

$$\frac{800 \text{ mL}}{24 \text{ h}} \diagdown \frac{\text{X mL}}{1 \text{ h}}$$

$$24\text{X} = 800$$

$$\frac{24\text{X}}{24} = \frac{800}{24}$$

$$\text{X} = 33.3 = 33 \text{ mL/h}$$

29.
$$\frac{20 \text{ g}}{500 \text{ mL}} \diagdown \frac{3 \text{ g}}{\text{X mL}}$$

$$20\text{X} = 1500$$

$$\frac{20\text{X}}{20} = \frac{1500}{20}$$

$$\text{X} = 75 \text{ mL}$$

$$\frac{75 \text{ mL}}{30 \text{ min}} = \frac{\text{X mL}}{60 \text{ min}}$$

$$30\text{X} = 4500$$

$$\frac{30\text{X}}{30} = \frac{4500}{30}$$

$$\text{X} = 150 \text{ mL/60 min or}$$
$$150 \text{ mL/h bolus infusion}$$

$$\frac{3 \text{ g}}{75 \text{ mL}} \diagdown \frac{2 \text{ g}}{\text{X mL}}$$

$$3\text{X} = 150$$

$$\frac{3\text{X}}{3} = \frac{150}{3}$$

$$\text{X} = 50 \text{ mL}; 2 \text{ g are contained in } 50 \text{ mL};$$
$$2 \text{ g/h are delivered by } 50 \text{ mL/h}$$
$$\text{continuous infusion}$$

30. 1) Convert: U → mU

$$\frac{1 \text{ U}}{1000 \text{ mU}} \diagdown \frac{5 \text{ U}}{\text{X mU}}$$

$$\text{X} = 15 \times 1000 = 15.000. = 15000 \text{ mU}$$

2)
$$\frac{15000 \text{ mU}}{500 \text{ mL}} \diagdown \frac{1 \text{ mU}}{\text{X mL}}$$

$$15000\text{X} = 500$$

$$\frac{15000\text{X}}{15000} = \frac{500}{15000}$$

$$\text{X} = 0.03 \text{ mL}; 1 \text{ mU/min is delivered}$$
$$\text{by } 0.03 \text{ mL/min}$$

3)
$$\frac{0.03 \text{ mL}}{1 \text{ min}} \diagdown \frac{\text{X mL}}{60 \text{ min}}$$

$$\text{X} = 0.03 \times 60 = 1.8 \text{ rounded to}$$
$$2 \text{ mL/60 min or } 2 \text{ mL/h}$$

Posttest 1 from pages 261–266.

1. O.U.
2. p.r.n.
3. four times a day
4. hour of sleep, at bedtime
5. intravenous piggyback
6. 37.2°C
7. 102.2°F
8. $\frac{1}{2}$ tab
9. $\frac{1}{2}$ tab
10. 2 tabs
11. 2 tabs
12. 7.5 mL
13. 2 caps
14. 1 tab
15. 1 tab
16. 3.5 mL
17. 3 tabs
18. 7.5 mL "Give $1\frac{1}{2}$ t by mouth every six hours."
19. 2 tabs
20. 0.8 mL
21. 1 mL
22. 1.3 mL
23. 0.7 mL
24. 0.5 mL
25. 0.6 mL
26. 2 mL
27. 0.5 mL
28. 1.3 mL
29. 0.8 mL
30. 0.8 mL
31. 0.4 mL
32. 3.7 mL; divided into 2 injections of 1.8 mL and 1.9 mL
33. 3.8 mL; divided into 2 injections of 1.9 mL each
34. 5 mL
35. 0.19 mL
36. 22.5 mL
37. $\frac{1}{2}$ t
38. 21 gtt/min
39. 38 mL/h
40. 1940 hours
41. 200 gtt/min, 43 gtt/min
42. 1.2 mL
43. 1024 mL
44. 0.5 mL
45. 7.5 mL
46. 50 mL
47. 0.6 mL
48. 15 mL
49. 1.6 mL
50. 0.61 mL
51. 12 mL/h
52. 50 gtt/min

53.

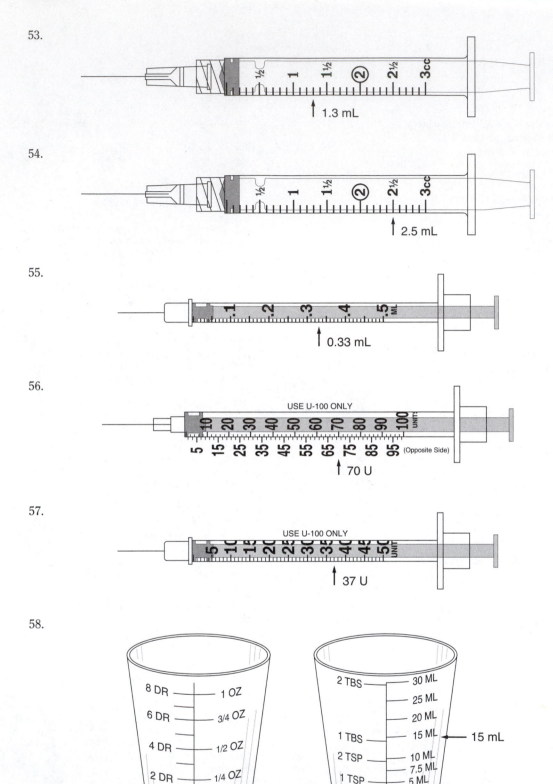

↑ 1.3 mL

54.

2½ cc

↑ 2.5 mL

55.

.1 .2 .3 .4 .5 ML

↑ 0.33 mL

56.

USE U-100 ONLY

5 10 20 30 40 50 60 70 80 90 100 UNITS
5 15 25 35 45 55 65 75 85 95 (Opposite Side)

↑ 70 U

57.

USE U-100 ONLY

5 10 15 20 25 30 35 40 45 50 UNIT

↑ 37 U

58.

8 DR — 1 OZ   2 TBS — 30 ML
6 DR — 3/4 OZ   25 ML
4 DR — 1/2 OZ   20 ML
                     1 TBS — 15 ML ← 15 mL
2 DR — 1/4 OZ   2 TSP — 10 ML
                     1 TSP — 7.5 ML
1 DR — 1/8 OZ   — 5 ML
                     1/2 TSP — 2.5 ML

59.

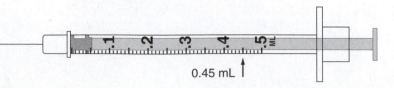

.1 .2 .3 .4 .5 ML

0.45 mL ↑

60.

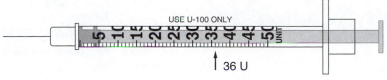

↑ 36 U

61. 3000–4500 mg a day
62. 7.5 mL
63. dextrose 5% and normal saline (sodium chloride 0.9%) with 20 millequivalents of potassium chloride per liter intravenous to run at a rate of 100 mL per hour
64. 10 mEq
65. 5 mL

Solutions—Posttest 1

6. $°C = \frac{°F - 32}{1.8}$

$°C = \frac{99 - 32}{1.8}$

$°C = \frac{67}{1.8}$

$°C = 37.2$

7. $°F = 1.8 \, °C + 32$

$°F = (1.8 \times 39) + 32$

$°F = 70.2 + 32$

$°F = 102.2$

8. $\frac{60 \text{ mg}}{1 \text{ tab}} \diagdown \frac{30 \text{ mg}}{X \text{ tab}}$

$60X = 30$

$\frac{60X}{60} = \frac{30}{60}$

$X = \frac{1}{2} \text{ tab}$

10. Convert: mg → mcg

$\frac{1 \text{ mg}}{1000 \text{ mcg}} \diagdown \frac{0.3 \text{ mg}}{X \text{ mcg}}$

$X = 0.3 \times 1000 = 0.300.$

$= 300 \text{ mcg}$

Order: 0.3 mg $\to$ 300 mcg

Supply: 150 mcg/tab

$\frac{150 \text{ mcg}}{1 \text{ tab}} \diagdown \frac{300 \text{ mcg}}{X \text{ tab}}$

$150X = 300$

$\frac{150X}{150} = \frac{300}{150}$

$X = 2 \text{ tabs}$

15. Convert: gr → mg

$\frac{\text{gr } 1}{60 \text{ mg}} \diagdown \frac{\text{gr } \frac{1}{5}}{X \text{ mg}}$

$X = 60 \times \frac{1}{5} = 12 \text{ mg}$

Order: gr $\frac{1}{5}$ $\to$ 12 mg

Supply: 12 mg

It is obvious you want to give 1 tablet.

18. $\frac{400 \text{ mg}}{5 \text{ mL}} \diagdown \frac{600 \text{ mg}}{X \text{ mL}}$

$400X = 3000$

$\frac{400X}{400} = \frac{3000}{400}$

$X = 7.5 \text{ mL}$

Convert 7.5 mL to teaspoons for discharge instructions.

$\frac{1 \text{ t}}{5 \text{ mL}} \diagdown \frac{X \text{ t}}{7.5 \text{ mL}}$

$5X = 7.5$

$\frac{5X}{5} = \frac{7.5}{5}$

$X = 1\frac{1}{2} \text{ t}$

20. Order: 12 mg

Convert: gr → mg

$\frac{\text{gr } 1}{60 \text{ mg}} \diagdown \frac{\text{gr } \frac{1}{4}}{X \text{ mg}}$

$X = 60 \times \frac{1}{4} = 15 \text{ mg}$

Supply: $\begin{cases} 15 \text{ mg} \\ \text{gr } \frac{1}{4} \text{ per 1 mL} \end{cases}$

$\frac{15 \text{ mg}}{1 \text{ mL}} \diagdown \frac{12 \text{ mg}}{X \text{ mL}}$

$15X = 12$

$\frac{15X}{15} = \frac{12}{15}$

$X = 0.8 \text{ mL}$

22. $\frac{75 \text{ mg}}{1.5 \text{ mL}} \diagdown \frac{65 \text{ mg}}{X \text{ mL}}$

$75X = 97.5$

$\frac{75X}{75} = \frac{97.5}{75}$

$X = 1.3 \text{ mL}$

28. $\frac{40 \text{ mg}}{1 \text{ mL}} \diagdown \frac{50 \text{ mg}}{X \text{ mL}}$

$40X = 50$

$\frac{40X}{40} = \frac{50}{40}$

$X = 1.25 = 1.3 \text{ mL}$

31. $\frac{25 \text{ mg}}{0.5 \text{ mL}} \diagdown \frac{20 \text{ mg}}{X \text{ mL}}$

$25X = 10$

$\frac{25X}{25} = \frac{10}{25}$

$X = 0.4 \text{ mL}$

33. $\frac{1 \text{ g}}{2.5 \text{ mL}} \diagdown \frac{1.5 \text{ g}}{X \text{ mL}}$

$X = 2.5 \times 1.5 = 3.75 = 3.8 \text{ mL}$

$\frac{3.8}{2} = 1.9 \text{ mL in each of 2 injections}$

34. Order: 1 mg

Supply: 1:5000 = 1 g:5000 mL = 1000 mg:5000 mL

$$\frac{1000 \text{ mg}}{5000 \text{ mL}} \diagdown \frac{1 \text{ mg}}{X \text{ mL}}$$

1000X = 5000

$$\frac{1000X}{1000} = \frac{5000}{1000}$$

X = 5 mL

35. Convert: g → kg

$$\frac{1 \text{ kg}}{1000 \text{ g}} \diagdown \frac{X \text{ kg}}{3000 \text{ g}}$$

1000X = 3000

$$\frac{1000X}{1000} = \frac{3000}{1000}$$

X = 3.000. = 3 kg

$$\frac{25 \text{ mg}}{1 \text{ kg}} \diagdown \frac{X \text{ mg}}{3 \text{ kg}}$$

X = 25 × 3 = 75 mg/day

$$\frac{75 \text{ mg}}{4 \text{ doses}} = 18.75 = 19 \text{ mg/dose}$$

$$\frac{100 \text{ mg}}{1 \text{ mL}} \diagdown \frac{19 \text{ mg}}{X \text{ mL}}$$

100X = 19

$$\frac{100X}{100} = \frac{19}{100}$$

X = 0.19 mL

38. $\frac{2000 \text{ mL}}{24 \text{ h}} = 83 \text{ mL/h}$

$$\frac{\text{mL/h}}{\text{Drop factor constant}} =$$

$\frac{83}{4} = 20.75 = 21 \text{ gtt/min}$

39. $\frac{10{,}000 \text{ U}}{500 \text{ mL}} \diagdown \frac{750 \text{ U}}{X \text{ mL}}$

10,000X = 375,000

$$\frac{10{,}000X}{10{,}000} = \frac{375{,}000}{10{,}000}$$

X = 37.5 mL = 38 mL; 750 U/h are delivered by 38 mL/h

40. $\frac{400 \text{ mL}}{X \text{ min}} \times 15 \text{ gtt/mL} = 24 \text{ gtt/min}$

$$\frac{6000}{X} \diagdown \frac{24}{1}$$

24X = 6000

$$\frac{24X}{24} = \frac{6000}{24}$$

X = 250 min

Convert: min → h

$$\frac{60 \text{ min}}{1 \text{ h}} = \frac{250 \text{ min}}{X \text{ h}}$$

60X = 250

$$\frac{60X}{60} = \frac{250}{60}$$

X = $4\frac{1}{6}$ h or 4 h and 10 min

IV should be discontinued @ 1940

41. Step 1. IV PB rate:

$$\frac{100 \text{ mL}}{\underset{1}{\cancel{30} \text{ min}}} \times \overset{2}{\cancel{60}} \text{ gtt/mL} = 200 \text{ gtt/min}$$

Step 2. IV PB time: q.4 h × 30 min = 6 × 30 = 180 min = 3 h

Step 3. IV PB volume: 100 mL × 6 = 600 mL

Step 4. Reg. IV volume: 1500 − 600 = 900 mL

Step 5. Reg. IV time: 24 − 3 = 21 h

Step 6. Reg. IV rate:

$$\text{mL/h} = \frac{900 \text{ mL}}{21 \text{ h}} = 43 \text{ mL/h}$$

$$\frac{\text{mL/h}}{\text{drop factor constant}} = \frac{43}{1} = 43 \text{ gtt/min}$$

43. $\frac{V}{T} \times C = R$

$$\frac{V \text{ mL}}{\underset{32}{\cancel{480} \text{ min}}} \times \overset{1}{\cancel{15}} \text{ gtt/mL} = 32 \text{ gtt/min}$$

$$\frac{V}{32} \diagdown \frac{32}{1}$$

V = 1024 mL

46. $\frac{500 \text{ mg}}{100 \text{ mL}} \diagdown \frac{250 \text{ mg}}{X \text{ mL}}$

500X = 25,000

$$\frac{500X}{500} = \frac{25{,}000}{500}$$

X = 50 mL

49. $0.8 \text{ m}^2 \times 2 \text{ mg/m}^2 = 1.6 \text{ mg}$

$$\frac{1 \text{ mg}}{1 \text{ mL}} \diagdown \frac{1.6 \text{ mg}}{X \text{ mL}}$$

X = 1.6 mL

50. Child's BSA = 0.52 m²

$$\frac{0.52 \text{ m}^2}{1.7 \text{ m}^2} \times 1000 \text{ mg} = 305.8 = 306 \text{ mg}$$

$$\frac{500 \text{ mg}}{1 \text{ mL}} \diagdown \frac{306 \text{ mg}}{X \text{ mL}}$$

500X = 306

$$\frac{500X}{500} = \frac{306}{500}$$

X = 0.61 mL

51. 1) Convert: mg → mcg

$$\frac{1 \text{ mg}}{1000 \text{ mcg}} \diagdown \frac{25 \text{ mg}}{X \text{ mcg}}$$

X = 25 × 1000 = 25.000. = 25,000 mcg

2) Convert: L → mL

1 L = 1000 mL

3) Calculate: mL/min

$$\frac{25{,}000 \text{ mcg}}{1000 \text{ mL}} \diagdown \frac{5 \text{ mcg}}{X \text{ mL}}$$

25,000X = 5000

$$\frac{25{,}000X}{25{,}000} = \frac{5000}{25{,}000}$$

X = 0.2 mL

5 mcg are contained in 0.2 mL.

5 mcg/min are delivered by a rate of 0.2 mL/min.

4) Calculate: mL/h

$$\frac{0.2 \text{ mL}}{1 \text{ min}} \diagdown \frac{X \text{ mL}}{60 \text{ min}}$$

X = 12 mL/60 min = 12 mL/h

52. $\dfrac{40 \text{ mEq}}{1000 \text{ mL}} \times \dfrac{2 \text{ mEq}}{X \text{ mL}}$

$40X = 2000$

$\dfrac{40X}{40} = \dfrac{2000}{40}$

$X = 50 \text{ mL/hr} = 50 \text{ gtt/min}$

61. 1) Calculate: minimum daily dosage

$\dfrac{200 \text{ mg}}{1 \text{ kg}} \times \dfrac{X \text{ mg}}{15 \text{ kg}}$

$X = 3000 \text{ mg/day}$

2) Calculate: maximum daily dosage

$\dfrac{3000 \text{ mg}}{1 \text{ kg}} \times \dfrac{X \text{ mg}}{15 \text{ kg}}$

$X = 4500 \text{ mg/day}$

62. $\dfrac{100 \text{ mg}}{1 \text{ mL}} \times \dfrac{750 \text{ mg}}{X \text{ mL}}$

$100X = 750$

$\dfrac{100X}{100} = \dfrac{750}{100}$

$X = 7.5 \text{ mL}$

64. $\dfrac{20 \text{ mEq}}{1000 \text{ mL}} \times \dfrac{X \text{ mEq}}{500 \text{ mL}}$

$1000X = 10{,}000$

$\dfrac{1000X}{1000} = \dfrac{10{,}000}{1000}$

$X = 10 \text{ mEq}$

65. $\dfrac{2 \text{ mEq}}{1 \text{ mL}} \times \dfrac{10 \text{ mEq}}{X \text{ mL}}$

$2X = 10$

$\dfrac{2X}{2} = \dfrac{10}{2}$

$X = 5 \text{ mL}$

Posttest 2 from pages 267–286.

1. 2 mL

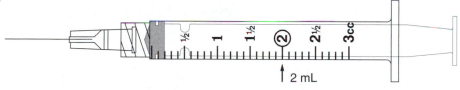

↑ 2 mL

2. 1 tablet
3. 2 capsules
4. SL = sublingual. The medication is to be administered under the tongue.
5. 1 mL

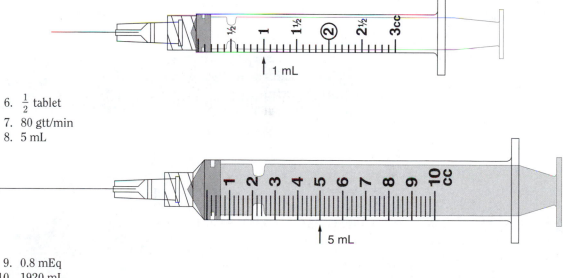

↑ 1 mL

6. $\frac{1}{2}$ tablet
7. 80 gtt/min
8. 5 mL

↑ 5 mL

9. 0.8 mEq
10. 1920 mL
11. 0500 hours on 9/4/xx
12. 2 tablets
13. 80 mL/h
14. digoxin and acetaminophen
15. 5 mL
16. 30 mL/h

17. 5 mL

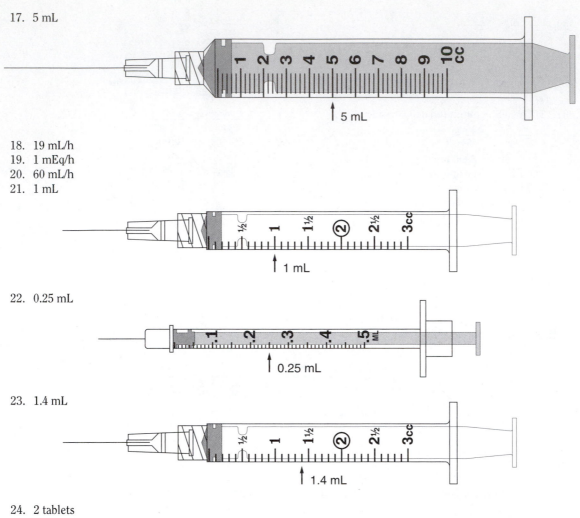

↑ 5 mL

18. 19 mL/h
19. 1 mEq/h
20. 60 mL/h
21. 1 mL

↑ 1 mL

22. 0.25 mL

↑ 0.25 mL

23. 1.4 mL

↑ 1.4 mL

24. 2 tablets

25. 1½ tablets

26. 19 mL; 5 mL; 45 mL; 5 mL (see drawing); 65 gtt/min

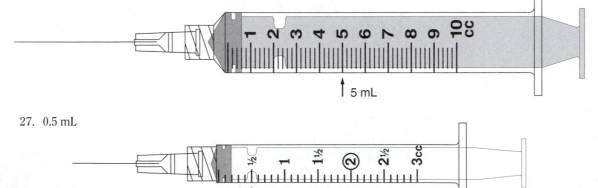

↑ 5 mL

27. 0.5 mL

↑ 0.5 mL

28. ½ tablet

29. 1.4 mL

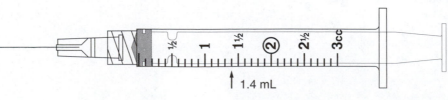

↑ 1.4 mL

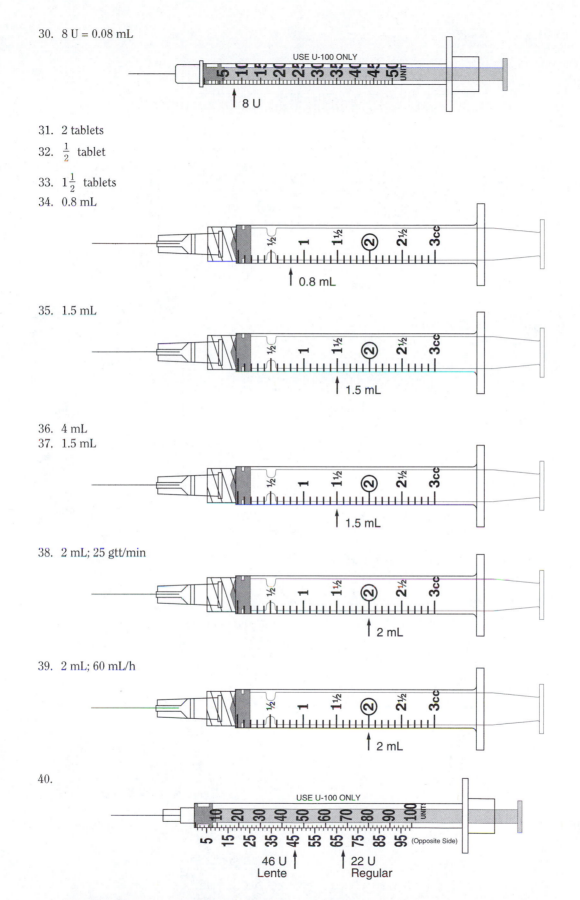

30. 8 U = 0.08 mL

USE U-100 ONLY

↑ 8 U

31. 2 tablets

32. $\frac{1}{2}$ tablet

33. $1\frac{1}{2}$ tablets

34. 0.8 mL

↑ 0.8 mL

35. 1.5 mL

↑ 1.5 mL

36. 4 mL

37. 1.5 mL

↑ 1.5 mL

38. 2 mL; 25 gtt/min

↑ 2 mL

39. 2 mL; 60 mL/h

↑ 2 mL

40.

USE U-100 ONLY

(Opposite Side)

46 U ↑   ↑ 22 U
Lente   Regular

41. Yes. Her temperature is 102.2°F. Tylenol is indicated for fever > 101°F every 4 hours. It has been 5 hours and 15 minutes since her last dose.

42. 2; 650 mg
43. One-half
44. Nubain; 0.2 mL

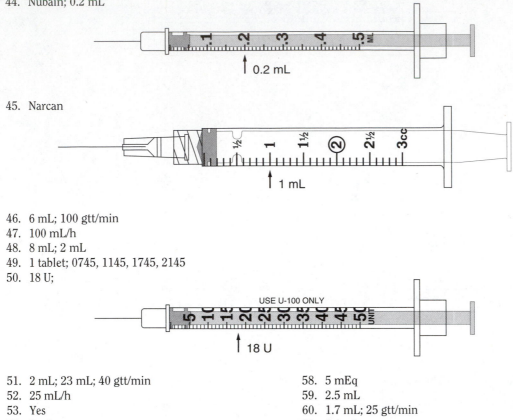

↑ 0.2 mL

45. Narcan

↑ 1 mL

46. 6 mL; 100 gtt/min
47. 100 mL/h
48. 8 mL; 2 mL
49. 1 tablet; 0745, 1145, 1745, 2145
50. 18 U;

USE U-100 ONLY

↑ 18 U

51. 2 mL; 23 mL; 40 gtt/min
52. 25 mL/h
53. Yes
54. 9 mL
55. Yes. The usual dosage is 20–40 mg/kg/day divided into 3 doses q.8h, which is equivalent to 47 mg– 93 mg per dose for a 15-lb. child.
56. 1 mL
57. 1 dropperful q. 8 h. Tell mother "every 8 hours."

58. 5 mEq
59. 2.5 mL
60. 1.7 mL; 25 gtt/min
61. 6.4 mL
62. 44 mL
63. 50 gtt/min
64. 50 gtt/min
65. 1200 mL

Solutions—Posttest 2

1. $\dfrac{10\ mg}{1\ mL} \diagdown \diagup \dfrac{20\ mg}{X\ mL}$

    $10X = 20$

    $\dfrac{10X}{10} = \dfrac{20}{10}$

    $X = 2\ mL$

2. $\dfrac{20\ mg}{1\ tab} \diagdown \diagup \dfrac{20\ mg}{X\ tab}$

    $20X = 20$

    $\dfrac{20X}{20} = \dfrac{20}{20}$

    $X = 1\ tab$

3. $\dfrac{6.5\ mg}{1\ cap} \diagdown \diagup \dfrac{13\ mg}{X\ cap}$

    $6.5X = 13$

    $\dfrac{6.5X}{6.5} = \dfrac{13}{6.5}$

    $X = 2\ capsules$

5. $\dfrac{0.25\ mg}{1\ mL} \diagdown \diagup \dfrac{0.25\ mg}{X\ mL}$

    $0.25X = 0.25$

    $\dfrac{0.25X}{0.25} = \dfrac{0.25}{0.25}$

    $X = 1\ mL$

6. $\dfrac{0.25\ mg}{1\ tab} \diagdown \diagup \dfrac{0.125\ mg}{X\ tab}$

    $0.25X = 0.125$

    $\dfrac{0.250X}{0.250} = \dfrac{0.125}{0.250}$

    $X = \frac{1}{2}\ tab/qd\ dose\ or\ \frac{1}{2}\ tab/24\ h$

7. $\dfrac{mL/h}{Drop\ factor\ constant} = \dfrac{80\ mL/h}{1} = 80\ gtt/min$

8. $\dfrac{30\ mEq}{15\ mL} \diagdown \diagup \dfrac{10\ mEq}{X\ mL}$

    $30X = 150$

    $\dfrac{30X}{30} = \dfrac{150}{30}$

    $X = 5\ mL$

9. $$\frac{10 \text{ mEq}}{1000 \text{ mL}} \diagup\!\!\!\!\!\diagdown \frac{X \text{ mEq}}{80 \text{ mL/h}}$$

$$1000X = 800$$

$$\frac{1000X}{1000} = \frac{800}{1000}$$

$$X = 0.8 \text{ mEq/h}$$

10. $$\frac{80 \text{ mL}}{1 \text{ h}} \diagup\!\!\!\!\!\diagdown \frac{X \text{ mL}}{24 \text{ h}}$$

$$X = 1920 \text{ mL}$$

11. $$\frac{1000 \text{ mL}}{80 \text{ mL/h}} = 12.5 \text{ h or } 12 \text{ h \& } 30 \text{ min}$$

$$1630 + 12 \text{ h and } 30 \text{ min} = 0500 \text{ on } 9/4/xx$$

12. $$\frac{325 \text{ mg}}{1 \text{ tab}} \diagup\!\!\!\!\!\diagdown \frac{650 \text{ mg}}{X \text{ tab}}$$

$$325X = 650$$

$$\frac{325X}{325} = \frac{650}{325}$$

$$X = 2 \text{ tablets}$$

13. mL/h = gtt/min when drop factor = 60 gtt/mL

15. $$\frac{10 \text{ mg}}{1 \text{ mL}} \diagup\!\!\!\!\!\diagdown \frac{50 \text{ mg}}{X \text{ mL}}$$

$$10X = 50$$

$$\frac{10X}{10} = \frac{50}{10}$$

$$X = 5 \text{ mL}$$

16. $$\frac{2 \text{ mg}}{1 \text{ min}} \diagup\!\!\!\!\!\diagdown \frac{X \text{ mg}}{60 \text{ min}}$$

$$X = 120 \text{ mg/60 min or } 120 \text{ mg/h}$$

$$\frac{2000 \text{ mg}}{500 \text{ mL}} \diagup\!\!\!\!\!\diagdown \frac{120 \text{ mg}}{X \text{ mL}}$$

$$2000X = 60,000$$

$$\frac{2000X}{2000} = \frac{60,000}{2000}$$

$$X = 30 \text{ mL}$$

30 mL/h delivers 120 mg/h

17. $$\frac{80 \text{ mg}}{1 \text{ mL}} \diagup\!\!\!\!\!\diagdown \frac{400 \text{ mg}}{X \text{ mL}}$$

$$80X = 400$$

$$\frac{80X}{80} = \frac{400}{80}$$

$$X = 5 \text{ mL}$$

18. 1) Convert: lb → kg

$$\frac{1 \text{ kg}}{2.2 \text{ lb}} \diagup\!\!\!\!\!\diagdown \frac{X \text{ kg}}{110 \text{ lb}}$$

$$2.2X = 110$$

$$\frac{2.2X}{2.2} = \frac{110}{2.2}$$

$$X = 50 \text{ kg}$$

2) Calculate: mcg/min

$$\frac{10 \text{ mcg/min}}{1 \text{ kg}} \diagup\!\!\!\!\!\diagdown \frac{X \text{ mcg/min}}{50 \text{ kg}}$$

$$X = 500 \text{ mcg/min}$$

3) Convert: mg → mcg

$$\frac{1 \text{ mg}}{1000 \text{ mcg}} \diagup\!\!\!\!\!\diagdown \frac{400 \text{ mg}}{X \text{ mcg}}$$

$$X = 400 \times 1000 = 400.000.$$

$$= 400,000 \text{ mcg}$$

4) Calculate: mL/min

$$\frac{400,000 \text{ mcg}}{250 \text{ mL}} \diagup\!\!\!\!\!\diagdown \frac{500 \text{ mcg}}{X \text{ mL}}$$

$$400,000X = 125,000$$

$$\frac{400,000X}{400,000} = \frac{125,000}{400,000}$$

$$X = 0.31 \text{ mL}$$

500 mcg are in 0.31 mL. The rate of 0.31 mL/min delivers 500 mcg/min.

5) Calculate: mL/h

$$\frac{0.31 \text{ mL}}{1 \text{ min}} \diagup\!\!\!\!\!\diagdown \frac{X \text{ mL}}{60 \text{ min}}$$

$$X = 18.6 \text{ mL/60 min or } 19 \text{ mL/h}$$

19. $$\frac{20 \text{ mEq}}{1000 \text{ mL}} \diagup\!\!\!\!\!\diagdown \frac{X \text{ mEq}}{50 \text{ mL}}$$

$$1000X = 1000$$

$$\frac{1000X}{1000} = \frac{1000}{1000}$$

$$X = 1 \text{ mEq}$$

At 50 mL/h, she receives 1 mEq/h.

20. $$\frac{2 \text{ mg/min}}{2 \text{ mL/h}} \diagup\!\!\!\!\!\diagdown \frac{4 \text{ mg/min}}{X \text{ mL/h}}$$

$$2X = 120$$

$$\frac{2X}{2} = \frac{120}{2}$$

$$X = 60 \text{ mL/h}$$

21. $$\frac{250 \text{ mg}}{5 \text{ mL}} \diagup\!\!\!\!\!\diagdown \frac{50 \text{ mg}}{X \text{ mL}}$$

$$250X = 250$$

$$\frac{250X}{250} = \frac{250}{250}$$

$$X = 1 \text{ mL}$$

22. $$\frac{50 \text{ mg}}{1 \text{ mL}} \diagup\!\!\!\!\!\diagdown \frac{12.5 \text{ mg}}{X \text{ mL}}$$

$$50X = 12.5$$

$$\frac{50X}{50} = \frac{12.5}{50}$$

$$X = 0.25 \text{ mL}$$

23. $$\frac{25 \text{ mg}}{1 \text{ mL}} \diagup\!\!\!\!\!\diagdown \frac{35 \text{ mg}}{X \text{ mL}}$$

$$25X = 35$$

$$\frac{25X}{25} = \frac{35}{25}$$

$$X = 1.4 \text{ mL}$$

24. $$\frac{200 \text{ mg}}{1 \text{ tab}} \diagup\!\!\!\!\!\diagdown \frac{400 \text{ mg}}{X \text{ tab}}$$

$$200X = 400$$

$$\frac{200X}{200} = \frac{400}{200}$$

$$X = 2 \text{ tablets}$$

25. $$\frac{5 \text{ mg}}{1 \text{ tab}} \diagup\!\!\!\!\!\diagdown \frac{7.5 \text{ mg}}{X \text{ tab}}$$

$$5X = 7.5$$

$$\frac{5X}{5} = \frac{7.5}{5}$$

$$X = 1\tfrac{1}{2} \text{ tablets}$$

26. $\dfrac{100 \text{ mg}}{1 \text{ mL}} \diagdown\hspace{-0.9em}\diagup \dfrac{500 \text{ mg}}{X \text{ mL}}$

    $100X = 500$

    $\dfrac{100X}{100} = \dfrac{500}{100}$

    $X = 5 \text{ mL}$

    $50 - 5 = 45 \text{ mL D}_5\text{W}$

    $50 \text{ mL D}_5\text{W} + 15 \text{ mL flush} = 65 \text{ mL}$

    $\dfrac{V}{T} \times C = R$

    $\dfrac{65 \text{ mL}}{\cancel{60} \text{ min}} \times \cancel{60}^{\,1} \text{ gtt/mL} = 65 \text{ gtt/min}$

27. $\dfrac{0.5 \text{ mg}}{2 \text{ mL}} \diagdown\hspace{-0.9em}\diagup \dfrac{0.125 \text{ mg}}{X \text{ mL}}$

    $0.5X = 0.250$

    $\dfrac{0.500X}{0.500} = \dfrac{0.250}{0.500}$

    $X = 0.5 \text{ mL}$

28. Convert: gr → mg

    $\dfrac{\text{gr } 1}{60 \text{ mg}} \diagdown\hspace{-0.9em}\diagup \dfrac{\text{gr } \frac{1}{8}}{X \text{ mg}}$

    $X = 7.5 \text{ mg}$

    $\dfrac{15 \text{ mg}}{1 \text{ tab}} \diagdown\hspace{-0.9em}\diagup \dfrac{7.5 \text{ mg}}{X \text{ tab}}$

    $15X = 7.5$

    $\dfrac{15X}{15} = \dfrac{7.5}{15}$

    $X = \frac{1}{2} \text{ tablet}$

29. $\dfrac{500 \text{ mg}}{2 \text{ mL}} \diagdown\hspace{-0.9em}\diagup \dfrac{350 \text{ mg}}{X \text{ mL}}$

    $500X = 700 \text{ mL}$

    $\dfrac{500X}{500} = \dfrac{700}{500}$

    $X = 1.4 \text{ mL}$

30. $\dfrac{100 \text{ U}}{1 \text{ mL}} \diagdown\hspace{-0.9em}\diagup \dfrac{8 \text{ U}}{X \text{ mL}}$

    $100X = 8$

    $\dfrac{100X}{100} = \dfrac{8}{100}$

    $X = 0.08 \text{ mL}$

31. $\dfrac{0.025 \text{ mg}}{1 \text{ tab}} \diagdown\hspace{-0.9em}\diagup \dfrac{0.05 \text{ mg}}{X \text{ tab}}$

    $0.025X = 0.05$

    $\dfrac{0.025X}{0.025} = \dfrac{0.050}{0.025}$

    $X = 2 \text{ tablets}$

32. $\dfrac{80 \text{ mg}}{1 \text{ tab}} \diagdown\hspace{-0.9em}\diagup \dfrac{40 \text{ mg}}{X \text{ tab}}$

    $80X = 40$

    $\dfrac{80X}{80} = \dfrac{40}{80}$

    $X = \frac{1}{2} \text{ tablet}$

33. $\dfrac{250 \text{ mg}}{1 \text{ tab}} \diagdown\hspace{-0.9em}\diagup \dfrac{375 \text{ mg}}{X \text{ tab}}$

    $250X = 375$

    $\dfrac{250X}{250} = \dfrac{375}{250}$

    $X = 1\frac{1}{2} \text{ tablets}$

34. $\dfrac{50 \text{ mg}}{1 \text{ mL}} \diagdown\hspace{-0.9em}\diagup \dfrac{40 \text{ mg}}{X \text{ mL}}$

    $50X = 40$

    $\dfrac{50X}{50} = \dfrac{40}{50}$

    $X = 0.8 \text{ mL}$

35. $\dfrac{2 \text{ mg}}{1 \text{ mL}} \diagdown\hspace{-0.9em}\diagup \dfrac{3 \text{ mg}}{X \text{ mL}}$

    $2X = 3$

    $\dfrac{2X}{2} = \dfrac{3}{2}$

    $X = 1.5 \text{ mL}$

36. $\dfrac{125 \text{ mg}}{5 \text{ mL}} \diagdown\hspace{-0.9em}\diagup \dfrac{100 \text{ mg}}{X \text{ mL}}$

    $125X = 500$

    $\dfrac{125X}{125} = \dfrac{500}{125}$

    $X = 4 \text{ mL}$

37. Convert: gr → mg

    $\dfrac{\text{gr } 1}{60 \text{ mg}} \diagdown\hspace{-0.9em}\diagup \dfrac{\text{gr } \frac{1}{100}}{X \text{ mg}}$

    $X = 0.6 \text{ mg}$

    $\dfrac{0.4 \text{ mg}}{1 \text{ mL}} \diagdown\hspace{-0.9em}\diagup \dfrac{0.6 \text{ mg}}{X \text{ mL}}$

    $0.4X = 0.6$

    $\dfrac{0.4X}{0.4} = \dfrac{0.6}{0.4}$

    $X = 1.5 \text{ mL}$

38. $\dfrac{250 \text{ mg}}{1 \text{ mL}} \diagdown\hspace{-0.9em}\diagup \dfrac{500 \text{ mg}}{X \text{ mL}}$

    $250X = 500$

    $\dfrac{250X}{250} = \dfrac{500}{250}$

    $X = 2 \text{ mL}$

    Compute: flow rate in gtt/min

    $\dfrac{V}{T} \times C = R$

    $\dfrac{50 \text{ mL}}{\cancel{30}^{\,2} \text{ min}} \times \dfrac{\cancel{15}^{\,1} \text{ gtt}}{\text{mL}} = 25 \text{ gtt/min}$

39. $\dfrac{5000 \text{ U}}{1 \text{ mL}} \diagdown\hspace{-0.9em}\diagup \dfrac{10,000 \text{ U}}{X \text{ mL}}$

    $5000X = 10,000$

    $\dfrac{5000X}{5000} = \dfrac{10,000}{5000}$

    $X = 2 \text{ mL}$

    $\dfrac{10,000 \text{ U}}{500 \text{ mL}} \diagdown\hspace{-0.9em}\diagup \dfrac{1200 \text{ U}}{X \text{ mL}}$

    $10,000X = 600,000$

    $\dfrac{10,000X}{10,000} = \dfrac{600,000}{10,000}$

    $X = 60 \text{ mL}$

    Each 60 mL contains 1200 U.

    The rate of 1200 U/h is therefore a rate of 60 mL/h.

40. $46 + 22 = 68 \text{ U total}$

41. $°\text{F} = 1.8 \, °\text{C} + 32$

    $°\text{F} = (1.8 \times 39) + 32$

    $°\text{F} = 70.2 + 32 = 102.2°$

43. $\dfrac{30 \text{ mg}}{60 \text{ mg}} = \dfrac{1}{2}$

44.
$$\frac{10\ mg}{1\ mL} \diagdown \frac{2\ mg}{X\ mL}$$
$$10X = 2$$
$$\frac{10X}{10} = \frac{2}{10}$$
$$X = 0.2\ mL$$

45.
$$\frac{0.4\ mg}{1\ mL} \diagdown \frac{0.4\ mg}{X\ mL}$$
It is obvious that X = 1 mL.

46.
$$\frac{250\ mg}{10\ mL} \diagdown \frac{150\ mg}{X\ mL}$$
$$250X = 1500$$
$$\frac{250X}{250} = \frac{1500}{250}$$
$$X = 6\ mL$$
$$\frac{V}{T} \times C = R$$
$$\frac{50\ mL}{30\ min} \times 60\ gtt/mL = 100\ gtt/min$$

47. gtt/min = mL/h when drop factor = 60 gtt/mL

48.
$$\frac{62.5\ mg}{1\ mL} \diagdown \frac{125\ mg}{X\ mL}$$
$$62.5X = 125$$
$$\frac{62.5X}{62.5} = \frac{125}{62.5}$$
$$X = 2\ mL$$

49.
$$\frac{1\ g}{1\ tab} \diagdown \frac{1\ g}{X\ tab}$$
It is obvious that X = 1 tablet. 0745, 1145, 1745, 2145

51.
$$\frac{1\ kg}{2.2\ lb} \diagdown \frac{X\ kg}{32\ lb}$$
$$2.2X = 32$$
$$\frac{2.2X}{2.2} = \frac{32}{2.2}$$
$$X = 14.55 = 15\ kg$$
$$\frac{15\ mg}{1\ kg} \diagdown \frac{X\ mg}{15\ kg}$$
$$X = 225\ mg/day$$
225 ÷ 3 = 75 mg or 2 mL (See label: 75 mg/2 mL)
25 mL – 2 mL = 23 mL
2 mL Kantrex + 23 mL D₅W
Buretrol delivers 60 gtt/mL.
25 mL solution + 15 mL flush = 40 mL
$$\frac{V}{T} \times C = R$$
$$\frac{40\ mL}{60\ min} \times 60\ gtt/mL = 40\ gtt/min$$

52.
$$\frac{250\ mg}{250\ mL} \diagdown \frac{25\ mg}{X\ mL}$$
It is obvious that X = 25 mL. 25 mL/h delivers 25 mg/h.

53.
$$\frac{1\ kg}{2.2\ lb} \diagdown \frac{X\ kg}{56\ lb}$$
$$2.2X = 56$$
$$\frac{2.2X}{2.2} = \frac{56}{2.2}$$
$$X = 25.45 = 25\ kg$$
$$\frac{1\ mg/h}{1\ kg} \diagdown \frac{X\ mg/h}{25\ kg}$$
$$X = 25\ mg/h$$

55.
$$\frac{1\ kg}{2.2\ lb} \diagdown \frac{X\ kg}{15\ lb}$$
$$2.2X = 15$$
$$\frac{2.2X}{2.2} = \frac{15}{2.2}$$
$$X = 6.82 = 7\ kg$$
Minimum dosage:
$$\frac{20\ mg}{1\ kg} \diagdown \frac{X\ mg}{7\ kg}$$
$$X = 140\ mg$$
$$\frac{140\ mg}{3\ doses} = 46.67 = 47\ mg/dose$$
Maximum dosage:
$$\frac{40\ mg}{1\ kg} \diagdown \frac{X\ mg}{7\ kg}$$
$$X = 280\ mg$$
$$\frac{280\ mg}{3\ doses} = 93\ mg/dose$$

56.
$$\frac{50\ mg}{1\ mL} \diagdown \frac{50\ mg}{X\ mL}$$
It is obvious that X = 1 mL.

57. 1 mL = 1 dropperful

58.
$$\frac{20\ mEq}{1000\ mL} \diagdown \frac{X\ mEq}{250\ mL}$$
$$1000X = 5000$$
$$\frac{1000X}{1000} = \frac{5000}{1000}$$
$$X = 5\ mEq$$

59.
$$\frac{2\ mEq}{1\ mL} \diagdown \frac{5\ mEq}{X\ mL}$$
$$2X = 5$$
$$\frac{2X}{2} = \frac{5}{2}$$
$$X = 2.5\ mL$$

60.
$$\frac{1\ kg}{2.2\ lb} \diagdown \frac{X\ kg}{110\ lb}$$
$$2.2X = 110$$
$$\frac{2.2X}{2.2} = \frac{110}{2.2}$$
$$X = 50\ kg$$
$$\frac{5\ mg}{1\ kg} \diagdown \frac{X\ mg}{50\ kg}$$
$$X = 250\ mg$$
$$\frac{300\ mg}{2\ mL} \diagdown \frac{250\ mg}{X\ mL}$$
$$300X = 500$$
$$\frac{300X}{300} = \frac{500}{300}$$
$$X = 1.67 = 1.7\ mL$$
Fluid rate in gtt/min
$$\frac{V}{T} \times C = R$$
$$\frac{50\ mL}{20\ min} \times \frac{10\ gtt/mL}{mL} = 25\ gtt/min$$

61.
$$\frac{1\ kg}{2.2\ lb} \diagdown \frac{X\ kg}{35\ lb}$$

$$2.2X = 35$$

$$\frac{2.2X}{2.2} = \frac{35}{2.2}$$

$$X = 15.91 = 16\ kg$$

$$\frac{20\ mg}{1\ kg} \diagup \frac{X\ mg}{16\ kg}$$

$$X = 320\ mg$$

$$\frac{500\ mg}{10\ mL} \diagdown \frac{320\ mg}{X\ mL}$$

$$500X = 3200$$

$$\frac{500X}{500} = \frac{3200}{500}$$

$$X = 6.4\ mL$$

62. 50 mL – 6.4 mL = 43.6 mL = 44 mL
Add 44 mL D$_5$W and 6.4 mL Vancocin to Buretrol.

63. Set the Buretrol rate at 50 gtt/min. Buretrol administers 60 gtt/mL; therefore, gtt/mL = gtt/min.

64. Resume the primary IV after Vancocin is infused at 50 gtt/min.

65. Jello:
$$\frac{\text{ʒ}1}{30\ mL} \diagdown \frac{\text{ʒ}4}{X\ mL}$$

$$X = 120\ mL$$

Water:
$$\frac{\text{ʒ}1}{30\ mL} \diagdown \frac{\text{ʒ}3}{X\ mL}$$

$$X = 90\ mL$$

$$90\ mL \times 2 = 180\ mL$$

Juice: pt 1 = 500 mL

IV:
$$\frac{50\ mL}{1\ h} \diagdown \frac{X\ mL}{8\ h}$$

$$X = 400\ mL$$

Total: 120
        180
        500
    +400 (Don't forget the IV fluids)
    1200 mL/8 h shift

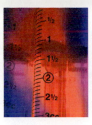

Index

With Pickar's *Dosage Calculations: A Ratio-Proportion Approach*, Delmar Publishers includes a comprehensive learning program on CD-ROM for Windows™. The CD-ROM is an interactive multimedia presentation that has been designed to enhance self-paced learning.

Features include:

- Complete text
- Tutorial to help you get started
- 300-word glossary
- Audio pronunciation of drug names
- Testing assessment tool with scoring capabilities
- Review questions with answers and rationales
- Practice problems with answers and rationales
- Critical thinking skills
- Animations

- Color photographs
- Drug labels
- Audio pronunciation of common sound-alike drug names
- Intuitive and attractive interface
- Help feature
- Toll-free technical support
- Plus Flash!™, an electronic flash card program

CD-ROM Set-up Instructions

Hardware Requirements

- 33 MHz 386 w/4 MB of RAM
- Recommend 486 w/8 MB of RAM
- Windows™ 3.1 or later; sound card

- VGA with 256 color display
- Double-spin CD-ROM drive
- 4 MB free disk space

Installation

Before you run the installation program, check the system requirements noted above. This program will take approximately 4 megabytes of disk space.

Windows™ 3.1

To install the *Dosage Calculations: A Ratio-Proportion Approach* CD-ROM, start Windows™. Insert the disk in the CD-ROM drive. From the Program Manager, click on "File," then "Run." Type "D:\SETUP" or "E:\SETUP" and press OK. The drive letter indicated depends on the drive designation for the computer's CD-ROM drive.

Windows™ 95

Insert the disk in the CD-ROM drive. Select "Start" and "Run." Type "D:\SETUP" or "E:\SETUP" and press OK. The drive letter indicated depends on the drive designation for your computer's CD-ROM drive. Installation of video playback software is not required in Windows™ 95.

Sound in Windows™ 3.1

If sound does not play while running the *Dosage Calculations: A Ratio-Proportion Approach* CD-ROM within Windows™ 3.1, check to be sure that your sound card is set up according to the manufacturer's instructions.

The MCI-CD Audio Driver must be installed. From the Main Group in Windows™ Program Manager, open Control Panel and select the "Drivers" option. Scroll through the installed drivers list. If [MCI] CD Audio is not installed, you will need your original Windows™ installation disks to proceed. Select "Add" and select the [MCI] CD audio driver from the list.

Technical Support

Call 1-800-824-5179 9:30 A.M. to 4:30 P.M. Eastern Standard Time *or*
Fax 1-800-880-9496 24 hrs. a day

Microsoft® is a registered trademark and Windows™ and Video for Windows™ are trademarks of Microsoft Corporation.
Flash!™ is a registered trademark of Delmar Publishers.

License Agreement for Delmar Publishers
an International Thomson Publishing company

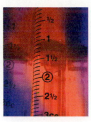

Index